BTEC national

Health & Social Care

Book 2

Series editors:
Beryl Stretch • Mary Whitehouse

Contributors:
Marilyn Billingham, David Herne,
Stuart McKie, Marjorie Snaith,
Beryl Stretch, Hilary Talman,
Sarah Wyatt

www.heinemann.co.uk
✓ Free online support
✓ Useful weblinks
✓ 24 hour online ordering

01865 888058

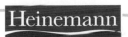
Heinemann

Heinemann is an imprint of Pearson Education Limited, a company incorporated in
England and Wales, having its registered office at Edinburgh Gate, Harlow, Essex, CM20 2JE.
Registered company number: 872828

www.heinemann.co.uk

Heinemann is a registered trademark of Pearson Education Limited

Text © Marilyn Billingham (Unit 19), David Herne (Units 12 and 20), Stuart McKie (Unit 11),
Marjorie Snaith (Unit 10), Beryl Stretch (Units 13 and 14), Hilary Talman (Unit 29), Sarah Wyatt
(Unit 9)

First published 2007

12 11 10 09
10 9 8 7 6 5 4

British Library Cataloguing in Publication Data is available
from the British Library on request

ISBN 978 0435 49916 7

Typeset and illustrated by 𝍂 Tek-Art, Croydon, Surrey, UK
Picture research by Zooid Pictures
Cover photo © Getty Images
Printed and bound in China (SWTC/04)

Website
Please note that the examples of websites suggested in this book were up to date at the time
of writing. It is essential for tutors to preview each site before using it to ensure that the URL is
still accurate and the content is appropriate. We suggest that tutors bookmark useful sites and
consider enabling students to access them through the school or college intranet.

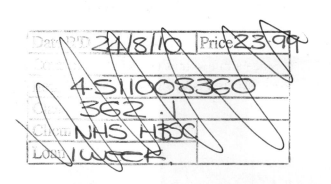
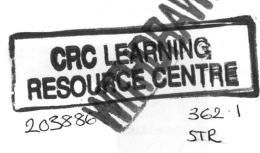

Contents

Acknowledgements

The publishers would like to thank:
The Connexions service for permission to show material from their website www.connexions-direct.com on page 52.
Stop The Traffik for permission to show a poster from their website www.stopthetraffik.org on page 57.
And the Alcohol Project, working with Lancashire County Council's School and Community Partnership Team and D2 Digital, for permission to use the images from their website www.lookoutalcohol.co.uk on page 289.

Photo credits
P2: © Harcourt Education Ltd / Jules Selmes; p4: © Harcourt Education Ltd / Martin Sookias / Mencap; p10: © Science Photo Library; p19: © Getty Images / Photodisc; p38: © Harcourt Education Ltd / Tudor Photography; p49: © Alamy / Jackie Chapman; p54: © Harcourt Education Ltd / Jules Selmes; p59: © Corbis / Jack Hollingsworth; p66: © Getty Images / Photodisc p70: © Harcourt Education Ltd / Jules Selmes; p80: © Science Photo Library; p83: © Alamy; p88: © Science Photo Library; p95: © Science Photo Library; p105: © Alamy; p114: © iStockPhoto.com / Nicolas Skaanild;

p121: © Alamy / SHOUT; p122: © Rex Features; p127: © Alamy / Photofusion Picture Library; p132: © Rex Features; p133: © Alamy / Johnny Come Lately; p137: © Getty Images / PhotoDisc; p156: © Harcourt Education Ltd / Jules Selmes; p202: © Science Photo Library / Deep Light Productions; p211: © Alamy / Edward Simons; p216: © Science Photo Library / Zephyr; p222: © Alamy / Janine Wiedel Photolibrary; p224: © Corbis; p225: © Science Photo Library / Jim Varney; p242: © Alamy / Andrew Parker; p249: © Getty Images / Leo Maguire; p255: © London Transport Museum; p268: © Alamy / Nick Emm; p276: © John Walmsley Education Photos; p288: © Ag MacKeith; p310: © Getty Images / Photodisc; p333: © TopFoto; p336: © Getty Images / Time Life Pictures / Nina Leen

The cover photograph is © Getty Images, and the photos in the icons are credited as follows: *Thinking points, Remember, Theory into Practice* and *Assessment* © Photos.com; *In context* and *Reflect* © Harcourt Ltd / Jules Selmes; and *Knowledge check*: Harcourt Ltd / Peter Morris

Introduction

Health and Social Care is a fascinating and growing area. You have chosen an excellent way to study it more closely and perhaps you will use this programme as a way into the professions, into higher education or straight into work. Or you may just be interested in the subject. Whatever helped you make your decision to do this course, welcome to the second BTEC National Health and Social Care course book.

This qualification is divided into several different pathways: Health and Social Care, Social Care, Health Studies or Health Sciences. Book 1 provides you with the core units that you will need for any of these pathways, plus four additional interesting and useful units which will fit into these programmes.

Book 2 gives you an additional nine units for your study and you will find details about the way these units fit into your specific programme on the table opposite.

The aim of these books is to provide a comprehensive source of information for your course. They follow the BTEC specification closely, so that you can easily see what you have covered and quickly find the information you need. Examples and case studies from health and social care are used to bring your course to life and make it enjoyable to study. We hope you will be encouraged to find your own examples of current practice too.

You will often be asked to carry out research for activities in the text, and this will develop your research skills and enable you to find many sources of useful health and social care information, particularly on the Internet.

In some units you will find information about different care settings and professionals which will be of great practical help to you in furthering career choices.

The books offer all the core texts for students on HND, foundation degree and first-year degree programmes. To help you plan your study, an overview of each unit and its outcomes is given at the beginning of each unit. There is a wealth of information in these two books that you will find useful for a long time in your training.

■ A note about language

There are many terms in use for people who receive care and people who give care so, to prevent any confusion, we have standardised the use of such terms in this book.

For general, non-specific contexts, we have used the term 'service user' for an individual receiving care and, specifically, for those in a care setting. We use the term 'patient' for those receiving care through health care settings, e.g. when attending the family doctor or a hospital, and the term 'client' in a counselling context.

Similarly, we have used the term 'carer' in an informal way and 'professional' for an individual who is specifically trained or working in a formal setting using a value-based system.

The units and the pathways

Whether you have enrolled to study for the BTEC National Award, Certificate or Diploma, along the pathway of Health & Social Care (H&SC), Social Care (SC), Health Studies (HS) or Health Sciences (HSc), this book provides all the core units you need, plus four further units to develop your understanding of your chosen field.

▼ **How each unit fits into each programme**

Unit and title	Core	Specialist		
Unit 9 Values and planning	Certificate SC Diploma SC	Award H&SC	Certificate H&SC	Diploma H&SC
Unit 10 Caring for children and young people	Cert SC Dip SC Dip HS	Award H&SC	Cert H&SC Cert HS Cert HSc	Dip H&SC Dip HSc
Unit 11 Supporting and protecting adults	Cert SC Dip SC Dip HS	Award H&SC	Cert H&SC Cert HS Cert HSc	Dip H&SC Dip HSc
Unit 12 Public health	Cert HS Dip HS	Award H&SC	Cert H&SC Cert SC Cert HSc	Dip H&SC Dip SC Dip HSc
Unit 13 Physiology of fluid balance	Cert HS Dip HS Cert HSc Dip HSc			
Unit 14 Physiological disorders	Cert HS Dip HS	Award H&SC	Cert H&SC Cert HSc	Dip H&SC Dip SC Dip HSc
Unit 19 Applied sociological perspectives			Cert H&SC Cert SC Cert HS Cert HSc	Dip H&SC Dip SC Dip HS Dip HSc
Unit 20 Health education		Award H&SC	Cert H&SC Cert SC Cert HS Cert HSc	Dip H&SC Dip SC Dip HS Dip HSc
Unit 29 Applied psychological perspectives			Cert H&SC Cert SC Cert HS Cert HSc	Dip H&SC Dip SC Dip HS Dip HSc

Guide to learning and assessment features

This book has a number of features to help you relate theory to practice, to reinforce your learning from both classwork and placements, and to help you to study independently. It also aims to help you gather evidence for assessment. You will find the following features identified in the sample spread below in each unit.

Your tutor should check that you have completed enough activities to meet all the assessment criteria for the unit, whether from this book or from other tasks.

Tutors and students should refer to the BTEC standards for the qualification for the full BTEC grading criteria for each unit (www.edexcel.org.uk).

Learning features

In context

Interesting examples of care situations are described in case studies to help you relate practice to theory. They will show you how the topics you are studying affect real people and their experience of health or social care.

Key terms

These define issues and vocabulary that have been used in the text and which are important for your understanding in relation to your studies and work in health and social care. They are gathered together in the glossary on page 500.

Reflect

These are opportunities for individual reflection on, or group discussions about, your experiences in a health and social care context. They will widen your knowledge and help you reflect on issues that impact on health and social care.

Remember!

These highlight important points to reinforce your learning or to give you practical tips.

Theory into practice

These practical activities allow you to apply theoretical knowledge to health and social care situations. Make sure you reinforce your learning by completing these activities as you work through each unit.

9.

In context

Surraya is a 'linkworker' at a busy hospital trust. She is based in the Department of Public Health Awareness and responds to staff who require her services. Today she is working in the ear, nose and throat department, translating some deaf awareness posters from English into Bengali. These will then be used in the waiting room.

Tomorrow, she will be working with the community midwife in some parenting classes – she will be interpreting the information for Bengali first-time expectant mothers.

1 What other kinds of health information are likely to need translation services?

2 What is the difference between interpretation and translation?

3 How do you think service users will feel about this service? What kind of worries may they have?

Cultural enrichment

It should be fairly obvious by now that, if all the benefits we have already explored (diverse food types, new languages, the arts etc) are available and accessed by everyone, we will be culturally enriched.

Key terms

Equality This means that individuals are all treated equally.

Rights This describes the roles and responsibilities attached to being an individual living and working within a wider society.

■ Tolerance

Tolerance doesn't just mean putting up with something or someone. It has a much wider meaning and it is important to recognise this. In society and in the workplace we do not have to be friends with everyone but we do have to behave at all times in a professional and caring manner, towards both our service users

Theory into practice

When you are at your work placement, look around and try to identify all the measures that have been taken to keep staff and service users safe. For example, carpets provide a non-slip surface for residents and remove the risks associated with spillages, which can lead to people slipping. Try to think of all the dangers that your service users would face if no measures had been taken to provide a safe environment. This will help you to realise how much thought goes into planning a safe environment for service users and staff.

For people to feel that they belong, there is a need for everyone's circumstances and background to be valued and respected. Alongside this lies a need for positive relationships between people from different backgrounds in all the social and economic places in which they might meet, for example, schools, workplaces and neighbourhoods.

Health and social care teams need to demonstrate social cohesion in the way individual members work together and support each other. As we have already said, most care teams are multicultural: it is important for these teams to support each other and to uphold the rights of every single member.

Reflect

What actions could be taken by a hospital trust to contribute towards a cohesive society at a local level?

Remember!

Visiting tradesman are experts in their trade, not care practice. They need to be made aware of the nature of the client group so that they do not unintentionally place people at risk.

Help with the Law

There is also an Appendix to this book which summarises key aspects of legislation that apply across several units. You should look at these whenever a piece of legislation is mentioned in the text of any of the units. This will help reinforce your learning about the key features of each Act and how the legislation relates to the theory and practice being discussed in the units. You will find the Legislation Appendix on our website: www.harcourt.co.uk/btechsc.

A number of health and social care professionals and teachers have contributed to this book to enable you to develop your knowledge. Each of them has expertise in a particular area and a wide teaching experience.

We do hope that you enjoy your course and find these books an excellent support for your studies. Good luck!

Beryl Stretch and Mary Whitehouse

Theory into practice

Write a short report describing either:

- how accessible your college Is for people who are wheelchair users, or
- how easy it is for wheelchair users to do their shopping in your local high street.

■ Iatrogenesis or 'doctor-generated' illness

Iatrogenesis refers to illness generated by medical activity and practice. It was a term introduced by Ivan Illich (1976) and was part of his more general attack on, and criticism of, industrialised society and its large bureaucratic institutions. However, it is still very much part of current debate. Particular areas of concern include the side-effects of drugs, the risks attached to medical drugs trials and concerns about infections spread within hospitals. Illich identified three major types of iatrogenisis:

- clinical iatrogenesis – the unwanted side-effects of medical intervention
- social iatrogenesis – medicine has gained so much power and status that people too quickly and easily place themselves in the hands of the professional and become mass consumers of medical products
- cultural iatrogenesis – society becomes over-concerned with perfect health, so making it difficult to develop positive attitudes towards impairment and to cope appropriately with death.

■ The clinical iceberg

Official statistics on levels of illness are sometimes called 'the clinical iceberg' because it is thought that the 'true' levels of illness are largely concealed; this is because people who are ill do not necessarily visit their doctor. This may be for a wide range of reasons.

Assessment activity 9.1

Describe different concepts of ill health.

1 Drawing on examples from your placement and from other life experiences, describe the different concepts of ill health introduced in this unit:

- disability
- iatrogenesis
- the sick role
- the clinical iceberg.

P1

Grading tip for P1

You can provide evidence of linking theory to practice by using well-chosen examples to illustrate concepts.

Take it further

Consider how concepts of ill health may help care workers in evaluating their own care practice.

Knowledge check

1 Explain what 'valuing diversity' means.
2 List the key aspects of the care value base.
3 Explain the consequences of making assumptions about people that are not based on fact.
4 List three ways of demonstrating respect for an individual.
5 Describe the purpose of a code of practice in the workplace.
6 List three ways of actively promoting anti-discriminatory practice.
7 Explain which circumstances would allow confidentiality to be broken.
8 List five benefits of diversity to society.

Unit 9 | Values and planning in social care   [3]

Assessment features

Activities and assessment practice

Activities are provided throughout each unit. These are linked to real situations and case studies and they can be used for practice before tackling the preparation for assessment.

Grading icons

Throughout the book you will see the **P**, **M** and **D** icons. These show you where the tasks fit in with the grading criteria. If you do these tasks you will be building up your evidence to achieve your desired qualification. If you are aiming for a Merit, make sure you complete all the Pass **P** and Merit **M** tasks. If you are aiming for a Distinction, you will also need to complete all the Distinction **D** tasks. **P1** means the first of the Pass criteria listed in the specification, **M1** the first of the Merit criteria, **D1** the first of the Distinction criteria, and so on.

Preparation for assessment

Each unit concludes with a full unit assessment, which taken as a whole fulfils all the unit requirements from Pass to Distinction. Each task is matched to the relevant criteria in the specification.

Knowledge checks

At the end of each unit is a set of quick questions to test your knowledge of the information you have been studying. Use these to check your progress, and also as a revision tool.

Values and planning in social care

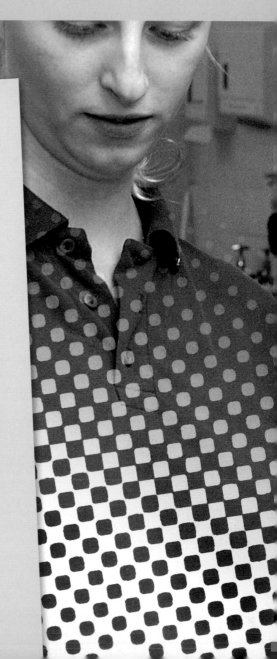

Introduction

In this unit you will begin to explore how each person is an individual. As individuals we are all very different and this has an impact on the way in which care services are both planned and delivered. You will develop an awareness of some of the ethics and values that are involved in health and social care and how we must be conscious of the diversity of people. Working within the health and social care sector, you will meet people who have very different needs. In this unit you will learn about some of the complex issues that you could become involved with. Care work regularly involves making difficult decisions, and through this unit you can start to investigate the different issues that can potentially occur and discuss ways of resolving them.

This unit links very closely with your vocational practice and you will be able to see how your learning in the classroom relates to your work-based learning. As your learning develops, you will be able to acknowledge good working practices taking place. You will understand why an appreciation of the Care Value Base is essential to being an effective care provider. Incorporated within the Care Value Base, you will see the importance of care planning and some of the ethical and legal boundaries involved when providing care for other people.

How you will be assessed

This unit is an internally assessed unit. You must complete all work set by your tutor to a minimum of the pass criteria in order to pass this unit.

Thinking points

Working in the health and social care sector will bring you into contact with many people who will potentially need your care and support. It is important that you treat each person as an individual with unique needs and personal circumstances. You may be faced with very similar scenarios but how you respond and care for each person can be very different.

The reasons why people need care can be varied and wide ranging. As a health and social care worker you may come into contact with individuals who could be dealing with the following issues:

- disability
- abuse by others
- serious injury
- addiction to substances that can affect behaviour
- a need for emotional as well as physical support.

Make a list of the types of qualities you think a person might need to work in health and care. Why is it so important to plan each person's care on an individual basis? How might workers ensure that each person that they care for feels involved in their care?

After completing this unit you should be able to achieve the following outcomes:

- Understand care planning principles and processes
- Understand the framework of legislation, policy and codes of practice that influence social care practice
- Understand the values that underpin social care practice
- Understand ethical principles in relation to social care.

Principles

When we think about care planning principles and processes it is vital that we first establish what a care relationship is. A care relationship has many facets and can be different for each person whose care we are involved in. There are some basic principles that should apply in all cases:

- respect for the individual concerned
- open communication
- remembering that the service user is at the centre of the care planning process at all times.

When applied, these principles can form the basis of a professional relationship which can develop between you and the service user. To enable the professional relationship to develop appropriately it is essential that you, the service provider, consider a series of processes that are involved within care planning.

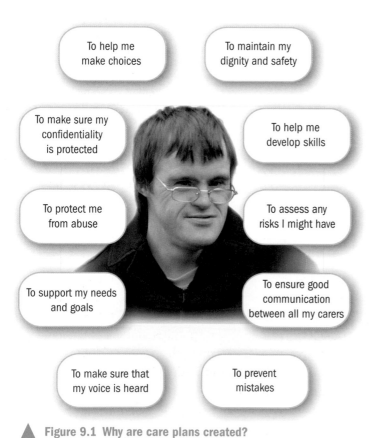

To help me make choices

To maintain my dignity and safety

To make sure my confidentiality is protected

To help me develop skills

To protect me from abuse

To assess any risks I might have

To support my needs and goals

To ensure good communication between all my carers

To make sure that my voice is heard

To prevent mistakes

▲ Figure 9.1 Why are care plans created?

[4] BTEC National | Health & Social Care | Book 2

The cycle of assessment refers to a way of determining the different needs of a service user. It is an extremely important part of setting up a care plan.

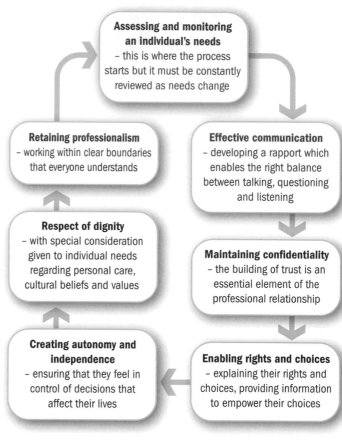

Assessing and monitoring an individual's needs – this is where the process starts but it must be constantly reviewed as needs change

Retaining professionalism – working within clear boundaries that everyone understands

Effective communication – developing a rapport which enables the right balance between talking, questioning and listening

Respect of dignity – with special consideration given to individual needs regarding personal care, cultural beliefs and values

Maintaining confidentiality – the building of trust is an essential element of the professional relationship

Creating autonomy and independence – ensuring that they feel in control of decisions that affect their lives

Enabling rights and choices – explaining their rights and choices, providing information to empower their choices

▲ Figure 9.2 Assessing the needs of the service user is an ongoing process.

The crucial element in the care planning process is the involvement of the service user. This might sound like an obvious statement but health and social care staff can be guilty of planning and providing the care that *they* think is needed rather than what the *service user* may perceive as being needed. The underlying philosophy of treating each person as an individual and creating choice must always be evident within the care planning process. The service user sits at the centre of the whole process and their perceived needs must be listened to.

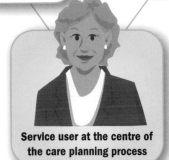

Social needs
- Communication needs and/or barriers
- Interactions with others
- meeting with others

Physical needs
- Personal care
- Aids and mobility
- Health provisions

Service user at the centre of the care planning process

Emotional needs
- Feeling and thoughts
- Religious/spiritual needs
- Personal relationships
- Aspirations/goals

Intellectual needs
- Learning activities
- Recreational activities
- Discussion
- Creative activities

 Figure 9.3 The service user must stay firmly at the centre of the care planning process.

Effective care planning should be aimed at empowering the service user. **Empowerment** is a skill that health and social care workers have to develop; it literally means giving the power back to someone who may feel as though they have no power in the circumstances, having become reliant on others to provide for them. Empowerment encourages the individual to make their own choices and to take control of the situation on their terms. People who are responsible for delivering care hold a great deal of power; this is the nature of the relationship in that the service user is vulnerable and dependent on you to provide the care needed. A skilled practitioner is able to guide the service user to become pro-active in making choices that they truly want or need, not just complying with what others may think are the best choices for them.

When an individual is unable to communicate their needs clearly, it is important that someone with the service user's best interests at heart advises the care provider when they are writing the care plan. This person is an **advocate.** Advocacy is a term used to describe a health or social care worker (or an appropriate other) who can speak or act on the service user's behalf. The role of an advocate is to make sure that a person's rights and interests are fairly represented. This doesn't have to be someone who works with the individual – it can be a family member, neighbour, friend or carer.

Key terms

Empowerment When an individual is encouraged to make decisions and to take control of their own life.

Advocate An independent representative who can speak or act on a service user's behalf, ensuring that their wishes are promoted and feelings made known.

Planning a person's care is an ongoing process. The care provider must talk through their needs with the service user and document this in a care plan. An important factor to remember is that people's needs and their care priorities can change. Care staff should review the service user's care plan on a regular basis to clearly document any progress that has been observed and alter the priorities within the plan if necessary. Care plans may be developed by one professional, for example, a nurse or care manager, or this can be a joint exercise by a multi-disciplinary team. A multi-disciplinary team refers to a group of people who may all be involved with the care of one person, i.e. social worker, nurse, physiotherapist and general practitioner (GP). It is essential that the service user is at the centre of the planning process for any care plan to be as effective as possible. We must remember first and foremost who the care plan is for – the service user *not* the service provider! The role of service users in their care planning is recognised in legislation such as the Children Act 1989, the NHS and Community Care Act 1990, the Carers (Recognition and Services) Act 1995.

The Children Act was reviewed in 2004 to incorporate the Every Child Matters government agenda.

SPRINGFIELD HEALTH SERVICES LIMITED
FRIARYHURST NURSING HOME
CARE PLAN

Isiah is around 25 years old. He was admitted to **A&E** when he was found by the road in extreme pain by passers-by. When questioned it became apparent that Isiah is an asylum seeker who speaks hardly any English. Investigations reveal that he has a broken pelvis and leg and is severely **dehydrated**.

Assessment

This process revealed both the physical problems Isiah has but also the language barrier and cultural differences.

Plan

Mobility

- Isiah will need surgery to correct his broken bones.
- Following surgery he will need to be moved regularly to prevent pressure sores.
- Isiah will need help to aid his rehabilitation to enable him to walk independently.

Language barrier

- Isiah speaks very little English.
- Locate a translator who can act as an advocate.
- Find out through the translator if he has any family members or friends we can contact.
- Establish if he has any previous medical history that the health care professionals need to know.

Pain control

- To make Isiah pain free.

Implement

Mobility

- Contact the surgical team to review Isiah and operate.
- After surgery use a special mattress that will relieve pressure areas.
- Start using a 'turning chart' to document every time he is turned.
- Liaise with the physiotherapy and occupational therapy teams so that they can plan a rehabilitation programme.

Language barrier

- Work closely with the translator to establish Isiah's needs.
- Use any information the translator can provide to improve care and treatment.

Pain control

- Administer regular painkillers as prescribed on Isiah's drug chart by the medical staff.
- Check pain levels using a **picture chart scale** to aid Isiah's understanding.

Review

- Check pressure areas twice daily to ensure the skin is intact.
- Liaise with the translator as often as is necessary – document outcomes daily.
- Check pain levels every two hours initially.
- Review and evaluate the care plan on a daily basis.

A care plan

This scenario is the type of situation you could find yourself involved in; a possible care plan is shown above.

Key terms

A&E The Accident and Emergency department of a hospital.

Dehydration Loss of fluid from the body due to causes like severe infection with sweating and vomiting, or spending long periods of time in hot conditions without drinking.

Picture chart scale Useful when there is a language barrier. For example, a patient with limited use of English can look at a row of faces from very smiley to very sad and point to the one that shows how they are feeling.

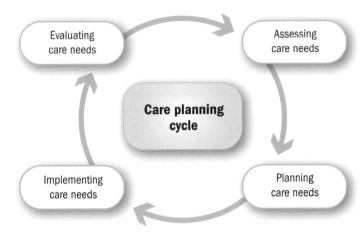

Figure 9.4 The care planning cycle.

In context

Martha, a care worker, has been involved in John's care for two weeks. John has reduced mobility following a **stroke** which he suffered two months ago. Martha is concentrating on improving John's ability so that he can be more independent. She has written a care plan that reflects this. John is becoming increasingly frustrated with Martha as he sees his priority as improving his speech which has been affected by the stroke.

1 **How has this difference in priorities between Martha and John come about?**

2 **Could this affect John's rehabilitation?**

3 **What are the potential problems that may arise in their professional relationship and how can the existing issues be resolved?**

Key terms

Stroke A cerebral vascular accident (CVA) is commonly referred to as a stroke. It is a bleed in the brain whose effect varies according to the severity of the bleed.

Needs

There are occasions when service users are not able to state their needs clearly. There could be lots of reasons for this. It may simply be that they are unsure of what their needs are: perhaps they have an injury or illness that prevents them from expressing their needs, or they may have difficulties with their communication skills.

Theory into practice

In small groups, identify five reasons why a person may not be able to communicate their needs to you. Try to think of experiences you have had on work placement, or with people you have encountered in everyday life. Discuss how you might help them to express themselves.

Reflect

Think about occasions when you felt powerless, as though you had no control over a situation or felt too intimidated to speak up for yourself. How did this make you feel at the time? How did you feel after the event? If it happened again, how might you react differently? Write this scenario down in a journal and be realistic about the amount of power you would really have if this happened again.

Some organisations provide advocates to act on behalf of service users. Section 2 of the Bristol Inquiry report, published in 2001, recommended that there should be representatives of patients' interests 'on the inside' of the NHS. The Labour government responded to these recommendations as part of the NHS plan (a 10-year programme initiated in 2000). Its vision is to create an NHS service in which the service user is at the centre of all health and care provision. The introduction and implementation of the Patient Advisory Liaison

Service (PALS) was the government's response to the recommendations made by the Bristol Inquiry. PALS are available within all NHS trusts and provide a number of services aimed wholly at empowering the service user. Some important services that PALS representatives offer include:

- providing confidential advice and support to service users, their families and carers
- information on the NHS and other health and social care related matters
- confidential assistance in resolving problems and concerns quickly and effectively.

Representatives from PALS act as advocates for service users, liaising with staff, managers and other agencies and organisations. They help to negotiate solutions and to bring about changes to the way that services are delivered.

Take it further

Look at the Bristol Inquiry report (www.bristol-inquiry. org.uk) and discuss the main recommendations for improving care. Do you think they are realistic? Can they work in real life?

Approaches

There are two recognised approaches within the care planning process: needs-led and service-led.

Needs-led and service-led approaches

Needs-led assessment was officially introduced by the NHS and Community Care Act in 1990. It is an assessment which starts by looking at a person's needs and works from there, rather than assessing with a particular service in mind. Needs-led care plans can be extremely complex.

In health and social care the term 'needs-led' is often invoked. This term can be quite misleading – it implies that the needs of the service user are focal, but, in fact, it may be the needs of the service being provided, that are truly being considered. The word 'need' is ambiguous: what it means to one person may be different from

what it means to another. *Need* is an extremely personal concept – as individuals we all perceive our needs very differently. Sometimes we get confused between the word 'need' and the word 'want'.

Reflect

What things can you think of that you need to survive? Now, think about what you really need to actually survive. A lot of the things we think we need, we actually want!

In its real sense, a needs-led care plan is a plan for a particular individual, not a care plan that could be used for any person with similar requirements. Care plans must also take account of the service available. It could be recommended that a person has a carer attend them at home three times a day. However, the service provided can only support one visit. Thus their care plan is compromised – it is service-led, not needs-led. Unfortunately, it is not always possible to put into effect a totally needs-led approach to care planning. The practical issue of resources has to be considered as well, and areas of necessity prioritised.

Potential conflicts

Resources

Resources are an ongoing source of conflict within health and social care. People can sometimes mistakenly link the term 'resources' just with money. Indeed, financial constraints are a constant consideration and organisations are always working within an allocated budget for each financial year (a financial year usually

Key terms

Resources These are things that are needed to enable the services to run, for example, money, staff, time, skills, accommodation and equipment.

runs from April to April). But other resources include the facilities available for use, staff numbers and staff skill levels.

The budget that health and social care providers are allocated each financial year is devolved from central government. Managers have to make difficult choices with regard to the services they provide with this allocated sum of money. There are statutory requirements to be met so that everyone can receive the services they are entitled to. In an ideal world we would all like to be able to deliver health and social care provision tailored to the exact needs and wants of every service user. However, this is not an option that is currently available. Therefore it is essential that realistic care plans are created. This involves explaining clearly to the service user the type of care delivery package they can expect to receive and why.

Rights of the service user

People who use and need service provision have a right to be informed of their rights and responsibilities. These include:

- a clear explanation to the service user and family members of which services can be supplied and why (so that they don't have unrealistic expectations and ask for services that are not available)
- an explanation of the way services are funded (this can help them understand the limitations of the service)
- an exploration of the issues regarding risk, both for the service user and the provider.

When discussing the care planning principles and processes you will often be trying to meet the needs

In context

Mrs Illich moved to England from Russia with her husband in 1962. They raised a family of one daughter and two sons, and she is now a widow and grandmother. She lives alone in a rented third-floor flat.

Mrs Illich recently suffered a stroke. This has affected her mobility and speech. Her daughter, Anna, visits every day but finds it hard with her own family commitments. Her sons live further away and cannot visit very often.

A social worker comes to assess the situation at the request of the family. Anna is unwell on the day of the assessment so one of Mrs Illich's sons, Markus, attends the meeting. The social worker asks Mrs Illich questions to help her assess the current situation; her son answers the questions as Mrs Illich's speech is slow and hard to understand as a result of the stroke. Markus is worried something will happen to his mother living alone and the burden of her care should not be left to his sister Anna. He feels the best course of action would be to place Mrs Illich in residential care.

- The social worker's job is to collect information and suggest a recommended course of action. What she wants shouldn't come into the equation.

- Mrs Illich's opinion isn't heard during the assessment; other people think they know what is best for her. She may be feeling worthless and that she is a burden to her daughter.
- Anna is in a difficult position. She might not want her mother to go into a home but she is unable to continue caring for her herself.
- Markus thinks he is acting in his mother's and sister's best interests; he may also be feeling guilty as he is unable to contribute towards his mother's care.

Situations like this are not unusual: there are many considerations that must be discussed. Mrs Illich's well-being and safety are central, but the feelings and needs of family members cannot be ignored. The service providers must also consider the potential risks involved if she remains at home by herself.

1 **Consider and list the options that are available to Mrs Illich and her family.**

2 **Devise a care plan that could help Mrs Illich to remain at home.**

3 **Whose rights, wishes and needs must be paramount? How can the service provider protect these rights?**

of several interested parties at once. The service user's needs come first (they are the most important person to be considered at all times), but the needs of family members and the risks involved to the service provider cannot be ignored.

Skills required

There are a range of skills that health and social care workers must use in building and enhancing good working relations with service users. Effective communication skills are essential when planning and implementing care plans. Often, as care providers, we have to respond to non-verbal cues: the service user may well be answering questions as they think they should be answered, rather than saying what they truly want. It is our responsibility to ask appropriate questions and to give the service user time to collect their thoughts and think about their responses. It is important to be open and unbiased to put a service user at their ease, and to use active listening. This is more than hearing what another person is saying, it is about valuing their opinion and ensuring they know their wishes will be respected.

It is important in any care plan that the service user feels comfortable and involved in the process. To make sure this happens, care workers have to be honest and respectful. It may not always be possible to cater for the ultimate needs of the individual, but we must always make sure that they clearly understand why that is and know that it is not a personal issue but merely due to the limited resources available.

It is possible to build a good working relationship with individuals in a very short space of time in health and social care. You must remember that a power balance exists in the relationship and be aware of the boundaries. Service users can become extremely reliant on staff who provide for their needs: the care provider may be the only other person that they come into contact with. Things are different for the care worker, who will have a range of people to cater for. It is important to establish that it is a working relationship, to be friendly and welcoming but to maintain a professional distance. A form of counselling is being established whereby one person (the service provider) is helping another person (the service user) to help themselves through the power of the care plan. Discussion about what is needed to go into the care plan is one aspect of care, but implementing the care plan (i.e. starting to use it) is essential to prove it is worthwhile.

Processes of care planning

A care plan is a systematic method that is produced as a formal document. The aim of the care plan is to assess the needs and risks of the individual concerned and make appropriate plans. The care plan document takes into careful consideration the needs of the person but also:

- the strategies needed to meet those needs
- the goals that are ultimately to be attained
- the realities of the service provision that is available.

A care plan is also essential for monitoring outcomes. Assessment and care planning are concerned with all areas of a person's life. In the past there has been an over-emphasis on the skills someone did or didn't have. However, we need to see and understand the person as an individual, not just as a collection of separate 'can do' and 'can't do' categories.

The Care Standards Act 2000 recognised the need for vulnerable adults to be protected, and the written documentation provided within a care plan can ensure that care is appropriate for the individual.

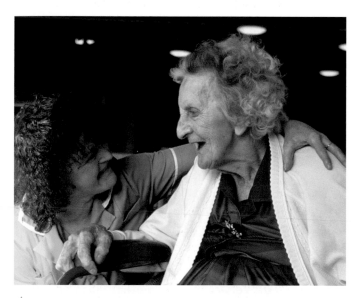

▲ **Effective communication skills are essential when care plans are being put together.**

The care planning cycle

The care planning and delivery process can be viewed as a circle:

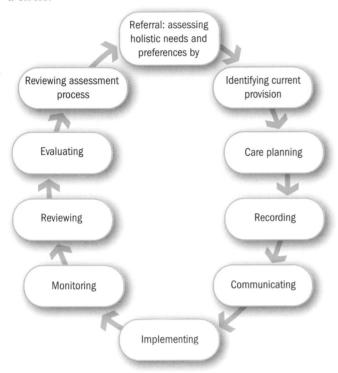

▲ Figure 9.5 The sequence of steps in a care plan.

The process of care planning starts at the point of *referral*. A referral means someone has an appointment arranged for a health and/or social assessment. There are two paths to referral:

- professional referral – a health and/or social care practitioner recognises the need for someone to be assessed by a specialist and refers them for assessment
- self-referral – an individual identifies their own need for intervention and support and refers themselves to the appropriate care provider.

Once a referral has been received, an assessment is then made. *Assessing holistic needs and preferences* is the process of objectively defining needs and viewing the person as a whole, i.e. taking into consideration not just their physical needs but also their intellectual, emotional, cultural, social and spiritual needs. It is a process involving the service user, their carers and relevant agencies. The process of assessment forms part of the White Paper *Caring for People*, published by the

Department of Health in 1990. Under the NHS and Community Care Act 1990, all assessments must be focused on the actual needs of the service user.

Reflect

Whenever we meet anyone we are subconsciously assessing them. We do this visually, verbally and by using our other senses. Think about the observations you make from the many encounters you have in one day.

- What do they look like? Are they tidy or unkempt?
- How are they behaving? Is this 'normal' behaviour or are they displaying signs of anxiety or distress?
- Are they speaking rationally or do they appear irrational?
- Is their behaviour appropriate to the setting you are currently in?

We constantly assess people and make judgements based on our assumptions. Within the formal assessment process in care planning it is important that we focus on the information we are being given that is factual not subjective and try not to prejudge it.

Once the assessment process is complete and needs have been identified, the next step is to link into the appropriate resources to meet those needs. Care planning is then a series of linked activities aimed at fulfilling the needs of the service user. For the vast majority of service users the aim will be to promote independence and to ensure full use of existing resources, i.e. *identifying current provision* and enhancing it. Priorities will be set within the care plan but they will be flexible as priorities can change, as can the needs of the service user. *Care plans* are documents that state the care provided to the service user. The *recording* of information on the care plan must be concise and accurate. When creating a care plan and setting desirable goals you must be able to justify your actions, *communicating* the objectives clearly. Be aware that you may be held accountable for the decisions made.

The person responsible for devising the care plan should also carry the responsibility for its implementation. The tasks of *implementation* include:

- determining the service user's participation
- agreeing the pace of implementation
- assessing the financial implications
- ensuring the service availability
- negotiating existing and new services
- revising the care plan as necessary
- establishing arrangements for monitoring.

Care planning requires careful *monitoring* at all stages. This ensures that the objectives set in the care plan are being achieved and that the care plan is adapted to meet the changing needs of the service user. Monitoring can be achieved in a variety of ways including observation, telephone calls, letters and home visits. Wherever possible the person responsible for the implementation of the care plan should also have responsibility for monitoring procedures. This helps to sustain the relationship with the service user and aids continuity.

Reviewing and *evaluating* the care plan is an ongoing process. It checks that care plan objectives are being met, allows evaluation of quality and cost provision and sets targets for review.

In summary, the care planning and delivery process is an ongoing process of *assessing holistic needs and preferences* – agreeing goals – providing care – reviewing effectiveness.

The General Social Care Council

The General Social Care Council (GSCC) is a government organisation set up in 2001 to enforce standards of conduct and practice within the social care workforce. The council ensures that service users, carers, practitioners, employers and the general public have confidence in the standards which are set for social care.

Take it further

Obtain a copy of the code of conduct of the General Social Care Council. What are the key areas concerned with? Does the code protect practitioners or service users? What are the implications if the code of conduct is not adhered to?

Multi-disciplinary/inter-agency working

The care planning and implementation process is not, and cannot be, delivered by one person alone. Working within the health and social care sector involves being part of a team of people. This is often referred to as inter-agency or multi-disciplinary working – involving health and social care staff, each with different skills, who work together to meet the needs of the service user.

Legislation and guidelines

Health and social care staff must work within the boundaries of legislation and guidelines. These are rules that must be followed to ensure that the best practice possible is received by the service user. Examples of the types of legislation that exist to protect both service users and service providers include:

- the Care Standards Act 2000
- the Children Act 2004
- Equal Opportunities legislation and policies
- General Social Care Council/Care Council for Wales/Northern Ireland codes of practice
- National Service Frameworks.

Assessment tools

Assessment tools are useful devices that are designed to improve the assessment process. The Department of Health defined assessment tools in 2002 as:

A collection of scales, questions and other information, to provide a rounded picture of an individual's needs and related circumstances.

Assessment tools are standardised systems that aim to provide an equal and fair approach. They are not just checklists that staff fill out (although that would be a useful starting point to collate information). Examples of assessment tools that could be used include:

- checklists
- forms
- diaries of both the service user and provider
- observations that have been noted.

The Social Care Institute of Excellence best practice guide states:

The standardised systems used within social work departments are usually not tools in the accepted sense, that are tested in terms of the quality or effectiveness of the information they provide about an individual's state. They are more often an administrative record, more likely to measure output and workload than outcome for an individual service user.

For some people the assessment process starts and ends with the forms or tools they fill out. This limits the value of the assessment process: they should be viewed as useful adjuncts to the assessment process rather than as the assessment process itself.

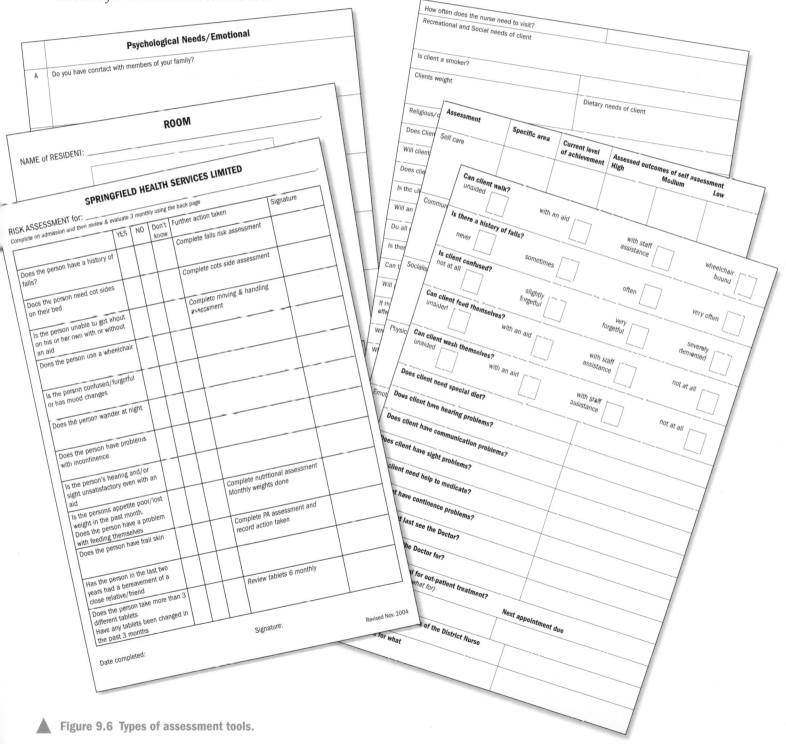

▲ **Figure 9.6 Types of assessment tools.**

Assessment tool	Description
Checklists	Checklists can be a series of criteria essential to the assessment process, used as an aid to ensure that they are all covered.
Forms	Forms are often essential documents that need to be completed so there is evidence of the information collected.
Diary of the care provider	This records meetings and who was present, and often a brief summary of the events that have taken place.
Diary of the service user	The service user's 'voice', providing evidence of the different agencies involved in their care, and their perception of the care they are receiving.
Questions	Open and closed questions are used in the assessment process to gain a full picture of the needs to be addressed.
Observations	Physical observations can be noted, i.e. blood pressure, temperature, weight, etc. Observations can also describe behaviour.
Personal history	A person's previous medical history, and their personal status, (i.e. relationships, carers, etc.) are central to their current assessment needs.
Flowcharts	These are useful tools to guide what other forms of assistance may be appropriate to the individual.
Discussions	Assessment should include a series of discussions involving all parties within the care process. This may also include network analysis (when professionals share information to enhance the support provided).

Table 9.1 Possible assessment forms and tools.

Assessment tools are not a finite list that must be used for every individual assessment – they are resources that can help inform the assessment process. If you make a very thorough assessment in the first instance, the care that is delivered subsequently should be of the highest standard. A list of the types of assessment tools that could be used is shown in the table above.

Theory into practice

When you next attend your work experience placement, ask to see the tools they use in their assessment process. Ask your supervisor how they incorporate the assessment tools into the assessment process. Do they always use the same tools, or do they inter-change them as is necessary? If possible try to observe an assessment taking place and witness assessment tools in practice.

Approaches to implementing care plans

Many different approaches can be used when implementing care plans. They are best regarded as **working documents,** in that all the care staff involved should have access to the plan and a place in its thorough implementation.

Key terms

Working document This is an ongoing piece of work that people add things to as circumstances change.

Key staff may have different approaches to the goals that have been set, i.e. the support worker could have a task-centred approach, focusing purely on the task they have been set to implement. An occupational therapist may have a very different agenda, identifying the behavioural needs of the service user and focusing the care plan around these needs. It is important, therefore, that that the key networks are integrated by the use of the care plan: identifying each other's skills and using them for the good of the service user concerned.

Never forget the significant role that the service user and their advocates play in the whole process. It can also be extremely useful to encourage the use of groups where others with similar needs can discuss and share experiences.

Finally, the service provider must always be careful not to misuse the power they hold within the relationship. They must never force anyone to accept anything against their wishes as this would be seen as an abuse of power.

Key people

There are a number of different key practitioners who help to deliver care provision within the health and social care sector.

- **Social workers** are qualified professionals who work with both individuals and families who are experiencing social difficulties. Social workers work with all age ranges and individuals with learning, physical and mental health impairments. They aim to help people come to terms with or solve issues; social

workers have statutory responsibilities especially in the area of child protection and have powers of control within this area.

- **Support workers** are not registered practitioners. However, they do provide essential support to the registered practitioners they work with, as well as to service users. Support workers provide direct support to a wide range of service users in their own homes and in hospital environments. This support enables people with a range of needs to maintain an independent or supported living situation.
- **Health visitors** are qualified nurses who have undertaken additional training. They monitor the growth and development of babies and young children, offering support and guidance to parents. They play a large part in child protection issues and health education. Health visitors can be the first practitioner to identify health and/or social care concerns with babies and young children and will refer to specialists as the need arises.
- **Occupational therapists** are registered practitioners who work with individuals to promote independent living. They ensure that capabilities are maximised and disability minimised. Occupational therapists can advise on equipment or home adaptations that might help the individual.
- **Domiciliary care workers** are health and social care service providers, for example, health care support workers who provide care in a person's own home.

Assessment activity 9.1

P1 Describe the processes of care planning with reference to care planning principles.

1. Describe the process of care planning, with reference to care planning principles, using diagrams to help your explanation.

Grading tip for P1

Identify the key elements involved within the care planning process and explain why each of them is important.

M1 Explain care planning principles.

2. Explain care planning principles and why it is important that we view each person that we care for as an individual.

Grading tip for M1

You need to provide a detailed explanation, evaluating care planning from an individual's perspective.

P2 Identify the importance of multi-disciplinary and inter-agency working on the care planning process.

3. List the health and social care workers who could be involved in the care planning and implementation process. Think about the roles they play and how their skills can enhance an individual's well-being.

Grading tip for P2

It would be useful to carry out some independent research to explore the different types of workers within health and social care. Compile your list in a table with brief descriptions of the roles.

M2 Use examples to explain how multi-disciplinary and inter-agency working can improve the care planning process.

4. What do the terms multi-disciplinary and inter-agency working mean?

Grading tip for M2

Your explanation should demonstrate in-depth understanding.

D1 Evaluate the role of multi-disciplinary and inter-agency working in social care.

5. Consider the potential consequences that could occur if multi-disciplinary and inter-agency working does not happen. How might this affect an individual's care experience?

Grading tip for D1

Analyse and evaluate the ways in which good working practices can be developed. This should be a detailed report including independent research.

Legislation

Legislation is the making of laws by parliament. Legislation determines the policy framework and reflects the different statutory rights of organisations, groups and individuals. Social care legislation protects service users, employers and employees. These laws protect against poor practice and standards and ensure everyone involved is clear about their rights. An example of recent legislation is the Care Standards Act 2000. This legislation was introduced to:

- establish a National Care Standards Commission
- make provision for the registration of children's homes, residential homes, independent clinics and hospitals, different care groups including fostering and voluntary adoption agencies.
- establish the General Social Care Council and the Care Council for Wales
- establish a Children's Commissioner for Wales
- make provision for registration, regulation and training for those providing childminding or day care
- make provision for the protection of children and vulnerable people
- amend the law for children looked after in schools and colleges.

Codes of practice

Health and social care services are strictly regulated and one of the ways regulation is provided is through the codes of practice that are in place. People who work in health and care need the right training and qualifications to perform within their roles; codes of practice are in place to guide and inform practitioners. Government responsibilities have now been devolved to the four countries of Great Britain (England, Scotland, Wales and Northern Ireland). The General Social Care Council/Care Councils for Wales and Northern Ireland all work within the same codes of practice. Although different organisations are responsible for regulating

standards, the regulatory framework is the same in all four countries.

The regulatory framework consists of:

- the professional councils that regulate practitioners and agree codes of professional practice
- the regulation and inspection bodies that regulate providers of health, care and early years provision
- the national standards that set out minimum levels of care and evidence-based practice against which organisations are measured.

Policy

Organisational policies are the mechanism through which legislation is delivered and implemented within the workplace. Policies implemented within the workplace cover areas such as:

- equal opportunity
- bullying and harassment
- confidentiality
- health and safety
- harm minimisation
- risk assessment.

Standards

It is through the National Minimum Standards that the values and principles of care are delivered. The Care Standards Act 2000 identified National Minimum Standards for a range of care services, which all service providers must meet.

National Minimum Standards apply to issues such as:

- staffing levels
- skills mix (this refers to different levels or expertise of staff, i.e. registered nurse and health care support worker)
- the necessary qualifications for practice
- the standards relating to the care and treatment of service user groups.

Assessment activity 9.2

P3 Use four examples to describe key aspects of legislation, policies and codes of practice that influence social care.

1   The following pieces of legislation have been important to the health and care sector's fundamental practice. From the list below choose four acts. Identify and summarise the key points of each chosen piece of legislation and produce a leaflet showing its importance. (For a full explanation of the law relating to Health and Social Care, see the Legislation Appendix on the website at www.harcourt.co.uk/btechsc.)   **P3**

- European Convention on Human Rights and Fundamental Freedoms 1950
- Health and Safety at Work Act 1974
- Mental Health Act 1983
- The Convention on the Rights of the Child 1989
- The Children Act 1989
- Race Relations (Amendment) Act 2000
- Disability Discrimination Act 1995
- Human Rights Act 1998
- Data Protection Act 1998
- Nursing and Residential Care Homes Regulations 1984 (Amended 2002)
- The Children Act 2004

Grading tip for P3

List the key points of each piece of legislation and add notes to describe how they affect social care.

M3 Explain the impact of legislation on the concept of care planning.

2   Look at one of the forms of legislation listed below. Explore how this legislation could impact on the care planning process. Prepare a handout or a Powerpoint presentation to summarise the key points and present this to your group. Make notes on two more laws based on others' presentations.

- Care Standards Act 2000
- Children Act 2004
- Equal Opportunities legislation and policies
- General Social Care Council/Care Council for Wales/Northern Ireland codes of practice
- National Service Frameworks.

Grading tip for M3

Your presentation needs to include reasons why you feel your chosen legislation could impact on the care planning process to justify your findings.

D2 Evaluate the effectiveness of current legislation in promoting care planning and multi-disciplinary/inter-agency working.

3   Using the legislation listed above, evaluate the effectiveness and importance of legislation when writing a care plan; analyse the importance of including multi-disciplinary and inter-agency working within your work. Develop a discussion/debate that clearly demonstrates your understanding of how legislation can protect both service users and service providers.

Grading tip for D2

Analysing is more detailed than an explanation – you need to consider different aspects and consider all sides of the discussion.

Values

Values form the very basis of a person's thoughts, feelings, beliefs and attitudes. They are closely linked to an individual's moral principles, the decisions that they make and the ways in which they behave.

Values are learned from an early age and the way that others feel and behave can influence us greatly, for example, children learn values from their earliest role models.

Values can be political, social, cultural, spiritual and moral. The way we express our values can be a very individual experience, for example:

- we may value the importance of family – these are our moral and cultural values
- we may highly regard the importance of freedom of speech – our political values

- for some, attending their place of worship and acknowledging religious festivals is significant – these are spiritual values
- some people are closer to their friends than family and this could be described as social values.

It is vital that you develop an understanding of the importance of these values and their potential impact within our diverse society.

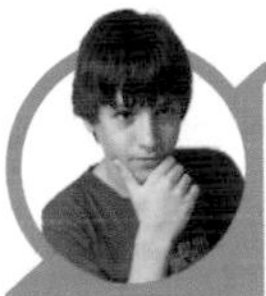

Reflect

Think about yourself and what values you hold. Try to consider each of the main areas and why these values mean so much to you. Who influenced you in holding them? If possible share your findings with someone else.

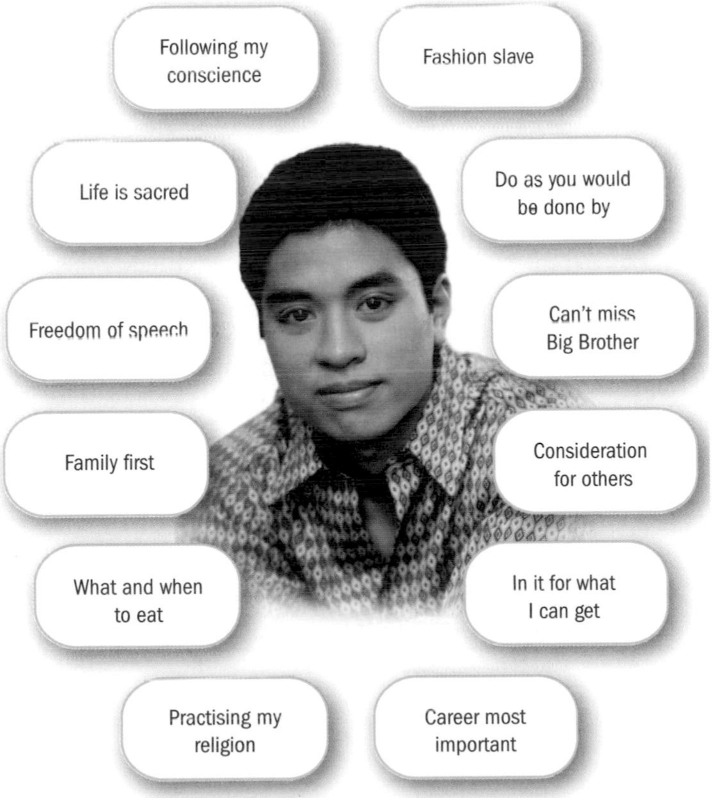

You will probably discover that your values are different from other people's. This is because we all have different influences in our lives that help to shape the value system that we believe in. There are no right or wrong answers necessarily, just differences of opinion. It is important that you begin to understand that different people can believe in different things from you. You don't have to agree with them but you should try to respect them.

Care Value Base

The Care Value Base is a name given to a framework which encourages and promotes good working practices in health and social care. The Care Value Base aims to help both service users and providers of health and social care by giving clear guidelines of acceptable or unacceptable practices and behaviours.

The Care Value Base is divided into three main areas. These are:

- to be aware of and acknowledge people's rights and responsibilities

Following my conscience

Fashion slave

Life is sacred

Do as you would be done by

Freedom of speech

Can't miss Big Brother

Family first

Consideration for others

What and when to eat

In it for what I can get

Practising my religion

Career most important

▲ **Figure 9.7 Different values.**

- to promote equality and diversity of individuals
- to maintain confidentiality.

The Care Value Base is incorporated into all health and social care work and qualifications, so it continually feeds into the workplace setting. All health and social care workers must consider the Care Value Base in every aspect of their work. Employers have a responsibility to ensure that all their staff uphold the Care Value Base and this means providing them with information and training.

Nowadays, service users are much more aware of how they should be treated by service providers. This is partly due to easy access to information on the Internet. As a result, they know far more about their rights to provision and confidently demand these rights are met. At times there can be some conflict between what service users *think* they should receive and what they are *actually entitled* to receive.

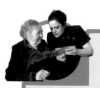

In context

Harry is living in residential care. He is 33 years old but has a debilitating neurological disorder which means that he is dependent on others for help with his physical needs. Mentally, he is extremely alert and is aware of what he wants. Recently, he has been refusing to change his clothes regularly, stating that the clothes he is wearing are clean enough.
It is clear to the staff involved in Harry's care that his clothes are soiled and other residents are complaining that he smells.

Using concepts from the Care Value Base identify:

1 **Harry's rights**
2 **the rights of the staff concerned**
3 **the rights of the other residents.**

Take it further

Can you suggest ways that the staff can manage this situation while protecting Harry's rights? If he continues to refuse to change his soiled clothes, what are the implications for his health and well-being?

1 List the different service providers and agencies that could become involved with Harry's care.

2 Use this research to develop a care plan with Harry's needs at the centre.

3 Consider the rights of both Harry and the service providers and the potential risks involved.

Codes of practice

To help health and social care staff, providers and users to implement the Care Value Base, employers have codes of practice and work-based policies. These are additional guidelines that have the Care Value Base embodied within them.

Codes of practice (also known as codes of conduct or codes of ethics) are used as a framework to guide practitioners on how to behave in the workplace. They ensure that members of staff are aware of the standards of behaviour that are expected of them at all times. They identify broad ethical principles on which core values and practices are based. Codes of conduct are produced from a range of sources including the government, professional bodies, non-governmental organisations and employers. They generally have a common underlying theme:

- They describe the basic rights of service users.
- They emphasise the need for respect of individuals.
- They stress the importance of confidentiality.

Registered practitioners have codes of practice guidelines that are specific to their profession.

Remember!

Registered practitioners are health and social care workers who have completed professional training and have qualified in a specialised role, for example, nurses.

Theory into practice

Registered nurses are governed by the Nursing and Midwifery Council (NMC) and they must comply with the code of conduct clearly laid out by the NMC.

Carry out some research into other health and social care practitioners, for example, doctors, physiotherapists, occupational therapists and social workers. Find out the names of the governing bodies of the different professions and compare their codes of conduct. How are they similar? How different?

Charters

Charters were implemented by the government in 1991 with the introduction of the Citizens' Charter. Its key principle was to improve public services and tailor them more to service users' needs. Since then, charters have been used by many of the key public and private sector services.

Charters are the way health authorities let the general public know what they can expect from their local services. They are freely available for members of the public to read, so that anyone who needs to use their local health and social care provision can find out what they are entitled to receive. Charters are not statements that are written in law so they do not entail legal obligations. However, they are taken very seriously and will often include advice for service users on how to complain if they feel their rights have been breached.

A residential care home may display a charter which states:

- the different kinds of accommodation available
- staff requirements

- costs and what they include
- a confidentiality policy.
- a complaints procedure

Theory into practice

Carry out some independent research into your local health and social care providers. Can you find any charters in your local area? Try looking in your local hospital, GP surgery and dental practice. See if you can think of any other local services that might have charters.

■ The Patients' Charter

In 1992 the Department of Health published its first charter, called the Patients' Charter. This charter clearly stated the rights to services that *all* service users are entitled to. The key points of this charter were that everyone has a right to:

- receive health care based on need rather than the ability to pay
- be registered with a general practitioner (GP)
- receive emergency treatment at any time (through a GP, the ambulance service and A&E departments)
- have their treatment fully explained to them by an appropriate practitioner and in a language they will understand
- complain if necessary and to have their complaint responded to.

Theory into practice

In small groups create a charter for the following work settings:

- a pre-school nursery
- a primary school
- a residential home
- a day centre for the elderly
- a hostel for young people.

In 2001, the Department of Health replaced the Patients' Charter with a new document entitled *Your Guide to the NHS*. This document was designed to focus on service users' expectations rather than rights. *Your Guide to the NHS* comments on what people can currently expect from the NHS and what improvements will be seen in the future. There are four main parts to the guide:

1   access to NHS services

2   hospital tests and treatment

3   ongoing care and support

4   concerns and complaints.

Now that codes of practice, charters and policies are available to the public, we might expect to understand a lot more about our **rights** and **expectations** when accessing health and social care provision. However, there does appear to still be an element of confusion among service users as to the difference between rights and expectations.

Key terms

Rights These are things that everyone is entitled to receive without question.

Expectations These are things that we would hope, expect or like to receive. We are not necessarily entitled to receive these things and have no right to demand them.

Policies

Policies and guidelines state how codes of practice and statutory requirements should be used within a health and social care setting. Most organisations will have their own policies written specifically to suit their workplace. They usually cover similar matters including staff training, bullying, harassment and equal opportunities at work.

Individual rights

What makes us individual?

Every single one of us is an individual and it is vital to remember that all people are distinct and vary from one another. We can look very similar to others (for example, our siblings) but our physical features are only one part of what makes us who we are.

Reflect

Think of a way to describe yourself, starting with the most general 'I am a man' or 'I am a woman'. So are many other people, so that doesn't identify you. 'I have dark hair and brown eyes'– so do lots of other people. Continue thinking of ways to describe yourself. Each time you think of another aspect, it will make you different from others around you, until finally you have come up with a description which applies to no one but you.

Each time you are tempted to react to people as part of a group, i.e. to stereotype, remember how long the task above took and how many descriptions you listed before you found one that uniquely identified you. Remember

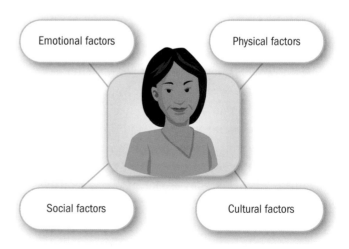

▲ Figure 9.8 **Factors that make you who you are.**

Factor	Examples
Physical factors	• Hair – colour, type (curly, straight, etc.) • Eyes – colour • Skin – tone • Height • Build • Any noticeable features you have
Social factors	How you get on with other people. • Do you like to be surrounded by others or to be on your own? • Do you make friends easily?
Emotional factors	How you express your feelings. • Are you a very calm person or do you become excited easily? • Do you cry easily?
Cultural factors	Your background. • Religion • Values • Family • The community you live in

Table 9.2 The factors that make you unique.

that each and every one of us is unique, irrespective of our need to receive health or social care.

Think about what makes you unique as an individual. There are a number of factors you should take into consideration. In addition to those listed in Table 9.2, there are other concepts to consider that make us individual; there are both concrete and abstract parts to our make-up that add to our individuality.

- **Concrete factors** – these are factual parts of us, things that have happened that shape who we are; experiences we have had, the lifestyle that we live and our backgrounds – how we have been raised to be who we are today.
- **Abstract factors** – these factors are more to do with our feelings about different things. They include likes and dislikes, ambitions, goals, personality and morality.

There are a number of different aspects that make us individuals and they can all influence how we feel about ourselves: this is known as our 'self-concept'. Self-concept can be divided into two areas:

- self-image – the way we see ourselves, or think others see us
- self-esteem – the way we feel about ourselves, or think others feel about us.

Many external factors can have a major effect on our self-image and self-esteem

Each person is a complex individual: this means that every service user that you encounter will be very different. They may share some characteristics with another person, for example, they may both have the same illness, or need similar social support, but their needs will be very different because they are individuals.

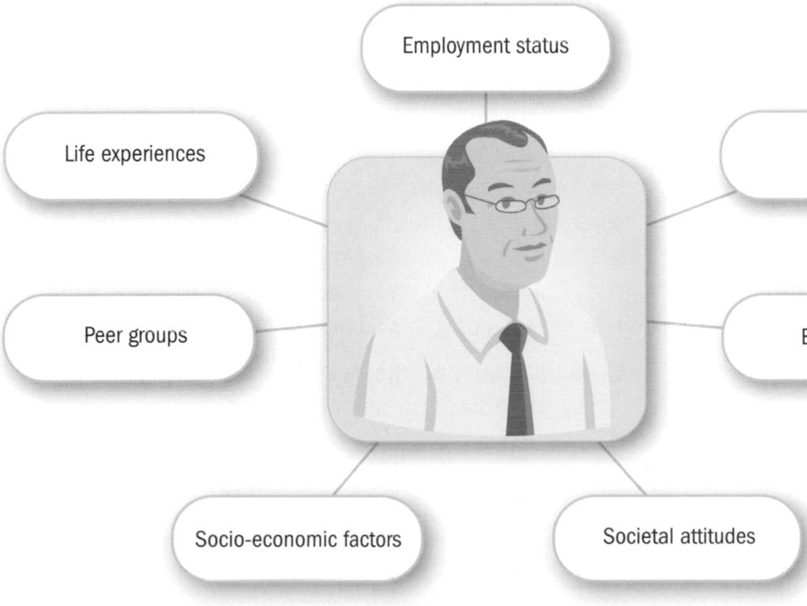

It is important that we always treat others in a dignified way. Think about how you would like to be treated: it would be important to you to both retain your dignity and be allowed privacy. As far as you can, you should treat others as you would like to be treated, respecting individual choices while taking account of personal needs – a vital aspect of care.

◀ **Figure 9.9 External factors that have an effect on our self-image and self-esteem.**

Service users have the right to access information about themselves, highlighting further the importance of respect, in both verbal and non-verbal exchanges. We must also enable people to communicate in a way which feels comfortable to them and not just to us. Sometimes we have to adapt our practices to accommodate our service users' needs in order to build a good working relationship.

Theory into practice

Mohammed is a 39-year-old self-employed builder. He is married and has four children under the age of 10. Peter is a 63-year-old retired businessman who lives with his sister. Both men have been admitted to hospital having experienced what they described as 'crushing' chest pains. The hospital staff are concerned that they have suffered heart attacks. Both men appear to be having the same experience; each is in a stable condition and they are both on the same hospital ward.

1   **What factors need to be considered when caring for both Mohammed and Peter?**

2   **Why might their own perception of the experience be very different from the other's?**

3   **Will the way they are treated have any impact on their health?**

Remember!

Heart attacks are known in medical terms as myocardial infarctions and can be shortened to MI.

Stereotyping

Stereotyping means making assumptions about groups of individuals based on a number of things including age, sex, race, nationality and sexuality. These assumptions can be positive or negative and are absorbed by children at a very young age. Later on, the media can also reinforce stereotypes, via magazines, television and newspapers.

Stereotyping can affect the standard of care that people receive. For example, a care worker who assumes that all elderly people are confused and forgetful might fail to involve them in decisions about food choices, meal times, clothing and personal care. They might assume that they would not remember anyway, and so not bother to ask. This could affect the service user's self-esteem, by making them feel worthless.

Prejudice

Prejudice means liking or disliking someone, not because of who they are, but because of their lifestyle or background. It involves pre-judging someone and forming an opinion about them without getting to know them as a person – an individual. Prejudice is usually wholly negative and can lead to discriminatory behaviour and practice. Again, this can have a negative effect on standards of care.

Of course, it works both ways – service users can be guilty of having prejudices about staff, as well as staff about service users.

Although service users have a right to the care they receive, people who work within the health and social care sector have rights too. This includes the right to refuse to care for someone who is abusive to them.

In context

Mike is 24 and has learning difficulties. He goes to his local genito-urinary clinic (an area in a hospital where people go to have checks on their sexual health) to book an appointment. The receptionist at the clinic tells Mike to speak to his carer and bring him or her along to book an appointment.

1   **What could be the outcome of sending Mike away without an appointment?**

2   **Why do you think the receptionist sent Mike away?**

3   **What prejudices were being shown by this behaviour?**

Discrimination

Discrimination is the result of stereotyping and prejudice. It occurs when a conscious decision is made to treat someone differently simply because they belong to a certain group. This can have a detrimental effect on the person being discriminated against and could ultimately affect the provision that they receive. The government has created legislation to try to remove discrimination. Anti-discrimination legislation covers areas such as disability, gender and race.

Discrimination is a part of the society that we live in: we all have prejudices and can stereotype individuals without being aware that we are doing it. It is part of the role of a health and social care worker to help to reduce the effects that discrimination can have on health and care standards. Always try to keep an open mind about people: treat them as individuals, and encourage others to do the same.

Reflect

Think about any prejudices that you have, or individuals that you might be tempted to stereotype. Where do these thoughts come from? Are there strong beliefs within your family that you have never questioned before? Have you had a negative experience which has resulted in these feelings? You do not have to share your findings with anyone else. Just be honest with yourself. By becoming aware of any prejudices that you have, you can then acknowledge that they exist within you. This helps you to explore why they exist and hopefully ensure you do not allow service users to know about them when you are caring for and supporting them.

Discrimination can exist in all areas of health and social care. Regardless of the labels that can be attached to a person, *everyone* is entitled to be treated *fairly and equally*. This must be without prejudice, focusing on the help and care needs that must be addressed, and nothing else. Feeling safe and free from harm is a fundamental right and not to be discriminated against

because of other factors when health and social care needs must be met. When you meet someone for the first time, approach them as a blank canvas, ignoring any associated labels and assessing the needs that require attention. We live within a diverse, multi-cultural society where the diverse needs of service users must be met as fully as possible, irrespective of age, gender, ethnicity, abilities, preferences and customs.

Workers' responsibilities

People who choose to work in the health and social care sector do so for various reasons. What they will all have in common is a deep concern for the rights and needs of other people, and a desire to help them. Health and social care workers are placed in extremely privileged positions – it is a huge responsibility to have access to, and work with, vulnerable individuals. Staff must be aware of the power that they hold and the responsibilities they have to the individuals they are caring for.

The Care Standards Act 2000 covers many health and social care areas and regulates the care standards that must be maintained. It regulates the issue of **accountability**. Members of staff are accountable for their actions in regard to service users at all times. They must be able to justify that the way they have behaved has been in the best interests of the person they are caring for. Furthermore, they must ensure that it is what the service user would want. Issues surrounding accountability are written into codes of conduct so that practitioners are clear about their responsibilities.

Key terms

Accountability Being responsible and required to account for your own conduct.

Communicating needs

To be sure that you are acting in the best interests of the service user, good communication skills are vital and communication takes many forms. Important considerations include:

- good listening skills
- written information that is clear and accurate
- enabling the service user to state their needs, views and preferences clearly.

A skilled care worker communicates intuitively, recognising and reading non-verbal signs and reacting appropriately. Good communication skills are central to developing a good relationship with a service user.

Some people find it harder to communicate their needs than others. It is part of the role of a care worker to promote equal opportunities for everyone to communicate in the best way they can. Our multi-cultural and diverse society can lead to difficulties in communicating, so we must find ways to adapt our practices to ensure all have equal rights, irrespective of potential barriers.

A great deal of work within the health and social care sector is based on trust. Service users place a great deal of trust in the staff that are involved in helping to care for them and this must be respected at all times. Care workers often have access to a lot of private details and it is essential that confidentiality is respected.

Confidentiality

Confidentiality means having respect for the privacy of any information about a service user. In 1997, a government review was held regarding the issues surrounding confidentiality. It resulted in the publication of a set of guidelines for staff to adhere to, named the Caldecott Principles. They include:

1. Justify the purpose – staff must be able to justify every proposed use or transfer of patient-identifiable information.

2. Do not use patient-identifiable information other than when absolutely necessary.

3. Use the minimum necessary patient-identifiable information.

4. Access to patient-identifiable information should be on a strict need-to-know basis.

5. All staff must be aware of the obligation to respect patient confidentiality.

6. Someone in each organisation should be responsible for ensuring that the organisation complies with legal requirements.

7. The legislative and administration protections described should leave service users feeling confident that they can rely on care practitioners to protect their personal information.

The Caldecott Principles clearly identify the importance of confidentiality with regard to caring for others and offer a purposeful framework for all staff to refer to for guidance.

If you think about what type of service user information you may have access to, you'll find that it includes:

- physical/mental health condition
- previous medical/social history
- family history – physical/social
- names and addresses
- medications – what is being taken now and what was previously
- personal experiences
- feelings/thoughts
- moral opinions
- risk-taking behaviours
- diet and rehabilitation regimes.

Take it further

Outline the action you would take in the following situations.

- Michael has had an appointment with the speech and language therapist. He wants to see the written report that has been made.
- Shanna wants to know the correct procedure for gaining access to her father's records as he is refusing to tell her anything.
- Michelle wants to know why Edward, who is diabetic, can't have strawberry gateau.
- Naseem wants to know the correct procedure for gaining access to her father's records as he has been diagnosed with dementia.
- Heidi tells you in confidence that she saves up her prescribed painkillers as her pain is much more severe at night – so she takes her daily allowance in one go before she goes to bed.

Theory into practice

Read the following scenarios and decide whether confidentiality has been breached. Give reasons for your answers.

Sarah, who works as a support worker, is out with friends having a meal in a restaurant. She is discussing an incident that happened at work the previous day. There had been a breakdown in communication with another individual and Sarah referred to this person as 'spiteful and dishonest'. Another diner overheard the conversation. Sarah did not mention any names.

Marnie is working as a support worker for social services. She receives a telephone call from a female who says she is the niece of one of Marnie's service users. She asks for details about her aunt's condition and well-being, stating that she would like to visit but needs to know how her aunt is first. Marnie informs the lady that her aunt's health is improving and that the medical staff are very happy with her.

Shakhira is travelling home from work on the bus when she meets an old work colleague, Max. They are thrilled to see each other as it is a long time since they last met. The course of the conversation naturally turns to the workplace; Max is keen to know how the service users from the day centre they both worked in are keeping. They talk about the service users and the colleagues that they both know – they only talk about good things and no subjects are touched on that could be regarded as detrimental to anyone's character.

This type of information can be damaging if it is disclosed to the wrong person so, as a health and social care worker, you must give full consideration before you share it with anyone. This privileged information is protected by the Data Protection Act 1998.

Confidential information is stored in numerous ways. It may be that you are verbally informed of something – sometimes a gesture such as a nod of the head can provide us with information. Much of the information that is held on service users is written, either by hand or electronically. Regardless of how the information is conveyed, the rules regarding confidentiality still apply.

Disclosure

You may find yourself in situations when service users want to disclose information to you; this can be because they feel they can trust you. It can be perceived as a compliment, showing that the service user feels comfortable with you and that you have made them feel valued. Staff must, however, be aware of the boundaries that exist concerning disclosure.

Disclosure is the revelation of information to another person. Sometimes a service user might want to tell you something in confidence. They might start the conversation by saying, 'You won't tell anyone what I say will you?' As a health and social care worker you are not in a position to make these promises. You cannot guarantee confidentiality until you know what a service user is going to say; you should inform the service user that you may be obliged to pass on information before they disclose.

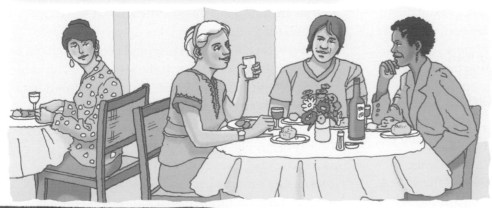

Figure 9.10 Has confidentiality been breached?

There are certain circumstances when it would be appropriate to breach a service user's confidentiality including:

- when a service user has given consent
- if there are exceptional circumstances
- if a court order has been issued
- if it is deemed that a service user or another person could be at risk.

Theory into practice

Lewis works in a day centre for service users with physical impairments. A service user called Rifa attends three days a week. Over a period of time Rifa has disclosed information to Lewis. Read the following statements and decide whether Lewis is in a position to maintain confidentiality or whether he should share Rifa's disclosure with an appropriate other.

- Rifa has decided to no longer take her medication as it makes her feel dizzy.
- Rifa had a baby before she was married who was adopted.
- Rifa went to her purse and discovered £20 was missing.
- Rifa doesn't like people with blonde hair.
- Rifa's carer shouts at her when she takes too long getting ready.

If the occasion ever arises when you feel that it is not appropriate to maintain confidentiality, you should always inform the service user first. They may actually be relieved that someone is taking control of the situation and can help resolve their dilemma. However, even if the service user is unhappy about you informing someone else, you are still obliged to. By informing the service user of your intentions, you are still maintaining their trust as you are being totally honest with them.

It is important that, if you do need to pass on confidential information, you seek out the most appropriate person. Confidential information must always be given on a need-to-know basis and these circumstances are no different. You need to decide if it

is an issue that needs dealing with urgently, or if it can wait. You must also choose the right time and place – try to make sure it is at a time when the person you need to speak to can give you their full attention and that the environment is private so the conversation cannot be overheard by others. Confidentiality is taken extremely seriously as a concept in health and social care and is written into codes of professional conduct and organisations' policies; if a staff member were to be found discussing a service user's details inappropriately, they could face disciplinary action.

There are some basic rules to remember when dealing with confidential information:

- Share information on a need-to-know basis only.
- Read your organisation's policy and follow the guidelines.
- If at all possible do not use names – choose an alternative means of identification, for example, numbers (which further protect anonymity).
- If unsure, ask a more senior member of staff for advice.

Storing confidential information

The storage of confidential information needs careful consideration. Sometimes information is written by hand but, with the increasing use of technology, this is becoming less common. Written information should always be kept in a locked unit and this can lead to storage problems. Handwriting can be difficult to read or the writing can fade with time, thus increasing the risk of mistakes being made.

Information technology has transformed the way in which personal information is stored. Computerised records are now widely used in health and social care. Computerised information takes up very little space and, if it is part of a network, several people can look at the available information at the same time. This is of benefit to both staff and service users, as records don't have to be physically transferred. The time saved on travel can be spent with the service user and the risk of information going missing in transit is reduced.

As we have said, all verbal, written and electronic information must be kept confidential. Therefore, the storage of such highly personal information must be considered carefully. The Data Protection Act 1998 protects service users' information. The act gives the same level of protection to electronic information as to information held in any other format. The act specifies that organisations that hold information about service users must be registered and comply with the principles of the act.

Organisations must install security measures so that only authorised and appropriate people can access confidential information. These security measures include appropriate training for staff and ensuring that passwords are in place. Staff using electronic technology also have a responsibility to protect information by:

- making sure the screen can only be seen by staff members
- never leaving the screen unattended

Theory into practice

List the types of information that could be stored in the following places:

- GP surgeries
- A&E departments
- medical records
- social services.

- not sharing passwords
- ensuring information is accurate and clear
- logging off when finished.

Assessment activity 9.3

P4 Describe the values that underpin social care practice.

1   Think about the three main areas for the Care Value Base (see below). Draw a mind map of what types of things you think might be under each of the areas. Break each bullet point down and make a list of words that you think might be linked to each one. **P4**

- to be aware of and acknowledge people's rights and responsibilities
- to promote equality and diversity of people as individuals
- to maintain confidentiality.

Grading tip for P4

You must make clear and relevant points to demonstrate a basic understanding.

9.4 Ethical principles and perspectives

Ethical principles

Working in the health and social care sector can be extremely complex. Individuals are diverse and vary in their values and beliefs – interactions within the working environment can give rise to many **moral** decisions and dilemmas on a regular, even daily, basis. Gaining an

Key terms

Morals The rules created by society that decide what is right and wrong, good or bad. Issues such as sexual behaviour, criminality and honesty are linked to moral values.

understanding of **ethics** and ethical principles can help when faced with difficult decisions.

Ethics has its roots within philosophy. Philosophers question our actions concerning the morally right course of action to take in different situations.

Key terms

Ethics The moral principles which guide a person's behaviour.

The concept of ethics is often linked to research. Researchers have to present their research ideas before an ethics committee which will determine if the proposal is ethically sound. In order to carry out experiments, researchers must prove that they are not causing unnecessary harm to anyone or deliberately deceiving. This is why very little research has been carried out in areas such as drugs for pregnant women or young children. It would be deemed unethical for pregnant women or young children to participate in drug trials – pregnant women would not only be taking risks with their own health, but with that of their unborn child too, and young children are unable to consent to participate in such trials.

Ethics can be described as the moral codes of practice. They encompass a large area including:

- behaviour or moral conduct – staff must be professional at all times; unprofessional behaviour such as direct prejudice or discrimination is not acceptable under any circumstances
- abstract issues such as legal, religious, social and personal opinions – these are often referred to as moral issues, for example, abortion and divorce
- moral debates that are raised within society with regard to professional practice, for example, euthanasia and genetic modelling.

Ethics in social care

Practitioners often work intuitively, using a sound moral conscience, i.e. identifying right from wrong and good from bad in a subconscious manner.

When faced with moral dilemmas, it is essential that staff can justify how the decision has been made. The following prompts can help staff to reach those decisions:

- Is the service user able to make a free choice?
- Do I respect their decision, irrespective of whether I approve or disapprove of it?
- Am I being non-discriminatory – respecting all concerned equally?
- Will I be doing good and preventing harm with this decision?
- Will I be telling the truth?
- Will I be minimising harm in the long term?
- Can I totally honour the promises and agreements that I make?

The most important ethical consideration for health and social care workers is to always act in the best interests of the service user. This principle underpins all health and social care work. There are four recognised sub-principles within the health and social care concept of ethics. They encompass the whole idea of acting in the best interests of someone you are working with. In the terminology of ethics they are referred to as:

- **non-maleficence** – never causing harm to an individual
- **beneficence** – doing good for the individual wherever possible
- **autonomy** – allowing an individual to plan their own actions and act on those plans
- **justice** – treating individuals fairly and equally and in accordance with their needs.

This might sound like common sense but, when dealing with complex ethical situations, these can be useful concepts to refer back to. There might be times when you will have to act in the best interests of a service user who could disagree with your actions or reasons for reaching your decision. They might not understand that, in the long term, you are supporting them, as you have a much wider perspective than they do at that particular time.

It is essential that all service users are treated with equal rights in these situations; in ethics the term used is *equity*. The principle of equity is that all users have equal access to, and benefit from, available services. Staff must be fair with both their time and the resources that are available, to ensure that users feel valued and worthwhile. Workers need to protect themselves so they cannot be accused of favouritism or discriminatory practice.

While it may be true that health and social care staff may *think* they are acting in the best interests of the service user, it is important to question whether this is indeed the case – it may be that they are really acting in their *own* best interests. Remember that all people are individuals and, just because you might not approve of their decisions, this does not make them wrong. It is essential that a carer protects and ensures freedom from harm; it is also essential that service users are empowered to have the freedom to act on their wishes. All adults should be afforded the same freedom, even if some of them rely on others to provide their care.

Benevolent oppression

People who are dependent on others have less power than their carers; they rely on staff allowing them to behave in the way they want to. Well-meaning staff often make decisions on the service user's behalf, or prevent them from risky behaviour, in the interests of safety. Although staff may believe they are acting in the best interests of the person they are caring for; they can end up being over-protective and smothering a person's freedom to act as an individual.

Examples of such 'benevolent oppression' include:

- not allowing people with disabilities to go out alone
- strapping people into wheelchairs in case they fall out
- limiting the alcohol intake of service users
- having set meal times
- leaving the toilet door open so that service users can be 'checked on'.

A loss of power or control can increase feelings of worthlessness. It can impact on self-image and self-esteem. Service users could respond to such negativity by becoming angry, frightened and frustrated – even prone to violent outbursts. Benevolent oppression compounds the idea that the service user is problematic or a burden to society.

Situations care workers may face

Conflicts of interest

As a member of staff in the health and social care sector, you will undoubtedly be faced with situations where there is a conflict of interest. Conflicts of interest occur when difficult decisions or dilemmas arise; the professional can be faced with complex issues and may have to make a decision after considering:

- all the facts
- all the potential risks
- their professional and legal responsibilities.

Over a period of time, staff who work within the health and social care sector will develop professional skills to help them cope with the ethical dilemmas that can arise. Although experience can be enormously beneficial, a sound basic understanding of the potential issues that you could encounter will be helpful.

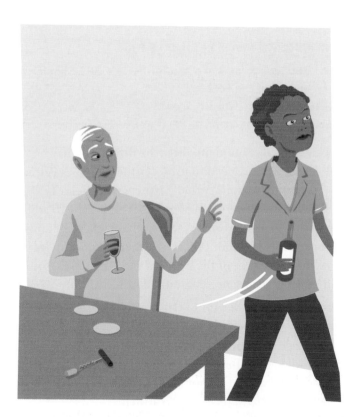

▲ Figure 9.11 Benevolent oppression in action!

Theory into practice

Read the following scenarios. Identify and explain the actions that you feel should be taken. Think of these from an ethical perspective and also consider values.

- Manisha is 14 years old and visits her GP because she has contracted a sexually transmitted infection. She asks that her parents are not informed.
- A man of approximately 25 years of age arrives in the A&E department. He has a shaved head and numerous body piercings and tattoos. He is bleeding heavily and refuses to reveal his name and address. He states that he will leave if the police are called.
- Danishe is 16 years old. He walks into a homeless shelter and explains that he has run away from home due to abuse. He asks that his family are not contacted or informed of his whereabouts.
- Suzy is 15 years of age and goes to see the school nurse complaining of a bad headache. When questioned Suzy discloses that she has taken some amphetamine tablets which she calls 'speed'. Suzy begs the nurse not to tell anyone.
- Laura is in hospital on a maternity ward, having given birth to her second child three days ago. Laura is reluctant to go home and when questioned reveals that her partner can be abusive, but she is too scared to tell anyone.

In context

Ben has attended his local genito-urinary clinic. He is seen by Dr Clark and, following counselling, has been told that he is HIV positive. During the counselling he is advised to contact all previous sexual partners and he is to start a course of treatment.

Ben has been with his partner Petra for 18 months. Petra is pregnant and the baby is due in two months. Prior to his relationship with Petra, Ben had a series of partners.

On a subsequent visit to the clinic it becomes clear to Dr Clark that Ben has not told Petra about his HIV status. Dr Clark is aware that their baby is due very soon. He tells Ben that Petra ought to be assessed to find out if she is HIV positive, and therefore if the baby is at risk, so that the necessary steps can be taken and treatment started. Ben adamantly refuses to tell Petra and says that if she is told without his consent he will stop attending the clinic and end his course of treatment.

1 **What should Dr Clark do? Can he legally inform Petra?**

2 **Ethically, should he inform Petra?**

3 **Can he inform Ben's and/or Petra's GP? Should he inform the GP?**

The types of ethical dilemmas you could face are not straightforward. A multitude of issues can arise, involving many different people and settings. These can include:

- service users and organisations
- service users and other service users
- service users and workers
- service users and relatives and friends
- resource issues.

The principle of respect for autonomy means that personal information should not be disclosed without consent. However, there are cases where consideration of the majority outweighs the minority, i.e. the need

to protect Ben's confidentiality (the minority) may be outweighed by the need to protect others such as Petra, the baby and previous sexual partners (the majority). In this case the autonomy of others is an issue – by not informing them, and so not telling the truth, their ability to make decisions about their treatment and lifestyles is at risk. The balance of the benefits and risks of disclosure and non-disclosure needs careful consideration.

If we think about Ben and Petra's situation, the harms of non-disclosure include:

- The risk that Petra may be HIV positive – if Petra is not told about Ben, she cannot take steps to be tested and so is harmed by not knowing her own HIV status and, potentially, receiving treatment.
- If Petra is HIV positive, but is not aware of the risk, she will not take steps to minimise the risks of

infection to her unborn child. The steps she could take would include receiving treatment during pregnancy, the baby being born by caesarean section, not breast feeding and prophylactic treatment.

- If Petra did later discover that there was a risk to her and her baby, and that she had not been informed, she could lose all trust in the health care system. Potentially this could place her and her baby at greater risk

- There are risks to Ben's previous sexual partners who could be contacted and informed.

- There is a risk that Ben could go on and infect future sexual partners.

The harms of disclosure include:

- If the clinic informs others without Ben's consent then, as a consequence, he might lose trust in Dr Clark and the health and social care services in general.

- Ben has stated that, if Petra is informed, he will end his course of treatment and sever contact with the clinic. The potential consequence of this would be a risk of relapse and severe health problems, possibly leading to death.

- Ben may be stigmatised by others and have difficulties with future employment opportunities due to discrimination.

Theory into practice

Carry out some independent research into the legal implications of this scenario. What would Dr Clark's code of professional conduct and governing body (the General Medical Council) advise? What would be the best decision to make morally?

Assessment activity 9.4

P5 Describe the ethical principles that underpin social care.

1. Think about the following questions within a whole class debate. Individually write a paragraph to answer the questions from your own perspective. Within your discussion consider why ethical principles are so important in the health and social care sector. **P5**

   - What behaviours would you consider to be risky?
   - Why should service users have the freedom to act on their wishes?
   - How would you react if a service user decided to participate in risky behaviour?

Grading tip for P5

Your discussion should focus on your own personal beliefs. Try to form a balanced argument to demonstrate your understanding.

M4 Explain the roles of individuals and organisations in relation to values and ethical practice.

2. Why is it so important that health and social care workers adhere strictly to ethical boundaries? What could be the potential consequences if workers and organisations chose to ignore ethical values and principles? **M4**

Grading tip for M4

A detailed explanation of your findings should be supported by examples to justify your statements.

Knowledge check

1 Why is it crucial that the service user is involved in the care planning process?

2 Who might you involve in planning an individual's care if a language barrier exists?

3 Describe what is meant by the term *resources* within the health and social care sector.

4 Peter's care plan was devised and implemented three weeks ago; can this be left as it is now?

5 What does the term *individual* mean?

6 Describe the difference between *confidentiality* and *disclosure*.

7 What is the most important ethical consideration that workers must abide by?

8 Whose needs must be taken into account when faced with ethical decision making?

9 Describe the term *conflict of interest*.

10 Why do health and social care workers need to be involved in ethical decision making?

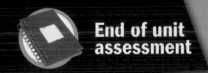
Preparation for assessment

Anthony is 28 and has cerebral palsy. He lives in supported housing with three other people and there are health care support workers present 24 hours a day. Anthony needs assistance with some of his activities of daily living and is reliant on a wheelchair for his mobility.

At times Anthony gets extremely frustrated with his lack of independence and his reliance on others for assistance. Sometimes he refuses to allow the care staff to help him with his hygiene needs. This has resulted in complaints from the other people in the house. Recently, when one of the carers was helping Anthony to shower, they noticed he had developed pressure sores which could become infected if left untreated.

Anthony is prone to violent outbursts where he throws items and uses offensive language. Recently, Anthony has been socialising with a new group of friends. He regularly drinks excessive amounts of alcohol and has become increasingly more abusive to the staff involved in his care.

There are concerns that Anthony's lifestyle is having a detrimental effect on his physical health. Furthermore, it is impacting on the other people living in the house as his violent outbursts are causing concern.

1   Anthony will need a care plan tailored to his individual needs. Describe the process that will lead to a suitable care plan **P1**

2   It is essential that Anthony is involved in decisions concerning his care and that his needs are taken into consideration. Consider and describe the different aspects of Anthony's life that will potentially be involved, and how legislation could impact on the care plan that is devised. **P4**, **M1**, **M3**

3   As Anthony lives in supported housing, key aspects of legislation will need to be observed and practised within the home. List four examples of the types of legislation concerned and explain how these could affect Anthony within his home. **P3**

4   Analyse the importance of multi-disciplinary and inter-agency working when devising, implementing and evaluating Anthony's care plan, remembering that current legislation must be included. **D2**

5   In addition to the support workers who are in attendance in Anthony's home, identify other health and social care workers who may be involved in his care. Provide examples to explain how these other workers can improve the care that Anthony receives. **P2**, **M2**

6   Anthony has been refusing assistance with some of his identified care needs. Consider how care workers might deal with the opposition they are facing. **P5**

7   Anthony is an adult and has the right to make decisions regarding his lifestyle. How may staff involved in Anthony's care empower Anthony so that he is sure he is making the right decisions for his health and well-being? **M4**, **D1**

Resources and further reading

Hendrick, J. (2004) *Law and Ethics* Cheltenham: Nelson Thornes

HM Government (1990) *Caring for People* London: HMSO

HM Government (2001) *Your Guide to the NHS: Getting the most from your National Health Service* London: HMSO

Holland, K., Hogg, C. (2001) *Cultural Awareness in Nursing and Health Care* London: Hodder Arnold

Nolan, Y. (2001) *Care S/NVQ Level 3* Oxford: Heinemann

Sussex, F., Scourfield, P. (2004) *Social Care Level 4* Oxford: Heinemann

Useful websites

Care Sector Skills Council
www.skillsforcareanddevelopment.org.uk

Department of Health
www.dh.gov.uk

Equal Opportunities Commission
www.eoc.org.uk

Health Care Sector Skills Council
www.skillsforhealth.org.uk

Social Care Institute for Excellence
www.scie.org.uk

Guardian newspaper
www.society.guardian.co.uk

Victoria Climbie inquiry
www.victoria-climbie-inquiry.org.uk

GRADING CRITERIA

To achieve a pass grade the evidence must show that the learner is able to:	To achieve a merit grade the evidence must show that, in addition to the pass criteria, the learner is able to:	To achieve a distinction grade the evidence must show that, in addition to the pass and merit criteria, the learner is able to:
P1 describe the processes of care planning with reference to care planning principles **Assessment activity 9.1 page 16**	**M1** explain care planning principles **Assessment activity 9.1 page 16**	
P2 identify the importance of multi-disciplinary and inter-agency working on the care planning process **Assessment activity 9.1 page 16**	**M2** use examples to explain how multi-disciplinary and inter-agency working can improve the care planning process **Assessment activity 9.1 page 16**	**D1** evaluate the role of multi-disciplinary and inter-agency working in social care **Assessment activity 9.1 page 16**
P3 use four examples to describe key aspects of legislation, policies and codes of practice that influence social care **Assessment activity 9.2 page 18**	**M3** explain the impact of legislation on the concept of care planning **Assessment activity 9.2 page 18**	**D2** evaluate the effectiveness of current legislation in promoting care planning and multi-disciplinary/inter-agency working. **Assessment activity 9.2 page 18**
P4 describe the values that underpin social care practice **Assessment activity 9.3 page 29**		
P5 describe ethical principles in relation to social care. **Assessment activity 9.4 page 33**	**M4** explain the roles of individuals and organisations in relation to values and ethical practice. **Assessment activity 9.4 page 33**	

Caring for children and young people

Introduction

Not all young people have the care and education they would wish for. There are various reasons for this, many of which are out of the hands of the young people themselves. This unit will explore the various reasons that children and young people might need to be looked after and the organisations that provide care for them. We will also consider the roles of the staff who work within those organisations and, in order to fully comprehend the issues involved, we will take a close look at the risks to children and young people caught up in abusive or exploitative situations. There will, additionally, be an opportunity to consider the strategies that might be used to minimise those risks.

How you will be assessed

You will be assessed through an assignment in which you will demonstrate your knowledge and understanding of the issues related to safeguarding children and young people. A variety of assessment tasks and case studies are included throughout this unit to help prepare you for this. They will also provide you with the information you need when developing strategies for supporting children, young people and their families within the current legislative framework.

After completing this unit you should be able to achieve the following outcomes:

- Understand why children and young people may need to be looked after
- Understand how care is provided for children and young people
- Understand the risks for children and young people of abusive and exploitative behaviour
- Know strategies to minimise the risk to children and young people of abusive and exploitative behaviour.

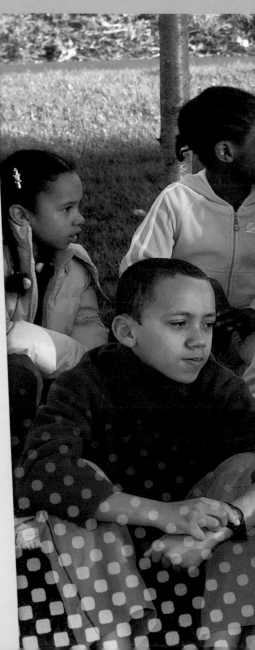

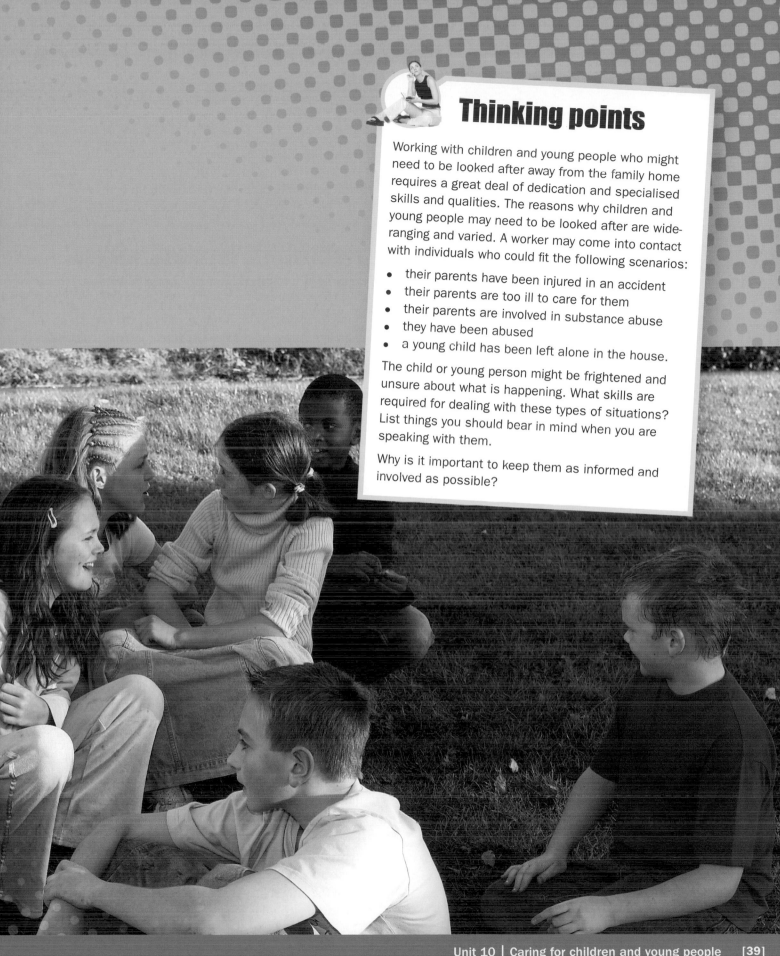

Thinking points

Working with children and young people who might need to be looked after away from the family home requires a great deal of dedication and specialised skills and qualities. The reasons why children and young people may need to be looked after are wide-ranging and varied. A worker may come into contact with individuals who could fit the following scenarios:

- their parents have been injured in an accident
- their parents are too ill to care for them
- their parents are involved in substance abuse
- they have been abused
- a young child has been left alone in the house.

The child or young person might be frightened and unsure about what is happening. What skills are required for dealing with these types of situations? List things you should bear in mind when you are speaking with them.

Why is it important to keep them as informed and involved as possible?

Looked-after children

There are a number of reasons why children may be looked after by people other than their own family. Those reasons may include family breakdown, bereavement, parental illness or incapacity of some kind or they may be linked to behavioural problems or even the child's own illness. These will be discussed in more detail later.

The imposition of a care order

It is the duty of each local authority to consider the welfare of all children. One of the main sections of the Children Acts of 1989 and 2004 is that they try to ensure that children are supported and kept within their family's home, if at all possible. However, if a child, for whatever reason, needs to live away from home and is cared for by a local authority, this child is known as being 'looked after'. Some children in this situation may have multiple behaviour problems and will often require individual support and care – some have been excluded from school and may have difficulty in developing relationships with other people. There are times when a care order needs to be imposed for the overall benefit of the child and their family. This means that social services, under the local authority, have the role of caring for the child or young person and making decisions for them.

Each local authority will endeavour to ensure that an appropriate placement is found for the length of time that the child or young person will need to be looked after. The ultimate goal is that the child will eventually return to live with his or her own family. This may not always be possible and in many cases a substitute family is required or the young person may have reached the age when they can move on to an independent life.

With the agreement of parents

There are times when parents realise that they are struggling with their parental responsibilities and that the child would benefit from a period of time away from the family home. Once the situation has improved the child often returns to the care of their parents.

Potential reasons why a child might be 'looked after'

Sometimes a child or young person might need to leave their home because of problems that are related either to their family or to themselves. This might be for a wide range of reasons, for example, the family may be unable to care for the child because of an accident or the child may present such difficult behaviour patterns that the family are unable to cope. The child or young person may be abused or exploited and might need to be cared for away from the family home for reasons of safety.

Family-related reasons

These could include bereavement, parental illness or incapacity (for example, mental health problems or substance misuse). We'll explore these in more detail below.

■ Bereavement and upheaval

Looked-after children are often very vulnerable as they have faced a great deal of upheaval and disruption in their lives. They may have been affected by damaging experiences such as abuse and rejection. There may have been traumatic experiences in their lives such as family bereavement and they may have learned to internalise their turbulent emotions. As a result, many of these individuals have great difficulty with their education and often fall behind the majority of children in their class. Their ability to concentrate is greatly reduced and they may display specific needs that must be addressed and met before progress can be made. However, school is often the only stable factor in the child's life – everything else except school is in turmoil.

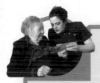

In context

John (aged 13) and his sister Sophie (aged 11) were having a day out with their parents. It had been a lovely day and they had ended it by playing family games and having a picnic by the river. They had gathered their belongings up and had packed the car ready for the homeward journey. They were almost home when another car sped across a junction and collided with them. John and Sophie could not remember much of the resulting chaos but when they reached the hospital, and after their initial treatment, they were told that their mother was very ill in intensive care, and would require hospitalisation for a number of weeks. Their father had not survived the crash.

1   **List three major aspects of John and Sophie's situation.**

2   **Suggest who might be involved in their short-term care, including any organisations.**

3   **Consider who might be involved in helping them with their rights.**

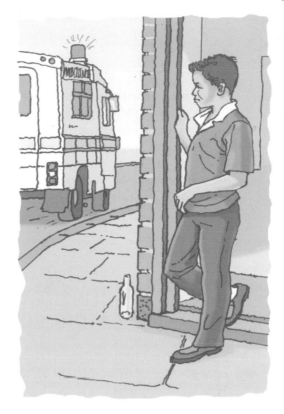

▲   **Figure 10.1 What is going to happen now?**

Reflect

Were your parents ever ill or did you need to be cared for by another member of your family, for example, a grandparent? Make a list of your feelings at that time.

■ Parental illness or family breakdown

The reasons why children and young people find themselves being looked after are varied. Their parents may be unwell or unable to cope and the child may return to the family home at some time in the future as this situation improves. Meanwhile, they may spend time with foster parents or in children's homes or in residential schools. The length of time they spend in this situation will vary according to circumstances. Family breakdown happens for a wide range of reasons, which include bereavement, parental illness, incapacity, mental health problems or even substance abuse. The family unit may break down totally because of violence and discord and the child require care that could be temporary or even permanent. A child who is being abused may need to be removed from that situation for their own safety and well-being. Such circumstances may result in their needing particularly sensitive care and later they may require therapy to help them come to terms with what has happened to them.

Child/young person-related reasons

A child or young person might need to leave their family home because of their own health problems, behavioural problems, learning difficulties or disability. It may also be because the child has committed an offence. Again, we'll explore these in more detail below.

■ Health problems

A child or young person themselves may have an illness or condition which makes it difficult for them to live in

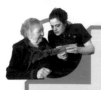

In context

Samelia is 11 years old and is blind. She has been looked after for most of her life in institutions and schools for the blind. Her parents feel that they cannot provide fully for her needs and that she benefits more by being away from them. She has a younger brother and sister who both live at home and attend their local primary school. The family visit her occasionally but their visits are becoming less regular and she rarely goes home as they feel that they cannot cater for her adequately. She is starting to feel isolated and alone.

1 List the advantages of specialised provision for Samelia.

2 List the disadvantages.

3 How might the emotional situation be more positive for her? What might help her feel less isolated?

a family home and so alternative arrangements must be made for long- or short-term care. The care required might be specific so that the child would benefit from the use of specialist resources, which may only be available outside the family home.

■ Behavioural problems

Some possible causes of changes in behaviour, which might lead to problems for children, young people and their families, are listed below.

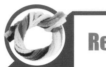

Remember!

The causes of anxiety in children may not always seem rational to an adult.

Stress	Many children suffer from stress, leading to poor school performance, and emotional and behavioural problems. Stress may be the result of an unstable home life or a feeling of being unloved. Their parents may not have the skills for bringing up children, or the child may feel that the demands for achievement and success are unrealistic.
Anxiety	Anxiety is quite common among children and young people. In fact, many anxiety disorders in an adult will have started in childhood. Chronic anxiety disorders require early diagnosis if they are to be treated in time. If they are left unrecognised, they may result in a disability, dysfunction and, in some cases, even suicide.
Depression	Childhood depression is a growing concern and may even lead to suicide. The reasons for depression are wide ranging and various. All individuals involved in the care of young people must be aware of the issues surrounding depression. The child or young person may become unresponsive, withdrawn and not seek the company of others. Without appropriate treatment depression can have serious consequences. Finding the root cause of depression may often be difficult and the young person may need counselling and therapy.
Obsessive–compulsive disorder	Children with obsessive–compulsive disorders are growing in number. In relation to other mental health issues, relatively little is known about this type of disorder. However, early recognition and the ensuing treatment will help to reduce the suffering they cause.
Phobias	Phobias often come under the heading of childhood anxiety disorders but they are now becoming so common that they may be dealt with as a separate issue. Panic disorders are also linked to phobias and these can be devastating as they can disable the normal life of the child. Once again early recognition and treatment are essential.

Table 10.1 Some reasons for behavioural change.

Learning difficulties

There are many families within the UK with children and young people who have learning difficulties. Some families are unable to cope with the challenges this presents, and may reject their child. In cases such as this, it can be more suitable if the child is looked after outside the family home. This may only be a temporary measure but in many cases, as the child requires specialist assistance, it may become a more permanent arrangement. Temporary **respite** care often allows the family time to relax and deal with their own needs so that they are better equipped when their child returns to the family home.

Key terms

Respite A break or a time of relief from the demands of care.

Remanded To be kept separate from society for a period of time in a young offenders' institution or a prison.

Disability

Children and young people with disabilities may be part of families with so many other demands on them that they find it problematic to cope with a child who has specific issues. Short-term respite care may be a possibility or there may need to be longer-term provision. If the family home cannot provide for the specialised needs of the individual, alternative care may be sought, which primarily benefits the child or young person.

Take it further

Carry out some research into the types of support and help available for families with children or young people who have disabilities. List the three that are the most important in your opinion. Discuss your findings with other people and agree on a revised list of three.

A child who has committed an offence

There are some young people who, for a variety of reasons, become caught up in a cycle of offending and breaking the law. The criminal activity and the involvement of the police may result in the young person's being **remanded** or detained. In general, the

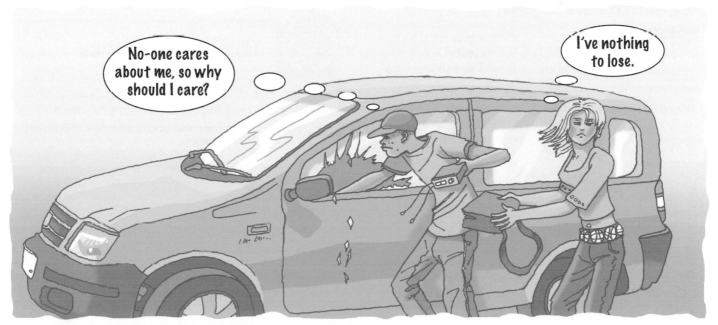

▲ Figure 10.2 Young people might offend because they want attention.

number of children and young people who are in care because they have been remanded or detained make up less than two per cent of the total that are looked after.

When a young person is remanded or detained it is usually as a result of criminal charges and a care order may be made on a short-term basis.

Assessment activity 10.1

P1 Describe the main reasons why children and young people may need to be looked after away from their families.

1   You have been asked to make an information booklet for potential carers of children and young people. Describe two family-related and two child-related reasons why they may need to be looked after away from their families. **P1**

Grading tip for P1

You should make this as interesting as possible by providing a hypothetical example. You could also illustrate it appropriately.

10.2 How care is provided for children and young people

Legislation/legal framework

It has been recognised for a long time that children and young people are vulnerable and are therefore greatly at risk of being abused and exploited. There is now a comprehensive legal framework in place to protect them. This is constantly being reviewed as the structure of society changes.

Theory into practice

In pairs, look at the five main points of *Every Child Matters* (*website on p. 78*). How might they have impact on the children and young people in education and care settings?

Legislation	Main provisions
United Nations Convention on the Rights of the Child 1989	This is an international agreement that considers the rights of all children and young people. It consists of 54 articles covering a range of rights. These include the right to be free from violence, the right to play, the right to express themselves and have their views taken into account. The convention also provides additional rights which ensure that those children and young people living away from home, and those who are disabled, are treated fairly and their specific needs are met..
Children Act 1989, 2004	The Children Act first became part of the legislative framework in 1989 and was initially designed to ensure that all local authorities were providing equal standards of provision to support children, young people and their families. The act includes the support of disabled children who, when they reach the age of 18, come under the NHS and Community Care Act 1990. The Children Act 2004 provides the legislation to accompany *Every Child Matters: Change for Children*, which considered all aspects of children's services. There were new statutory duties for local authorities and support was provided to help them implement it swiftly.
Human Rights Act 1998	The Human Rights Act came into force in England and Wales in 2000. It incorporated the European Convention on Human Rights into the national legislative framework. It enables children, young people and adults to seek protection of their rights both at national level and internationally, through the European Court of Human Rights in Strasbourg.
Data Protection Act 1998	The Data Protection Act prevents personal information from being misused, while protecting the safe use of data for legitimate reasons. There are eight principles to ensure that personal information is: • fairly and lawfully processed • processed for limited purposes • adequate, relevant and not excessive • accurate • not kept longer than necessary • processed in accordance with your rights • kept secure • not transferred abroad without adequate protection.
Framework for the Assessment of Children in Need and their Parents 2000	This Framework was introduced for the specific purpose of securing the well-being of children and young people at vulnerable times during their lives. It provides a framework and guidance for the understanding and assessment of children and their families. Many families require help to resolve their problems. It is important for people in this situation, that sensitive assessments are made and support strategies are put in place. The assessment will identify the needs of the child or young person and this may be the first stage of a much longer process of support and possible intervention.
Every Child Matters 2003	*Every Child Matters: Change for Children* considers the well-being of children and young people from birth to 19. There are five principles that are at the heart of this legislation and they apply to every child, whatever their background or circumstances. The aim is that all children should: • be healthy • stay safe • enjoy and achieve • make a positive contribution • experience economic well-being. All groups and organisations working with children and young people must work together to protect children from harm and help them achieve their goals in life. Information will be gathered concerning vulnerable groups, so that support strategies can be put in place if necessary. Children and young people will have their voices heard and be involved in decision-making processes. There are a number of initiatives which will enable their views to be taken into account. The first Children's Commissioner for England was appointed in 2005 to help give children and young people an input into government.

Table 10.2 Legislation in place to protect children and young people (more details on Legislation Appendix at www.harcourt.co.uk/btechsc).

Alternative forms of care

A wide range of care possibilities are open to families and some of these are listed in the table below.

Type of care	Characteristics
Temporary/permanent	Care can be arranged on either a temporary or permanent basis but there are a number of assessments and procedures to be completed before the care of a child or young person becomes permanent. An example of this may be in the case of a child who has been in foster care for a considerable time and whose natural parents are deemed to be incapable of the care of a minor.
Foster care	Foster care is often short-term but can become long-term as circumstances change. Foster carers are checked by the local authority to ensure that they are suitable and competent to provide care in their own homes Foster carers need to be adaptable as they may be caring for a baby one day and an eight-year-old a week later. Sometimes children and young people in foster care can present very complex and difficult problems.
Respite care	Respite care is usually decided in advance and is a short-term arrangement. Often the child or young person has learning difficulties and/or disabilities and the family need a break. Respite care consists of a child spending some time in a residential establishment which caters for their specific needs.
Adoption	Adoption is a formal and legal process in which the child or young person becomes a permanent member of a family other than their natural birth family. Sometimes parents relinquish all responsibility for a child and offer that child or young person for adoption. Adoption can also follow the death of the child's natural parents.
Residential childcare	Children and young people may be taken into residential care for a variety of reasons. It may be part of the respite arrangements for a family unit or a temporary emergency situation in an abusive or exploitive family situation. Residential childcare may be arranged for children and young people with behavioural difficulties so that specialised staff are available to interact with, and provide for, the individual needs of the person.

Table 10.3 Possible forms of care.

In context

Shabir is two years old and lives with her mother in a town in the north of England. There are no other relatives in the area and her father died in an accident shortly after her birth. Recently, they were out in the town shopping when Shabir's mother collapsed and they were both taken to the local hospital. After diagnosis it became clear that her mother had to be admitted and would be in hospital for at least three weeks and would then need a considerable period of time for convalescence.

1   What are the possible care arrangements for Shabir?

2   Compare two different types of care that might be provided.

3   How might the stress of the situation be lessened for her mother? How might the stress of the situation be lessened for Shabir, bearing in mind that her needs are paramount?

Planning for care in partnership with the child/young person, parents and other agencies

It is in the child's or young person's best interests that any care provisions are established and organised, whenever possible, in a mutually acceptable way. In some cases the family and parents have requested support and help, which might be on a short-term basis. The possibilities of successful and positive outcomes are greatly increased if all parties (including other agencies involved) can agree on the partnership arrangements for the mutual care and support for the child or young person.

Organisation of care provision

Care for children and young people is provided by the following agencies:

- central and local government
- the voluntary sector
- private providers
- provision for young offenders.

These are all explored below.

Central government

There are a number of departments and services within central government as detailed below.

Department of Health	This is the government department responsible for public health issues. It monitors and regulates the NHS. It aims to provide for public health and well-being by providing easily accessible services and highly qualified and dedicated staff.
National Health Service (NHS)	The NHS is involved in all situations which have a health bias and these may include children and young people who have learning difficulties or disabilities. There is a duty of care in providing the appropriate resources and assistance for the family. The staff will work very closely with other agencies and a multi-disciplinary team may be involved in the overall care plan for the individual.
National Service Framework for Children, Young People and Maternity Services	The National Service Framework was established in 2004 and set the standards for children's health, social services and other related services. It promotes an integrated approach to multi-agency working when supporting children, young people and their families. The death of eight-year-old Victoria Climbie in 2000 was one of the reasons why the National Framework came into being. These guidelines mean that there is a more cohesive and inter-connected approach, especially when dealing with vulnerable children and young people.

Table 10.4 Departments and services within central government.

In context

The Smithson family consists of Mr Smithson, who works in a local factory, Mrs Smithson, who works part-time some evenings at a local shop, but who is at home during the day, and their three children, Amelia, Jason and Alan. Amelia is the youngest and has just had her first birthday. Jason is eight, attends the local school and has cerebral palsy. Alan is the oldest and, at thirteen, is finding school life quite difficult as he is being bullied.

Mr and Mrs Smithson spend an evening out together, having arranged childcare for the children. They have taken a taxi to the restaurant but it is involved in a road traffic accident. They are not badly injured but will need to spend some days in hospital.

Consider each child separately and make informed suggestions for the following, giving reasons for your answers.

1   **Which organisations might be involved for Amelia in this situation?**

2   **Which organisations might be involved for Jason?**

3   **Which organisations might be involved for Alan?**

Local government

Each local authority has a duty of care for children and young people and may become involved in all cases where they are at risk of not being cared for appropriately. They will provide help and assistance for families and in many cases will work in partnership providing human and other resources to keep the family together. However, there are other times when the authority must intervene for the good of the child. This might mean providing temporary care until a parent recovers from an accident or illness or it may involve removing the child to a place of safety until a danger is reduced or eliminated.

Integrated services	Integrated children's services plan to provide the best start in life for children. They will draw together all the services provided, especially for those with special and specific needs. They will include education, health, social services and youth justice and will produce objectives for a more integrated approach.
Children's services	The Children Act 2004 introduced legislation to protect children and young people to a greater degree. Children's services deal with the education, health and social care issues related to children, young people and their families. They aim to provide an integrated approach and all the services provided are subject to inspection under the Children Act 2004.
Children's trusts	Children's trusts bring together all the services in an area that link with children and young people and assist with the improvement of those services to meet the outcomes of *Every Child Matters*. They help to develop integrated approaches for all services and assist with sharing decisions and resources.
Children's centres	Children's centres are part of the Sure Start programme (see below). They provide a range of services for children and their families throughout the ante-natal period until the child begins statutory education. They provide early years education programmes on a flexible basis, family support, child and family health services as well as support for those with special needs.
Early Years Foundation stage	The Early Years Foundation stage will come into being in 2008 although many providers are implementing it earlier. It is a framework that covers the curriculum for children from birth to five years and replaces the Birth to Three Matters Framework and the Foundation Stage Curriculum. It provides a more integrated approach to early years and is structured in a cohesive manner.
Sure Start	Sure Start is a government programme designed to ensure that every child has the best start in life. Sure Start centres provide support care and advice for children and parents. They provide early years education, childcare services, health advice and information together with support for parents, which may include training, courses, information sessions and workshops.
Nursery provision	Private nurseries usually cater for children from 0 to 4. Other nursery provision is part of the local education service and may be in a nursery school or part of an early years unit in a primary school. There will be a qualified teacher in charge of the class with other early years workers operating alongside. They will all follow a structured curriculum such as the Early Years Foundation Stage.
Extended schools	Many schools provide an extended day with 'wrap around provision'. This may include breakfast clubs and after school programmes and homework clubs. The extra care and provision helps working parents and supports the children by meeting their needs in various ways.
Connexions partnerships	Connexions is a public service which works in partnership with other organisations (for example, colleges) and is designed specifically for young people. It provides advice and support, in the main for young people aged 13–19, but this age increases to 25 if the individual has learning difficulties and/or disabilities.

Table 10.5 Services provided by local government.

Voluntary sector – pre-school provision

Pre-school provision covers a range of services, some provided by volunteers, for example, carer and toddler groups and play provision in church halls or local community centres. The leaders of these groups may have some training but many have not and, as long as the parents or carers do not leave their children, then there is no legal requirement that they should.

Reflect

Did you attend any pre-school provision or a nursery? Can you remember what you enjoyed most about the experience? What did you enjoy least about it?

Private providers – nurseries

Private nurseries usually cater for children from birth up to the age of four (although many three- and four-year-olds attend local authority nurseries). Staff are trained in early years and there may be some members of staff who are working towards a recognised qualification. The

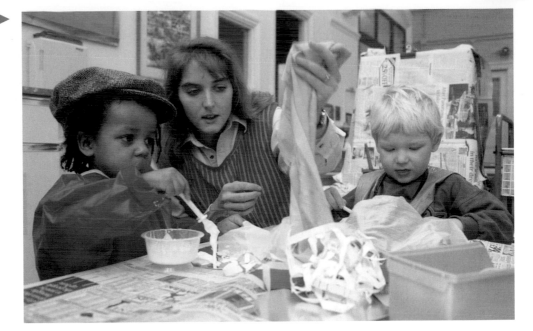

Early years provision covers children from birth to five years old. ▶

arrangements for childcare are usually made on an individual basis between the nursery and the family as the provision required will vary considerably. The family will pay a fee based on the number of hours or sessions the child attends.

Young offenders

Secure children's homes are provided for children who are at risk to themselves and/or others. The children are often educated within the homes, which are usually residential, and the workers are specially trained to provide for the needs of the individuals who are there.

Young offender institutions are designed to provide secure accommodation for young people who have been remanded in custody or who have been sentenced by the courts. The main aims are to help the young people prepare for life back in society and to educate and equip them so that they are less likely to re-offend.

Take it further

Carry out some research to find out more about the range of voluntary organisations, charities and not-for-profit organisations in your area. You might like to work in pairs or small groups for this activity.

Job roles

Within the organisations mentioned there will be various job roles. Some of these are documented below.

Director of Children's Services

After the Children Act 2004, every local authority had to appoint a Director of Children's Services. The person in this role would be responsible for the delivery of education, health and social service programmes and duties within the authority. Additionally, they would be responsible for developing a more integrated service.

Social workers

Trained and qualified social workers support families with children who present problems and difficulties in a wide range of areas. They often work as part of a **multi-disciplinary team** to provide a comprehensive support framework.

Key terms

Multi-disciplinary team A team of professionals drawn from a range of disciplines or services, for example, health care, education and social services, all working together towards a common goal.

Foster parents

Foster parents accept children and young people into their homes and provide family care for the individual. The care offered may be emergency care where immediate help is required. They work closely with the social service departments in providing secure and reliable care.

Theory into practice

In pairs, make a list of the qualities you feel are necessary for anyone wishing to be a foster parent.

Support workers

Support workers may work alongside social and other workers so that a greater level of support can be given to families that require it. The support worker might liaise with other agencies and assist the family unit in a variety of ways.

Residential care staff

Residential care staff provide full-time care for children and young people in residential care homes. Many of the children and young people present complex and differing needs and the residential care staff need to be versatile and flexible in approach to the differing situations.

Tutors

Tutors and teachers in educational establishments are involved in teaching but they also have extra responsibilities for the general care and well-being of the child. They may provide extra support where required as well as information about a range of children's services and support groups. They can also be a valuable link between agencies such as Connexions, and can assist with career and training choices.

Lecturers

Lecturers will be involved in the education of young people in further and higher education establishments. In addition, in line with the government agenda on work with 14-year-old pupils, many colleges are providing courses and training for students who are younger than those traditionally involved in college education. The lecturer will be an expert in a particular field of education and will deliver appropriate programmes suitable for the young people involved.

Nurses

Nurses may give children and young people medical care when they have been injured in some way, and they may also be involved in home visits as part of follow-up programmes. There are nurses who are specially trained to care for the health of the younger sector of society.

Take it further

Nursing is a profession that appeals to a wide range of individuals. Working in small groups, gather information about as many branches of nursing as you can that might be involved in work with children and young people. Produce an information sheet in which you itemise each one – you could also illustrate it.

Health visitors

Health visitors visit every family when a baby is born, once the specialist skills of the midwife are no longer required. The health visitor is a nurse with further qualifications in other aspects of childcare who visits the family in their home to provide advice and support on a wide range of situations. Many families only require the support of a health visitor for a relatively short time after the birth of a baby, but there are an increasing number of families who require additional support and advice for a longer period of time.

Educational psychologists

There are specialist psychology services that work with children and young people. This may be within the education system where they will provide advice and support in the face of complex difficulties. Educational psychologists also work with parents and families and provide support for multi-agency working.

Counsellors

Children and young people who have had traumatic experiences may benefit from counselling. The British Association for Counselling and Psychotherapy recognises that counselling for children and young people requires different skills from those adopted for adults. Counselling for Children and Young People is a division of the British Association for Counselling and Psychotherapy.

Nursing/health care/social care assistants

This group includes people working towards a qualification in a specific area, who are working as an assistant in their specialised area. They will work closely with the nursing/health care/social care staff to provide a comprehensive service in the support of children and young people together with their parents and families.

Education welfare officers

The education welfare officer generally deals with children and young people at school who present issues such as poor attendance. Their role is sometimes looked upon as a schools' social worker. They will work with school staff and families to investigate why problems occur and to try to identify possible solutions. They will be able to advise parents of their legal responsibilities and be involved in multi-agency provision in resolving issues. They may give advice on the statementing process for children with special educational needs, or on child protection issues.

In context

John, who is 11 years old, lives at home with his mother, who has a number of problems. She has been involved with substance abuse for a few years and is often inebriated when John comes home from school. He tends to look after himself most of the time and is often the carer for his mother. There are some days when he does not go to school as he is worried about her and feels that he needs to be at home. However, there are times when the situation improves and so does his attendance. The school is aware, to some extent, about the situation, but his school work is suffering and things have reached the point when others must be involved.

1 Who else might the school involve?

2 What could they do to try to help the family?

3 Suggest some possible outcomes for this situation.

Learning mentors

Learning mentors are individuals who will work with children and young people, primarily within the school situation, to provide extra support and help for pupils. This may be on a whole class, small group or individual basis and they will work alongside the teacher in the classroom to build up skills and confidence in young learners.

Play therapists

Play therapists are usually individuals who have undertaken specialist training in play therapy, which can be used as a diagnostic tool for children who have suffered stress or trauma, or as a form of treatment. Children and young people may have had experiences which they find very difficult to deal with in the usual way. They may not have the maturity of language to be able to explain what has happened. While working with an experienced play therapist they can find ways of expressing themselves and dealing with their problems in a safe and secure environment and in a way which meets their individual needs.

Play workers

Play work is a specialist area of provision, usually working with children and young people aged 4–16. The values and principle of play work are such that they enable children and young people to indulge in free play and take control of their own situations. Play workers work in a range of settings outside statutory education and may be involved in play schemes, play buses, out-of-school clubs, adventure playgrounds, breakfast clubs, etc.

Connexions advisers

These people work within the Connexions service to provide advice and support for children and young people in the 13–19 age group (extended to 25 for individuals with learning difficulties and/or disabilities). They will advise on a whole range of issues from personal factors to pointers towards education, training and employment.

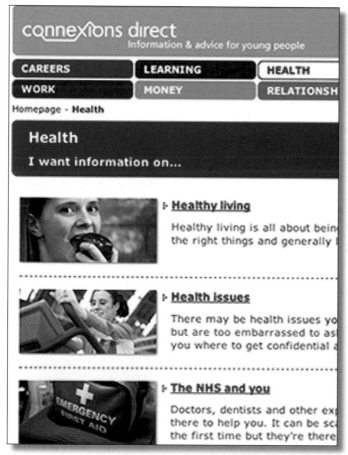

▲ The Connexions website. Pay it a visit to research the range of information it offers.

Early years workers

Early years workers work with children from birth to eight in a range of settings which may include private day nurseries, local authority nurseries, family centres, hospitals and crèches. They understand the needs of young children and will be able to provide appropriate and relevant experiences to aid their overall development.

Youth workers

Youth workers work with children and young people, usually between the ages of 13 and 19. They may work in youth centres, clubs, schools, etc. and may work as part of a youth offending team. However, some work in less traditional ways as detached youth workers, trying to engage with young people who might be more at risk in the community. They may be involved in delivering programmes, supporting young people, working with parents and community groups and undertaking other activities as and when required.

Youth justice workers

Youth justice workers are involved in the youth justice system and have an important role in helping young people to achieve the five outcomes as laid down in *Every Child Matters* (see page 45). They usually work as part of a multi-disciplinary team to establish positive outcomes for young people and their families.

Prison officers

Prison officers work within the prison service and are responsible for caring for young people serving custodial sentences or on remand. Their role includes trying to establish a professional relationship with the goal of rehabilitation. They need to maintain a healthy and safe environment, which includes training and education, so that the individual will be better equipped on release.

Assessment activity 10.2

P2 Identify the current relevant legislation affecting the care of children and young people.

1   You will need to cover the main aspects of current legislation, providing hypothetical examples of its implementation.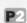

Grading tip for P2

You might like to devise an appropriate scenario and identify how the legislative framework can provide safety and support for children, young people and their families.

M1 Analyse how policies and procedures help children/young people and their families whilst the child is being looked after.

2   You should ask to see the policies and procedures in your placement. Consider the detail and determine whether they safeguard and support the child and the family. **M1**

Grading tip for M1

'Analyse' means to study and explore. You will need to consider any positive or negative impact on the child/young person or the family, for example, the assessment of needs, support given and consideration of health and education needs.

D1 Evaluate the legislative rights of the child/young person and the rights of their families, bearing in mind that the needs of the child/young person are paramount.

3   Using the legislation you have identified for P2, describe how far the legislation protects the rights of the child/young person and the family. You will then need to judge whether the needs of the child/young person are always a prime consideration. **D1**

Grading tip for D1

When evaluating the legislative rights of the child/young person and their families, it will be necessary to consider the value that legislation can have on a situation in safeguarding the needs of the child/young person and if there are any potential conflicts.

P3 Describe health and social care service provision for looked-after children and young people.

4   You will need to describe a range of services and should draw on experience from any placements or visits you have made. **P3**

Grading tip for P3

You will need to state what the provision is, for example, nursery and then provide some explanation about the purpose or function it has in the care of children and young people.

M2 Compare the care provided by at least two different organisations offering care to children and young people.

5   Compare two different organisations that provide care for children and young people. You might like to interview members of staff to gain insight into the provision. **M2**

Grading tip for M2

'Compare' means to look at the similarities and the differences and you will need to be able to say what the two organisations have in common and how they differ in the individual care of the child or the young person.

Child protection must always be at the front of the mind of anyone who is working with children and young people. However, while considering this important aspect of work in the sector, it must always be remembered that children do sustain bruises and minor injuries during the normal rough and tumble of play activities. It is important to listen to children and take note of their body language and general behaviour and appearance.

Risk of abuse

Abuse can happen to children both within and outside the family. It can also happen within a care setting. These issues are explored below.

Abuse within the family

The majority of children are not at risk of abuse within their own family but there are situations that increase the risk. External stresses and strains on a family may

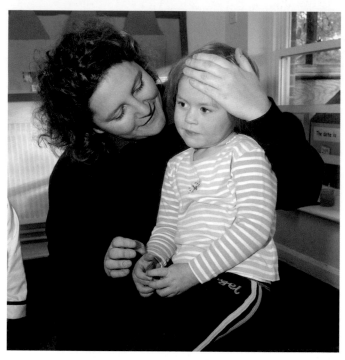

▲ Children need the support of someone who listens to what they are saying.

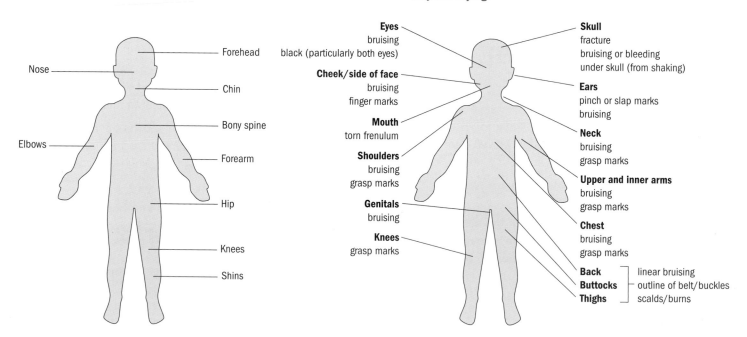

Common sites of accidental injuries

Nose —
Forehead
Chin
Bony spine
Elbows —
Forearm
Hip
Knees
Shins

Non-accidental injuries

Eyes
bruising
black (particularly both eyes)

Cheek/side of face
bruising
finger marks

Mouth
torn frenulum

Shoulders
bruising
grasp marks

Genitals
bruising

Knees
grasp marks

Skull
fracture
bruising or bleeding
under skull (from shaking)

Ears
pinch or slap marks
bruising

Neck
bruising
grasp marks

Upper and inner arms
bruising
grasp marks

Chest
bruising
grasp marks

Back — linear bruising
Buttocks — outline of belt/buckles
Thighs — scalds/burns

▲ **Figure 10.4 Accidental and non-accidental injuries.**

cause one or both parents to react in anger and the child might suffer as a result. There are individuals who have volatile personalities and react adversely to the youngest or most vulnerable members of the family unit. There are instances of parents who lack the appropriate parenting skills and are unable to look after children who may be neglected and malnourished as a result. Instances of abuse within the family home can cover the whole range of abusive situations, for example, physical, emotional, sexual and neglect.

Abuse outside the family

Child abuse occurring outside the family home can be more common, while neglect is more common within the family. Other adults and relatives can be responsible for the child being abused or other children or young people may perpetrate the abuse through bullying or harassment.

Abuse in a care setting

There have been a number of high-profile cases when child abuse has occurred within a care setting. Although these cases are relatively rare they make major headlines in the press. However, there are many more cases of abuse in these situations including the whole range of abusive situations, but especially instances of bullying and harassment.

Theory into practice

There are times when a person working with children and young people might wonder if there is more to a situation than meets the eye. A child attends a nursery, school or other childcare setting with:

- grazes on both knees
- bruises on both upper arms
- small bruises on both cheeks
- a grazed elbow.

Which of these might indicate an abusive situation? What would you do first? What would you do next?

The risk of exploitation

There is a risk that children may be exploited via visual, written and electronic forms of communication and media. Nowadays a wider range of children is more at risk of coming into contact with unsuitable forms of communication. Much of this is because of advances in technology and this in turn means that children, young people and families have easier access to inappropriate materials. Parents have a responsibility to monitor the types of DVDs and Internet sites their children can access. However, there are families that allow children to watch films intended for a much older audience and many children are now very familiar with Internet chat rooms. They may not realise that other people may use these to groom children and young people for their own purposes.

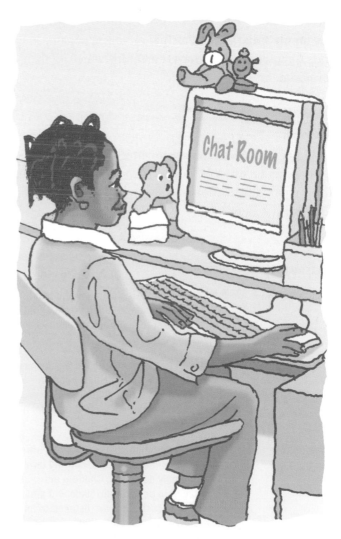

▲ Figure 10.5 Is she learning or being exploited?

Family functioning

The family situation that a child or young person finds themselves in can have a great influence on their development.

Family types

Child rearing styles can have an effect on the developmental processes a child experiences. Styles vary from one family to another but can be broken down into three main groups

Parenting styles	Attitudes
Authoritarian	Parents rearing their children in this way will expect them to do everything they are told and to conform to decisions made on their behalf.
Permissive	Parents rearing their children in this fashion will allow them a great deal of freedom. They may consider that children will break any rules that are in place, so it is better not to have many rules at all.
Authoritative	Parents rearing their children like this will allow them to make choices, and will involve them in family decisions. Children are encouraged to act as individuals and are respected as such. They are listened to and decisions are explained to them.

Table 10.6 Three styles of parenting.

Partnership arrangements

Partnership arrangements within a family can vary considerably but there are usually two adult partners living together with the children as a family unit. The partners may both be the biological parents of the children or the family unit may be a reconstituted one. The parents in a **reconstituted family** may be gay or lesbian and the children might be from previous relationships or adopted.

Key terms

Reconstituted family This is usually two adults, one or both with children of their own from another relationship, living together as one family.

The changing face of the family

The concept of family life has changed considerably over the years. Family units can be made up in a number of different ways and the children will have various types of relationships within those units. As well as conventional two-parent families, children may live with one biological parent and have visitation rights with the other and both parents may have other family units of their own. Some children will live with their mother and grandparents while others are in a reconstituted family. Anyone working with children and young people must be aware of the background and culture of the individuals in their care.

Social disadvantage

Many families are disadvantaged and this adds stresses and strains to the family unit, which may contribute to abusive or exploitive situations. Families in poor housing and on low income may find it difficult to buy nourishing food and the children may be in poor health and be very demanding. Children who are not well may be frustrated and want more attention. They may be unreasonable in their wants and their moods may vary considerably because they are generally feeling ill and are unhappy.

Different concepts of discipline

Discipline differs greatly from one family to the next and has close links with parenting styles. Some parents will impose sanctions while others resort to more physical forms of punishment.

Abuse within families

As mentioned above, abuse can occur within families when stresses and strains become overpowering. Children and young people do not read the warning signs as an adult might and so become caught up in an abusive situation. However, there are families where abuse is deliberate and planned and, because the adult is powerful and threatening, this type of situation can continue for a considerable period of time.

Cultural variations

There are cultural variations on the upbringing of children and you should note that this is not always linked to race. In some families, girls and boys are treated in different ways, for example, a girl's place is to serve the other members of the family. In some cultures the female is not valued in the same way as the male and this can lead to bullying and harassment within the home.

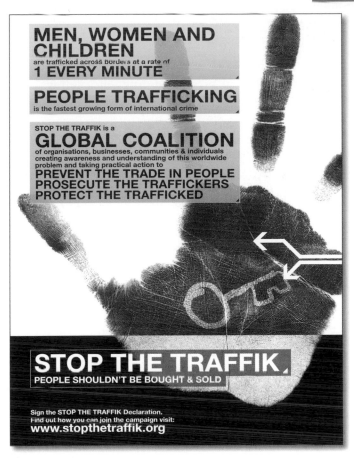

▲ Figure 10.6 'Stop the Traffik' publicity material. Start your research with their website.

Take it further

Stop the Traffik is involved with trying to stop the traffic in human beings across the world. Many people are surprised that human trafficking happens in the UK. Carry out some research into this movement of vulnerable people, especially the young. Report your findings to other members of your group.

Predisposing factors (the abuser)

There are a number of factors which need to be taken into consideration when studying abusive behaviour, in relation to both the abuser and the abused. These predisposing factors may help explain why abuse occurs and alert carers to the possibility of abuse. The factors outlined overleaf relate to the abuser.

Substance abuse

There are a number of substances that might be abused, for example, alcohol, prescribed drugs, illegal drugs and solvents. These may change the user's perceptions and lead to altered behaviour, which in turn can become abusive. If the individual has become dependent on substances, and the supply is stopped, then that can also have a detrimental effect on behaviour resulting in violent emotional and/or physical outbursts.

A lack of knowledge about children's needs

A number of adults lack parenting skills to such an extent that they have little understanding about the needs of the child. If children do not receive the care and attention that they need and crave, then they will alter their behaviour so that they do receive attention of some kind (even negative attention). This may then turn into an abusive situation as parents feel that they cannot cope and become angry with the child.

Theory into practice

Not all parents know about childcare and child development. In small groups, discuss the pros and cons of parenting classes being an obligatory part of the curriculum in schools and prepare a short report to present to the other members of the class.

A lack of attachment

Some parents find it difficult to form close attachments with their child and this can be for a number of reasons. Some babies are not very easy to relate to and seem to cry a lot – a young mother may find this difficult to cope with. Occasionally the parents are very young and not mature enough for the situation they find themselves in and devolve the responsibility of the child to others, for example, the child's grandparents. Separation and illness also contribute to attachment difficulties.

A lack of role models

Bad role models and childhood abuse can lead to unsound foundations for family life. Victims may base their family relationships on their own dysfunctional ones, or they may recognise that their childhood was flawed but have no model for a good family life.

Reflect

Who were your role models when you were younger? What lasting influences have they had on your life?

Social problems

There are a number of people who have difficulty relating to others in society or whose behaviour can be considered as anti-social. Such people will experience difficulty when trying to raise children as their pattern of behaviour is damaged in some way. Occasionally there is an underlying anger which must be dealt with before the individual can develop meaningful relationships.

Mental illness

Mental illness varies considerably in type and severity but if parents have been diagnosed as having some form of mental illness then their ability to raise a family may be brought into question. It is common for parents with mental illness or instability to have social workers attached to the family so that they can be supported and the children monitored and helped.

Personality

The personality of the individual must always be considered in cases of child abuse as some adults have violent tempers or a desire for absolute control. In extreme cases they may be diagnosed with a personality disorder, which may need further investigation and treatment before the family can function normally.

Predisposing factors (the abused child/young person)

There are a number of predisposing factors that can be looked at in relation to the abused child or young person. These are explored below.

Disability

Disability in a child or young person can lead to frustration on their part and for their parents. The whole situation can be extremely demanding and can, in some cases, lead to abuse of one kind or another. The family may require support from different agencies and may benefit from respite care on a regular basis.

Pre-maturity

Some children and young people appear to be very mature for their age and this can in turn lead to some difficult and abusive situations. Relationships, sometimes of a sexual nature, can develop before the individual is mature enough to deal with the emotional feelings. There is an ongoing debate as to whether the media has some responsibility for promoting clothes and makeup, etc., which could be seen as sexually provocative when worn by young people.

Types of abuse

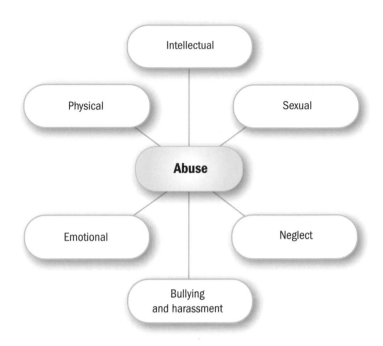

▲ **Figure 10.7 Types of abuse.**

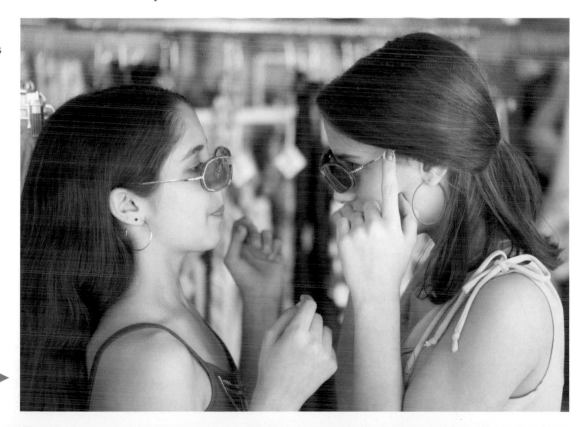

▶ Children need time to experiment and grow up at their own pace!

Physical abuse

When considering physical abuse you should always remember that children do suffer bruises and scratches in general play. However, early years workers must be aware of the signs of physical abuse, which includes hitting, nipping, burning and inflicting physical harm of any kind.

Sexual abuse

Sexual abuse can take a number of different forms.

Sexual abuse	Indications
Inappropriate touching	Adults will often hold a child's hand or cuddle them especially when they are upset. The touching becomes inappropriate when it is unwanted or directed in a sexual way, for example, touching the bottom or the genitals.
Inappropriate language	Children should never be subjected to language and conversation which is inappropriate or of a sexual nature. The innocence of childhood should be respected and protected at all times.
Inappropriate sexual advances	This will include inappropriate touching and kissing and speaking with children about intimate issues.
Looking at children in an inappropriate way	While there are many people who enjoy watching children play in all innocence, some will watch children at play in parks and nursery gardens with malicious intent.
Showing children inappropriate pictures	This type of behaviour is designed to eventually engage children in sexual activity.
Talking with children in an inappropriate way	Engaging children in manipulative conversation may be designed to lull them into a sense of security, which will lead to a more intimate relationship.

Table 10.7 The different forms of sexual abuse.

Emotional abuse

Emotional abuse (including aspects of effect on intellectual development)	
Constant shouting	Shouting at children all the time will inevitably destroy their self-esteem and make them unwilling to participate or engage in any conversation with the abuser.
Dominating adults	If the child is totally dominated then the developmental process can be impaired. For example, the child may be held back from developing normally as they are not allowed to 'get dirty' or indulge in messy play.
Threatening behaviour	Children who are threatened in systematic ways will be withdrawn and lack confidence in their own abilities. If the threats start suddenly then the child's behaviour will change and the early years care and education worker should be aware of this.
Belittling and undermining	Systematic belittling will destroy a child's self-esteem and they will lack confidence, which will mean that they will be reluctant to attempt anything new.
Verbal abuse	This is often a mixture of belittling, undermining and shouting. It all has the effect of destroying the spirit and tenacity of the child.

Table 10.8 The different forms of emotional abuse.

Neglect

Signs of neglect may include:
- inappropriate clothing
- dirty or smelly
- unkempt appearance
- underweight – always hungry
- skin irritations
- withdrawn
- isolated
- dejected
- low self-esteem
- listless.

Be on the lookout for such children as, while the neglect may not be deliberate, the family need help in developing the necessary skills to raise children effectively.

In context

Sally is 12 years old and has recently started attending a new school. She has had difficulty fitting in and there is a small group of other girls who have begun to follow Sally and call her names. Sometimes they jostle against her, pretending that it is an accident, whereas it is more purposeful. She found her books defaced and torn and she feels very much alone. She told her brother who said she was being silly and to forget about it. She eventually confided in a support worker in school.

1 What do you think the support worker would do after hearing Sally's story?

2 What strategies might the school recommend in order to alleviate the situation?

3 What support do you think Sally would need?

Bullying and harassment

Other young people often carry out bullying and harassment of young people and children. However, this is not an exclusive group and often adults bully children and young people in an exploitative manner. Bullying may take many forms and some of these are indicated below.

Many children and young people manage to hide the fact that they are being bullied. They may feel that it is their fault and that they have brought the situation upon themselves. They are often reluctant to tell other people, as they feel vulnerable and intimidated.

Indicators of abuse

There are a number of indicators of physical abuse that you will need to be aware of. In many cases each one, taken separately, may carry with it an innocent explanation. However, they should never be ignored and should warrant some further investigation. The tables which follow provide only a range of indicators and are not totally exhaustive.

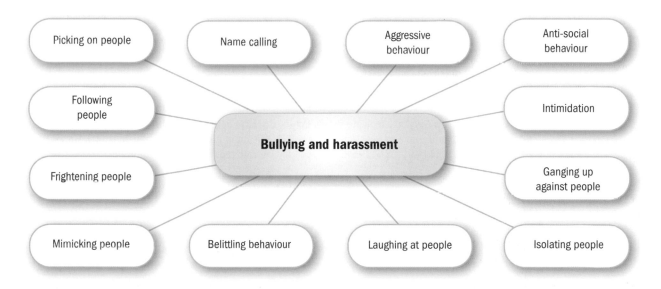

▲ Figure 10.8 Types of bullying and harassment.

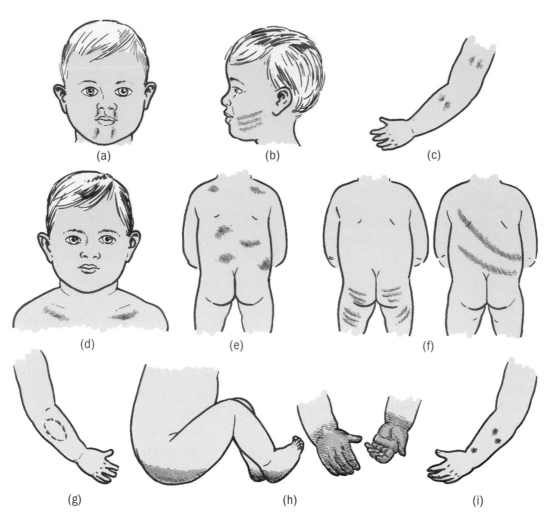

▲ Figure 10.9 Indicators of physical abuse.
(a) facial squeezing, (b) diffuse facial bruising, (c) pinch marks, (d) grip marks, (e) body bruising, (f) identifiable lesions, (g) bite marks, (h) burns or scalds, (i) cigarette burns.

Physical

Physical abuse	
Bruising	Systematically inflicting pain and injury on a child or young person is abhorrent but there are individuals who will methodically punch, beat and damage children. Children who are treated in this way will have multiple bruises, possibly fractures and tissue or organ damage and this may even lead to death.
Burns	Small round burns will usually indicate marks from a cigarette or other such item. Burns of all types are extremely painful and prone to infection and they are inflicted in a particularly malicious way. Hands or feet may be placed in hot liquid as a punishment and such injuries will require medical attention.
Unexplained injuries	Sometimes non-accidental injury occurs because of stresses and strains in the family situation. However, there are occasions when children are systematically abused and ill-treated and it is vital that the care and education practitioner is alert to and aware of the signs and symptoms.
Soreness	Soreness might be a sign of bruising or underlying fractures as a result of abuse. Tenderness and soreness occur at times in the life of every child but when this occurs on a regular basis or persists then the situation requires investigation.
Infections	A child who is continually ill or has regular infections may be a child who is not receiving the care and attention or nutrients to build up the immune system and this could be a physical sign of neglect.

Underweight	Children are weighed at regular times throughout their lives. It is one of the first things that happens after the birth and continues with every medical check throughout childhood. If a child does not progress at the recognised rate then further tests may be carried out to see if there is an underlying cause. One such reason may be that the child is not receiving the right types of nutrients to grow at the established rate.
Poor personal hygiene	Neglect is often the cause of poor personal hygiene and the child may be wearing clothes that are dirty and too big or too small. There will be other signs and symptoms to alert carers of the situation.
Failure to thrive	Failure to thrive is an accumulation of the signs and symptoms that indicate child abuse. Further investigation is required if the child is failing to meet the accepted norms of development.

Table 10.9 Physical signs of abuse.

Behaviour

All types of abuse will lead to a change in the child's behaviour, as they have been subjected to things that a young person should never have to experience. Each child copes with their trauma in their own way as they feel that they are helpless and cannot stop whatever is happening to them.

Behaviour	
Withdrawal	A child who suddenly shows signs of withdrawal is displaying signs that something is bothering them and this could be an indicator of abuse or exploitive behaviour.
Aggression	Some children are more aggressive than others but if a child begins to display aggressive behaviour when previously they did not, then this will be an indication that the child is disturbed about something.
Distress	When a child feels safe and secure they may let down their defences and become distressed over relatively stress free situations. This often indicates that the child is under some degree of stress.
Rocking/head banging	This type of repetitive behaviour is an indication that the child is disturbed about issues that they feel unable to talk freely about.
Hunger	Some children appear to be extremely greedy when presented with snacks or other items of food. This may be an indication that the child is not receiving adequate nutrition at home.
Reluctance to go home	Children who are being abused in any way may show a reluctance to go home, especially if the abuser is in the house. The child may not put their fears into words but may try to find excuses to avoid the family home.
Low self-esteem	Low self-esteem can result in patterns of undesirable behaviour, which may manifest itself in emotional problems, unhappiness, depression, robbery or even violence. Wherever and whenever possible adults should take the opportunity to build a child's self-esteem.
Developmental delay	Children who are being abused or exploited are unhappy and will not be able to function on a higher intellectual plane, which may result in an apparent developmental delay. Maslow's Hierarchy of Needs determines that individuals will not be able to function at higher levels until their fundamental needs are met.

Table 10.10 Changes in behaviour as a result of abuse.

Theory into practice

Consider a child who has been abused. List the emotions they might be feeling. How might their behaviour change? List three activities that you think would help a child to build up relationships with other children.

Consequences of abuse

The consequences of abuse are far reaching and have a long-term effect on the individual. Children and young people who have been abused may have difficulties with mental health, social behaviour, low self-esteem, forming relationships and in their general emotional development. Some children do go on to form meaningful relationships, but there is a risk that they may become abusers themselves.

Type of abuse	Possible consequences
Emotional	A child who has been subjected to regular emotional abuse may have extremely low self-esteem and could enter into further abusive situations in adulthood. They may not reach their full potential as they may have been belittled and under-valued, making them feel unable to take on roles of responsibility.
Social	Many people who have suffered abuse find that there are long-term effects in social relationships. Children who have been abused sexually may find it difficult to form any intimate relationships as they grow older. They may be unable to trust another person with their innermost thoughts and feelings.
Physical	If a child has been subjected to consistent physical abuse, then the damage that may have been caused could have effects that last for the rest of their lives. Children who have been punched or kicked violently may have sustained internal damage, which could affect normal bodily function. Fractured bones that have not been healed properly may result in a deformity or impaired used of a limb.

Table 10.10 The possible consequences of abuse.

Models of abuse

Several models of abuse have been put forward in an attempt to categorise and explain why abuse takes place. Each may explain some aspects of abuse but none seems to cover all the aspects. The main theories are listed below.

Model of abuse	Characteristics
Medical model	There is a view that child abuse is a disease with specific signs and symptoms. If this view is accepted then, as with other medical conditions, it indicates that there will be treatment for it and that it can be 'cured'. This tends to be a simplistic approach and does not take into account the complexities of many cases of abuse.
Sociological model	This model concentrates on the changing society in which we live and how these changes have affected family functioning. Unemployment, low wages, poor housing, disadvantage and poor health are all seen to contribute to abusive situations. However, statistics show that abuse occurs across the spectrum and that abuse also occurs in families with high income, good housing, etc.
Psychological model	This model focuses on family functioning and how people relate to each other within the family unit. It gives great consideration to family breakdown and dysfunction but advocates that these situations can be improved by therapy and that abuse can be prevented or reduced in this way.
Feminist	This model focuses more on the power relationships between men and women within a family and asserts that most abusers are male. While this argument might be considered to be strong in the case of sexual abuse, it is recognised that some 10 per cent of abusers are female and the victims of abuse are both male and female.

Table 10.11 Models of abuse.

Theory Into practice

Victoria Climbie was eight years old when she tragically died in February 2000. This case of child abuse became very famous. Carry out some research into this event. Which theoretical models do you think might link with this case? Explain the reasons for your choice.

Recognising abuse when children/young people cannot communicate

Health, care and education workers need to be aware of the signs and symptoms of abuse. It may be that the child is so young that they cannot communicate their fears and feelings or may not have developed the knowledge that certain adult behaviour is inappropriate. It is in cases such as this that the physical signs of abuse and neglect may be the main indicators that things are not as they should be.

Children who depend on other forms of communication, for example, signing and using **inclusive technology**, may find it more difficult to let others know of their feelings and what is happening to them.

Key terms

Inclusive technology A range of technological communication aids primarily for individuals with learning difficulties and/or disabilities.

If a child or young person with learning difficulties and/or disabilities displays changes in behaviour, other warning signs need to be observed carefully in order to determine the underlying problem. This may be something that is quite innocent but it should never be ignored.

Assessment activity 10.3

P4 Describe signs and symptoms of child abuse.

1   Produce a leaflet about child protection for trainees who wish to work with children and young people. In your leaflet, you should explain what child abuse, including exploitation, is and describe how it might be recognised.

Grading tip for P4

You might find it useful to describe the signs and symptoms under the different headings, for example, physical, emotional, etc. Remember 'signs' are what you can see and 'symptoms' are what the individual feels.

There are a number of strategies that can help to protect children and young people from being abused or exploited. The strategies listed below are some that are used to minimise the risks and to help children and young people realise that they have the right to be safe, secure and free from harm.

Person-centred approach

It is important always to remember that the child or young person is at the centre and that they are the people who need to be empowered and supported so they can take control of their lives. They should be encouraged to develop strategies that will enable them to avoid situations that put them at risk. They also need be helped to be strong enough to seek appropriate support and guidance if they find themselves in an adverse situation.

Providing active support

Support needs to be readily available and practical when people are in need. It may be useful to have someone who will listen but children also need those who can provide the necessary support and be pro-active in a practical way.

You should endeavour to increase the children's self-confidence and raise their self-esteem so that they are resilient and empowered. Children and young people who know they are valued and loved, and who are used to making decisions, are more likely to refuse unwanted advances and less likely to be drawn into exploitative situations.

Sharing information and not keeping secrets

It is important to encourage children and young people to have open relationships with people so that they can share information. They also need to realise the difference between bad secrets and good secrets. Good secrets are usually only to be kept from one or two people, for example, a present for someone's birthday or a surprise outing, but they can be shared with other people. Bad secrets are usually those which are to be kept from everyone else except the people directly involved, for example, inappropriate pictures, words or touching.

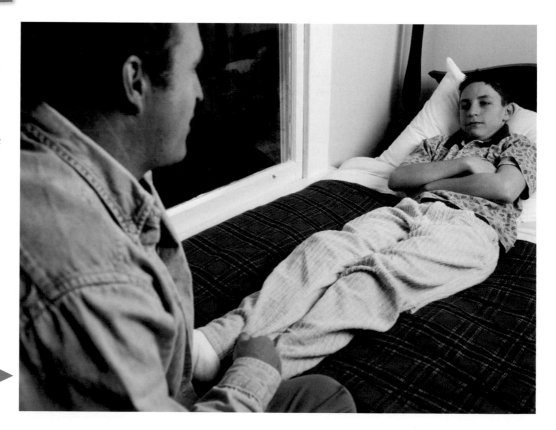

Figure 10.11 Children need someone to confide in.

Children need people to confide in so that they can express their concerns and fears.

In context

Samantha is four years old and attends an early years setting. When she was talking to Jane, one of the early years workers, she said that she had a secret and that daddy had said that it was their special secret. Jane became concerned but tried to remain calm. She had been taught about child protection issues when she was a student, but this was the first time she felt her training might be needed. She wished she had paid more attention and she also regretted not reading the policies of the setting more thoroughly. However, she asked Samantha if she wanted to share her secret and the little girl asked Jane not to tell anyone and Jane agreed. Samantha then went on to explain that it would soon be her mum's birthday and that she and her daddy were going to take her out for the day and buy a special present, but it was a special secret just between the two of them.

1 **How do you feel Jane dealt with the situation?**

2 **What would you do differently?**

3 **What could Jane do to improve her professional development?**

Providing information to children according to their age, needs and abilities

Children and young people need to be aware of their bodies, how they function and how to respect them and keep them safe. As they grow older they need to be aware of the emotions that might affect them as they mature. They should also be aware of the changes in their bodies and how these changes may affect other people. As children and young people mature they are exposed to strong peer pressure and adult images in the media. They should be aware of the dangers of early or inappropriate relationships and understand how to ensure their safety.

In some cases, children and young people may also need to be aware of infections and diseases associated with abusive and exploitive situations. This includes conditions affecting wounds and injuries but more often the transmission of diseases associated with sexual activity. There are a variety of sexually transmitted diseases including herpes, syphilis, gonorrhoea and chlamydia. These must be treated quickly as they may have long-term effects leading to infertility and other conditions.

Working with parents and families

Whenever possible, it is important to work closely with the parents and families of children and young people. In this way a sense of trust and respect can be encouraged together with a feeling that everyone is working together for the good of the child.

Theory into practice

In pairs, discuss how a childcare and education worker can try to develop a good relationship with parents. Prioritise three main points and share these with another group.

Involving parents in the assessment of children's needs

In many cases parents have vital information about the specific needs of their children and about any problems or difficulties they may be trying to come to terms with. Assessment of a child's needs must involve their parents in order to gain an overall picture of the situation.

Helping parents to recognise the significance and value of their contributions

Parents must be made aware of the importance and significance of their contribution to the assessment

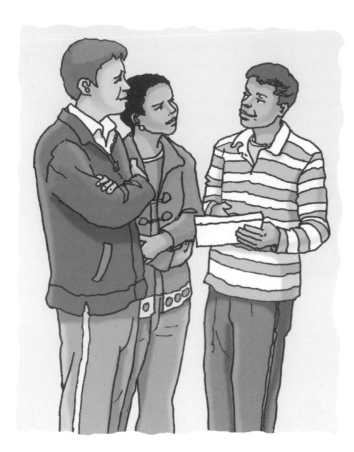

Figure 10.12 It is important to develop good communication skills.

process and they must feel valued. In some cases the parents must share a responsibility for the situation but, if the family is to be supported as a whole, then all contributions must be valued and parents' feelings respected.

Encouraging the development of parenting skills

Parenting skills do not always come naturally to people, especially if they have been raised in a family situation where those skills are lacking. There are many courses available on developing parenting skills, but people do not like to admit that they need help in this area. Those working with children and young people can help parents to improve parenting skills by developing meaningful relationships with them and spending time talking about children and young people.

Procedures where abuse is suspected or confirmed

Policies of the setting

It is important that all people working with children and young people in a care and education setting are aware of, and have read, the policies of the setting. These should be available and easily accessible and many settings ask individuals to sign to show that they have read the policies. This safeguards the organisation and the staff and ensures that a common practice is used in all cases.

Reflect

You should have been shown the policies and procedures of your setting. It may now be the right time to refresh your memory.

Safe working practices that protect children/young people and adults who work with them

Within any setting there will inevitably be a number of policies and procedures and staff need to be aware of these. They will include equal opportunities, health and safety, behaviour and child protection. There will be a number of other policies written to safeguard the children, young people, staff and visitors from danger and to ensure safe practice throughout the setting. It is important to be aware of the content of the policies and procedures so that everyone knows what to do in any situation.

Whistle blowing

Many settings have now also adopted a whistle blowing policy so that if any inappropriate behaviour is observed among the staff it can be reported in an appropriate way, which will trigger an investigation. The person reporting the situation will be supported and protected but they must be aware that they may need to be interviewed by the police, etc., if necessary.

Lines of reporting

The policy of the setting will specify the lines of reporting in cases where abuse is suspected or confirmed. It is important that these procedures are strictly adhered to or the case could be severely compromised. Within a care and education setting the procedures would be to report to the line manager or person in charge of the setting, who will then contact appropriate people in authority. All information should be recorded factually as this may be required as evidence later.

Accurate reporting

It is important that reporting and recording of information is accurate and factual and without any speculation at all. All written reports should be re-read carefully to ensure there is no ambiguity and that all information is fully recorded, is true and without any judgemental phrases or statements.

Security of records

All records must be safely and securely stored, with access only available to those with a right to know. Confidentiality is paramount in these instances and breaking it in this type of situation could, in severe cases, lead to police involvement and even prosecution, as these records may be used in court appearances if criminal proceedings ensue.

Remember!

It is important that all documents are stored in a secure, locked cabinet and are only available to those people who are allowed access to them.

The sequence of events leading to registration on the child protection register

In the first instance, cases of suspected or confirmed abuse should be reported to the line manager. Many establishments have a nominated child protection officer or manager and, wherever possible, cases of actual or suspected abuse or neglect will initially be referred to this person. They will in turn contact the area child protection team, who will initiate an investigation or, in cases where the child might be deemed to be in danger, involve social services or the police so that the individual may be removed to a place of safety. The police have trained child protection officers who will help with the investigation. The child should never be left in a dangerous situation and may be removed to a place of safety. After investigation a child protection conference will be convened, taking all the evidence into consideration, and a decision will be made whether the child needs to be recorded on a child protection register. In severe cases there may also be criminal charges brought against the perpetrators of the abuse. The child protection register is confidential and only people from the main areas of those working with children (for example, health, education, social services, etc.) have access to it. It contains the names of all children who are thought to be at risk of abuse and it alerts all agencies to work together for the safety and protection of those children and young people

Roles and responsibilities

Following the policies and procedures of the setting

All people involved in the care and education of children and young people have a responsibility to follow the policies and procedures of the setting. This is especially important in the cases of abuse and neglect as failure to do so may endanger the child further or may even be detrimental to the case against the perpetrators. Children who disclose should be supported but not questioned by untrained people as it may negate any evidence gleaned.

Observation

Systematic observation of children and young people within the setting is good practice as it helps ensure that planning is linked to the needs of the individual and that development is monitored and recorded. As a result of these observations, it could be noticed that a child's behaviour has altered or that there are unaccountable marks on their body, etc. It may be through observation that staff are alerted to a potentially abusive or exploitive situation, which warrants further investigation.

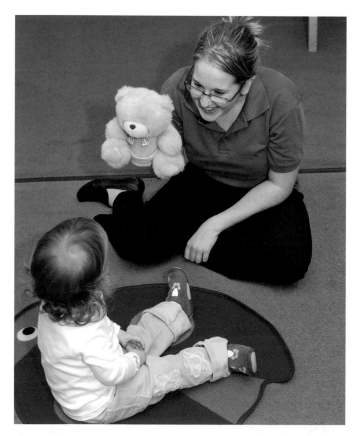

▲ Figure 10.13 Intelligent observation helps to keep a child safe.

Appropriate recording and reporting

Observations should be kept confidential within the setting and access only given to those who have reason to need it, for example, a line manager, educational psychologist, social services, the police, etc. All records and reports should contain facts and not uninformed judgements. These may be used in case conferences later so should always be dated and signed.

Recognising signs and symptoms of abuse

The signs and symptoms of abuse have been covered earlier in this unit but most care and education settings provide in-service training on child protection issues. Many local authorities also require employees to undertake appropriate training as part of a continuous professional development programme. It is essential that everyone is aware of the signs and symptoms of abuse so that immediate action can be taken to ensure the safety of the child.

Knowing how to respond following disclosure

If a child discloses sensitive information, which raises concerns about their safety, then the policy of the setting should be followed immediately. The child should be believed and supported and the procedures implemented straightaway. This is why it is so important to be aware of the content of policies and procedures because, while it may be rare to implement them, when it is required it is vitally important that they are followed implicitly.

Maintaining confidentiality according to the policies of the setting

The policy of the setting will include information about the code of confidentiality to be followed. There is a legal obligation to divulge information to the area child protection team and the police but all information should be kept confidential and not given to anyone without due cause. Passing information to other parties could jeopardise the safety of the child and any ensuing legal procedures.

Disclosure

To disclose information is to tell another person about an incident or event. The word *disclosure* is usually linked to sensitive information often connected to cases of abuse and exploitation.

- *Direct disclosure* occurs when the child or young person informs someone directly that they have been abused or exploited and may begin as a comment that requires further investigation.
- *Indirect disclosure* often involves a third party, who may have information which, added to comments from the child, rings alarm bells. Staff may observe behaviour which might be indicative of abuse or the child may be sexually aware and act in a way that is inappropriate. The child or young person may make a statement or comment which alerts the listener to potential problems.

Listening carefully and attentively

When a child or young person indicates that something is wrong, the adult must listen carefully and not interpret words incorrectly. Listening carefully is an indication that you are taking what the child or young person says seriously and that you are not shocked. It is important not to show disgust or shock as the child will only be more reluctant to disclose if you do.

Communicating at the child/young person's own pace

The child or young person should be supported and there should be no added pressure to hurry things along.

It may have taken a great deal of courage to reach the point of disclosure and the child should be allowed to determine the pace of the proceedings. If they feel rushed they may also feel uncomfortable and as if they are being judged, so it is vital that they are able to control the situation. Remember, they may have been threatened with untold horrors if they tell anyone about their abuse and they will feel extremely vulnerable.

Taking the child or young person seriously

The child or young person should be kept as calm as possible and it should be evident to them that they are being taken seriously. It may be extremely traumatic for a child to disclose sensitive information about themselves and they have obviously put a great deal of trust in the person they are talking to. In the majority of cases children will not be able to make up the things they disclose and their word should always be treated with the utmost gravity.

Reassuring and supporting the child/young person

The child or young person should receive the support and reassurance that they require and will need to be assured that they are not at fault or to blame for anything that has happened.

Unconditional acceptance

It is important that the child is accepted, no matter what they have said, as they will already feel that they are in some way to blame or have brought the situation upon themselves by their actions or behaviour. The term *unconditional acceptance* is used to convey a message that whatever has happened, and in whatever way, that child or young person is a valued person without blame and will be supported and accepted whatever happens.

Boundaries of confidentiality

While confidentiality is to be respected in most cases, there are exceptions in the case of abusive situations. There is a legal responsibility to pass information to the authorities investigating the case and these may include a number of different agencies, for example, area child protection teams, police, social services, etc.

Following the correct procedures of the setting promptly

The procedures of the setting are in place to safeguard all involved and it is important that they are followed correctly and promptly. If the procedures are followed then no one can be blamed if the outcome is not as desired.

Theory into practice

If you are in placement, check that you know the reporting procedures to follow if you suspect a child is at risk of abuse.

Dealing with your own feelings and emotions

Once someone is involved in a child protection case they will have their own feelings to deal with and these may be very strong. They may feel that they have begun proceedings that they no longer have control over and they may have strong negative feelings against members of the child's family. It is necessary for these feelings to be addressed and in some cases a debriefing exercise is beneficial. In others it may be deemed appropriate to undertake sessions with a counsellor who may help the individual rationalise and deal with their emotions.

Support for children/young people who disclose

Once a child has disclosed what is happening, there are authorities and agencies which can protect and support them. It is necessary to make sure that the truth is told and that means the child must be sensitively encouraged to talk about what has been happening to them. The information needs to be passed on to the relevant authorities so that the allegations can be investigated.

The area child protection team, as part of the local authority social services, will be involved, as will the police who will lead the investigation.

Empowering children and young people

Children and young people should be given strategies which will empower them in abusive and exploitive situations. Lessons or programmes, specifically designed to address some of the issues related to abuse in a sensitive way, are often used by settings and the individuals should be encouraged to understand that it is OK to say 'no' and to be aware of what is unacceptable or inappropriate behaviour by others.

Theory into practice

Think of an activity or topic that will help children to be more aware of dangers or exploitation.

Unconditional acceptance for the child/young person

It is often extremely difficult for children to disclose as they may feel that no one will believe them. Again, it is essential that workers in the sector believe what the child or young person is saying. It may be partial or full disclosure but the individual must never be made to feel insecure or that they are not believed. Unconditional acceptance is an important aspect as the child may feel dirty, useless and unloved and they must be shown respect and love for them as an individual and for the courage they have demonstrated in disclosing.

Awareness of the potential impact on the child/young person and other family members

There will always be some impact on the child and on other members of the family because of the very nature of the situation but this will be more traumatic if the abuser is a member of the nuclear family. In cases where someone outside the nuclear family has abused the child or young person, then the family can be a strong and powerful support for them. There are support mechanisms in place which will help families come to terms with abusive and exploitive situations, for example, individual or whole family counselling and play therapy for younger members.

Counteracting possible stereotyping

It is important that people do not fall into the trap of stereotyping. A family may be poor but that does not mean that they will be neglectful. It is important that any stereotyping is counteracted immediately or it will prove to be detrimental for the family and for the child or young person involved.

Alleviating the effects of abuse

Encouraging expression of feeling

Children and young people who have suffered abuse may have had to override their natural feelings and keep their emotions blocked for a considerable period of time. They need the opportunity to express their feelings openly. They may feel a loss of control as some of the feelings which have been repressed are likely to be very strong and unusually powerful and, because of this, they will need a lot of support.

Improving self-image

Children who have been abused will inevitably have a poor self-image and may need help in developing a more positive view of themselves. People go through stages where they feel that, in some way, they deserve what has happened to them or that they have encouraged it or been at fault in some way. They will need to be reassured that this is not the case and they need to be supported through the difficult times and encouraged when they are feeling more positive.

Building self-esteem and confidence

Praise and encouragement are positive tools in the hands of dedicated people who work with children and young people. Children who have been through traumatic events will need a great deal of positive reinforcement in order to build up self-esteem and confidence. Many individuals feel used and unworthy of respect and it can take a long time to build up positive relationships and trust. Workers in this sector must have a sensitive and supportive nature as well as needing to be calm and patient.

■ Play therapy

Play therapy is used to both diagnose and treat children and young people who have been through traumatic experiences in their lives. They are able to live out their fears and express emotions in safe and secure environments with staff who are highly trained and who can support them in times of need.

■ Counselling

Counselling (as has been noted earlier in the unit) is an important service that is provided for all people involved in cases of abuse. There are specially trained personnel who are equipped to offer counselling specifically for the young.

The role of voluntary organisations

There are a number of charities and voluntary organisations that help children and young people at risk. These may be the first point of contact for anyone who suffers abuse or who is aware of abusive situations. Organisations such as the NSPCC have specific campaigns to involve all members of the public in trying to stop child abuse. Other organisations provide telephone contact for anyone seeking advice, for example, Childline. All these have an important role to play in supporting the authorities and those in abusive situations.

Sources of information and support

Benefits of a multi-professional, multi-disciplinary approach

Every Child Matters was concerned with all agencies working together as a multi-disciplinary workforce for the well-being of children and young people and this became part of the legislation in the Children Act 2004. After the devastating revelations of the Victoria Climbie case, it was deemed to be vitally important that all agencies involved in cases such as this work together and keep each other informed. In this way it is hoped that the errors of that case will not be repeated.

Common assessment framework

There is a common assessment framework that also ensures that all agencies are informed about the details of cases under review and being assessed. *Framework for the Assessment of Children in Need and their Families* (2000) endeavours to ensure that all interested parties are involved and informed throughout the process.

Co-operation with other professionals

It is important that all professionals involved in the care and education of a child or young person are involved in, or informed of, the assessment of such children. Case conferences or interviews may be implemented so that all relevant information is gathered and so that appropriate decisions are made for the good and well-being of the child.

Sharing information

Sharing information is one of the strengths of working as part of a multi-disciplinary team but it is important to be aware of the codes of confidentiality. It is usual that information, even of a sensitive nature, is shared amongst professionals, with the welfare of the child at the heart of the proceedings.

Boundaries of confidentiality

Legislation dictates the boundaries of confidentiality in the cases of abusive and exploitive behaviour. However, it is important that, within those constraints, the confidential policy of the setting is strictly adhered to: failure to do so may call into question the reliability of personnel involved.

Other professionals involved

There may be a wide range of professionals involved with children and young people who have been exploited or abused. These have been mentioned previously in this unit but it is vital that all people working with a child or young person do so with integrity and sensitivity.

Community support networks

Community support networks have been set up to provide links with agencies, which can provide specific support for anyone with difficulties or problems. They provide information about a wide range of expertise which may be beneficial for families with children and young people.

Assessment activity 10.4

P5 Describe appropriate responses where child abuse is suspected or confirmed, making reference to current legislation and policies.

1 Describe the order of events once abuse is suspected or confirmed and, in doing so, you should make reference to the policies and procedures that are in place and how they comply with current legislation. **P5**

Grading tip for P5

You might like to include a chart of events to provide a simpler visualisation of the process.

M3 Explain strategies and methods to minimise the risk to children and young people where abuse is suspected or confirmed.

3 You will need to provide more detail, giving reasons why these methods might be used for the support of children/young people and their families.

Grading tip for M3

It may be useful to consider strategies individually and provide a reasoned explanation for the implementation of each one.

P6 Identify the strategies and methods of supporting children, young people and their families where abuse is suspected or confirmed.

2 When identifying and describing the strategies, it will be necessary to consider short-term support and longer-term support and actions to alleviate the affects of abuse. **P6**

Grading tip for P6

It may be useful to refer to a case study or hypothetical situation in order to illustrate your meaning.

D2 Evaluate a range of strategies and methods to support children/young people and their families where abuse is suspected or confirmed.

4 You will need to provide a range of strategies and methods and then consider their strengths and weaknesses with regard to their potential effectiveness.

Grading tip for D2

It would be beneficial if you could make reference to any current research you have carried out relating to this topic.

Knowledge check

1 Why might a child or young person be looked after?

2 Why is it important to have a robust legislative framework for the care of children and young people?

3 What type of care for children and young people might be classed as temporary?

4 What is the role of local government in providing care for children and young people?

5 What is the role of a foster parent?

6 What are the signs and symptoms of physical abuse?

7 Give an example of peer abuse.

8 How might a child or young person be at risk of electronic exploitation?

9 Why is it important to follow the policies and procedures of the setting?

10 Why is it important to support and reassure the child or young person who discloses that they have been in an abusive situation?

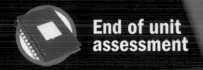
Preparation for assessment

You will need to demonstrate an understanding of this unit for your own development but you may also need to be able to explain this to other workers in the field.

1 In order to help you collect evidence for the unit outcomes, you should carry out some individual research into the reasons why children and young people might need to be cared for away from their families. It may be useful to interview members of staff in your placement who may have experience of the children they provide care for, being looked after by others. You will need to keep in mind that factors outside the family unit may have an influence on the care of the child or young person, for example, accident or bereavement. Other factors will include disability, behaviour and abusive situations.

Once you have carried out your research, you should describe the main reasons why children and young people may be looked after away from their families. **P1**

2 Your research will, in addition, include the relevant and current legislation relating to the assessment of children and their families. You will need to demonstrate knowledge of the legal framework for safeguarding children and young people. **P2**

3 When you are in placement you should be aware of the policies and procedures relating to the safety and welfare of children. It would be beneficial to ask to read these so that you can identify the relevance of these in the legal framework. Analysis of these, and how they help the child/young person and their family while being looked after, would give you evidence for **M1**.

4 An evaluation, considering the strengths and weaknesses, weighing the rights of the child/young person and their family against the needs of the ididividual, will provide you with the evidence for **D1**.

5 Try to interview staff from a range of settings to draw up a picture of the provision available when children and young people need to be looked after. You will need to describe a range of services in order to meet the requirements for **P3**.

6 Consider two different organisations in more detail and compare their provision. You will need to look at aspects that are similar and provide detail of where they vary and how they meet the differing needs of the child or young person. **M2**

7 Discussing abusive situations is always very difficult but, in order to provide overall care for children and young people, it is necessary for you to know about the types of abuse and how you might recognise the signs and symptoms. You will need to be able to describe the signs and symptoms of abuse under each of the main headings, i.e. physical, sexual, emotional, neglect and bullying. **P4**

8 An interview with your placement supervisor may provide you with the information required to describe the appropriate responses where child abuse is suspected or confirmed. You will need to explain the sequence of events and which other agencies might be involved in the process. **P5**

9 You will need to consider the support mechanisms that might be used to support children/young people and their families. Many of these will be used by your placement in making children aware of their rights and ensuring they have an awareness of their body and what is appropriate and what is not. The difference between good and bad is often covered in a setting, for example, good/bad secrets, good/bad touching. You will need to able to identify a range of methods of support and strategies in order to meet the requirements of the pass criteria. In order to meet the higher grades you will need to provide a

more detailed explanation of why the strategies you have identified might be used and you might like to further evaluate those methods and strategies giving due consideration to their strengths and weaknesses.

 P6, M3, D2

Resources and further reading

Beckett, C. (2003) *Child Protection: An Introduction* London: Sage Publications

Department of Health (2000) *Framework for the Assessment of Children in Need and their Families*, London: HMSO

Hobart, C., Franknel, J. (2005) *Good Practice in Child Protection* Cheltenham: Nelson Thornes

Lindon, J. (2003) *Child Protection* London: Hodder and Stoughton

Munro, E. (2002) *Effective Child Protection* London: Sage Publications

Useful websites

Childline
www.childline.org.uk

Every Child Matters
www.everychildmatters.gov.uk

Kidscape
www.kidscape.org.uk

Local authority websites, for example:
www.cambridgeshire.gov.uk

National Children's Bureau
www.ncb.org.uk

NSPCC
www.nspcc.org.uk

Parentline
www.parentlineplus.org.uk

Save the Children
www.savethechildren.org.uk

Stop the Traffik
www.stopthetraffik.org/resources

GRADING CRITERIA

To achieve a pass grade the evidence must show that the learner is able to:	To achieve a merit grade the evidence must show that, in addition to the pass criteria, the learner is able to:	To achieve a distinction grade the evidence must show that, in addition to the pass and merit criteria, the learner is able to:
P1 describe the main reasons why children and young people may need to be looked after away from their families **Assessment activity 10.1 page 44**		
P2 identify the current relevant legislation affecting the care of children and young people **Assessment activity 10.2 page 53**	**M1** analyse how policies and procedures help children/young people and their families whilst the child is being looked after **Assessment activity 10.2 page 53**	**D1** evaluate the legislative rights of the child/young person and the rights of their families, bearing in mind that the needs of the child/young person are paramount **Assessment activity 10.2 page 53**
P3 describe health and social care service provision for looked-after children and young people **Assessment activity 10.2 page 53**	**M2** compare the care provided by at least two different organisations offering care to children and young people **Assessment activity 10.2 page 53**	
P4 describe signs and symptoms of child abuse **Assessment activity 10.3 page 65**		
P5 describe appropriate responses where child abuse is suspected or confirmed, making reference to current legislation and policies **Assessment activity 10.4 page 75**		
P6 identify the strategies and methods of supporting children, young people and their families where abuse is suspected or confirmed. **Assessment activity 10.4 page 75**	**M3** explain strategies and methods to minimise the risk to children and young people where abuse is suspected or confirmed. **Assessment activity 10.4 page 75**	**D2** evaluate a range of strategies and methods to support children/young people and their families where abuse is suspected or confirmed. **Assessment activity 10.4 page 75**

Supporting and protecting adults

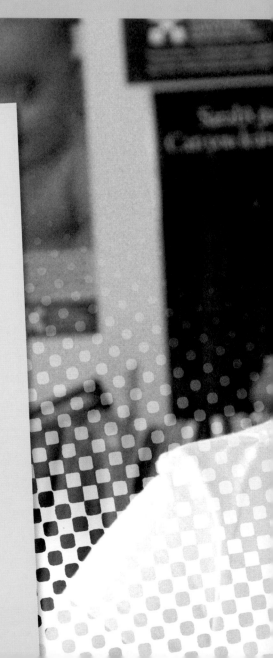

Introduction

In this unit, you will explore issues relating to vulnerable adults and their needs. Child protection, which raises similar issues, has a high profile and a long history as a recognised area of concern, going back to the times when children worked in factories, mines and as chimney sweeps. However, it is only since the 1980s that the protection of vulnerable adults has started to produce similar concerns and a developing profile.

In this unit, you will learn how to develop supportive relationships with adults who are users of health and social care services. Many of these people tend to be vulnerable in a range of specific and different ways.

You will also investigate the various forms of abuse and the signs, or indicators, that it has taken place. You will examine the kinds of abuse that might occur in the various different health and social care environments, and consider ways it can be reduced. You will look at ways agencies, professionals and service users can all work together to reduce the likelihood of abuse.

How you will be assessed

Your tutor will assess this unit internally. The range of activities, case studies and opportunities to think through issues presented in this chapter will further your understanding of the need for care and support of the vulnerable people with whom the health and social care services have contact, and help you prepare for your assessed assignment.

Thinking points

This unit introduces you to an area of concern that the general public have become aware of in the last 25 years. It links in with issues raised in, among others, Unit 2: *Equality, diversity and rights* (in Book 1) and Unit 10: *Caring for children and young people*.

You may also find it resonates with your own experience of being vulnerable, at home, school or in the local community, at various times in your life. If you find that some of the issues or situations in this chapter are upsetting, for whatever reason, make sure you discuss them with your tutor, college nurse, counsellor or whoever you feel most comfortable with. Understanding our own feelings is the first step towards helping others.

The term 'vulnerable adults' is usually understood to mean frail older people or people with learning disabilities. However, anyone who is unable to look after themselves effectively falls into this category. Who do you think these might be? Jot down some other groups of people who may be vulnerable because of their care needs.

Here are some examples to get you started:

- patients in hospital recovering from an operation
- people with mental health problems living in a hostel
- disabled people with mobility problems living alone
- people with drug or alcohol addictions
- teenagers who have had their drinks 'spiked' on a Saturday night out.

All these are vulnerable. We will be considering 'vulnerability' in the broadest of terms.

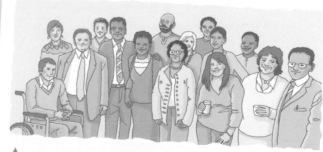

▲ **Figure 11.1 Can you tell who is vulnerable?**

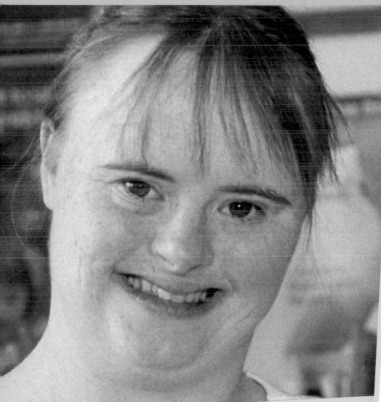

After completing this unit you should be able to achieve the following outcomes:

- Know how to develop supportive relationships with adult users of health and social care services
- Understand types of abuse and indicators of abuse in health and social care contexts
- Understand the potential for abuse in health and social care contexts
- Understand working strategies to minimise abuse.

As someone who is thinking of a career in health or social care, you will need to develop the skills to form professional supportive relationships with service users and their families. However, before you can develop such skills, you need a basic understanding of the elements that make up such a relationship. It is from this understanding that skills can grow.

Supportive

Relationships come in all shapes and sizes. Below is a mind map that shows some of the different types of relationships you have and who you have them with.

Each type of relationship has a different expectation – there are different degrees of emotion, involvement and behaviour. For example, you are likely to behave, feel and act differently as a daughter or a son from how you are as a student in school or college! The type of relationship between an adult service user and a health or social care professional can also vary greatly but there is likely to be a certain commonality in the support and approach offered. This approach is humanistic in nature and emphasises the unique importance and value of each individual.

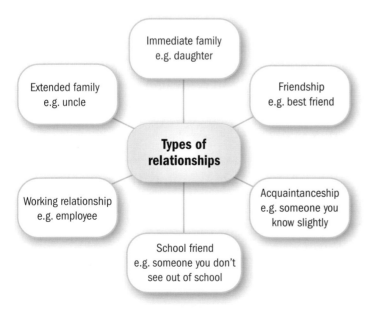

▲ Figure 11.2 Relationships come in all shapes and sizes!

The **humanistic approach** focuses on treating people with dignity, respect and as unique individuals – humans – who have individual needs.

Key terms

Humanistic approach Treating people with dignity, respect and as unique individuals with individual needs.

Core conditions These are the essential ingredients for a person-centred approach.

Theory into practice

You and your friend are involved in a car accident and are admitted to hospital. You are in the same ward and have each fractured a similar bone in the right leg. Are your needs likely to be the same as your friend's? In what way might they differ? How would you want to be treated by the nursing staff in terms of approach and care? Briefly research the NHS Plan 2000 and identify what approach is central to the plan in terms of patient care.

(See www.nhsia.nhs/uk/nhsplan/summary.htm)

The humanistic approach has been developed in recent times through the work of psychologists such as Carl Rogers and Gerald Egan. They stressed the importance of the individual's own experience and that the service user, not the professional, is the 'expert' on themselves. It is through a supportive, enabling professional relationship that individuals can be empowered to help themselves. For example, the General Medical Council, in its guidelines to doctors, requires them to 'make the care of your patient your first concern'.

Rogers identified the **core conditions** for such relationships as being:

- **empathy** – the ability to 'see' and understand the situation through the eyes of the person who is experiencing it – 'walking in their shoes'
- **congruence** – to be genuine, transparent and real – not acting as the expert but as a person
- **unconditional positive regard** – respecting and valuing the individual and appreciating them as a person – being non-judgemental about them as individuals.

Egan also emphasised the importance of:

- **active listening** – focusing carefully on what a person is saying so they know they are being listened to
- **flexibility in approach** – responding to what the person says rather than following your own agenda or what you want to say.

The person-centred approach has been applied to health and social care settings through the development and use of the Care Value Base by staff (fostering service users' rights; fostering equality and diversity and maintaining confidentiality) and the introduction of the National Minimal Standards (identified in the Care Standards Act 2000).

The person-centred approach is also part of the government's white paper *Valuing People: A New Strategy for Learning Disability* (2001) in which the four key features of person-centred planning are spelt out. These are:

- rights
- independence
- choice
- inclusion.

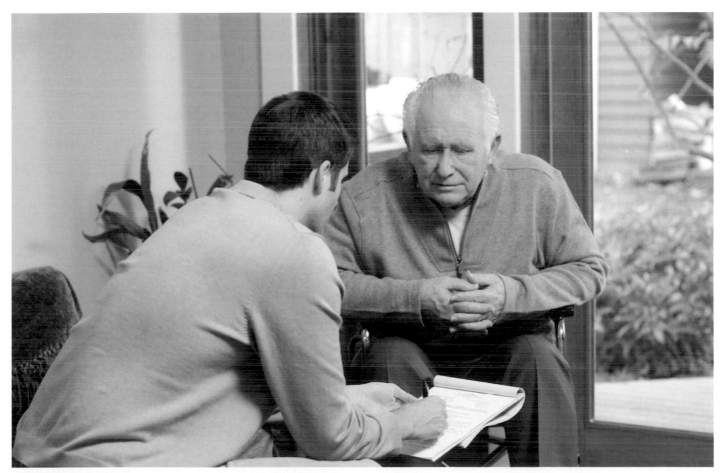

▲ Being listened to.

Reflect

Consider a close relationship you have with a friend. In what way do the three core conditions (empathy, congruence and unconditional positive regard) exist in the relationship? Give examples of each. If these conditions did not exist, how would the relationship be affected?

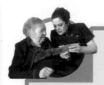

In context

Nancy is 70 and has just moved into a care home. She has had a stroke which has left her paralysed down one side and needs help with day-to-day activities, for example, washing, toileting, getting dressed, etc. Her husband, who was her main carer, recently died.

Her sons and daughters arranged for her to move into the care home without discussing it with her. She feels she was rushed into making the decision. She has difficulty speaking clearly and finds the staff often ignore her. When she is taken to the toilet the door is often left open so they can check that 'everything is alright'. At meal times she is given the same as everyone else even though she is a vegetarian. She is told to eat the vegetables and leave the meat. She has been given the nickname of 'the veggie' by some of the staff. One member of staff discussed her occasional incontinence with her in the TV lounge, while others were within hearing.

She is unhappy about the way she has been treated.

1   **Identify which elements of a supportive relationship are not being applied and the likely effects on Nancy.**

2   **Explain what should happen so that she feels respected and supported.**

3   **Produce a set of guidelines for new members of staff on how new residents should be treated.**

Supportive professional relationships with adult service users should include the following:

Element	Example
Helping	Willingness to assist: collecting a prescription from the doctor
Enabling	Removing an obstacle: moving chairs out of the way so that a wheelchair user can propel themselves to a table
Empowering	Giving the power to make decisions relating to own life: involving the service user in planning their care package
Making choices	Being able to exercise own preferences from a range of options: doctor explaining the different types of treatment available so patient can decide on their treatment of choice
Maintaining privacy	Ensuring an individual has their own space regardless of circumstances: making sure the screens are securely around a patient's bed when carrying out a medical examination in hospital
Confidentiality	Protecting information that has been given on trust: not leaving files around for residents to read
Advocacy	Speaking on behalf of someone who cannot do so for themselves: making a complaint on behalf of an older person who is confused
Promoting rights	Ensuring an individual's rights are not compromised because of their care needs: people with learning disabilities also have the right to make choices
Non-judgemental	Having an open mind about an individual: not stereotyping people based on what others have told you

Table 11.1 Elements within a supportive professional relationship.

Relationships

Being supportive towards adult users of health and social care services involves the establishment of a professional relationship between the service user and the member of staff. This relationship will differ from a personal friendship in a number of ways.

A relationship implies a connection between people. A professional relationship concerns the connection between a service user and a carer provider that has certain defined and understood boundaries and expectations. These are clearly spelt out for professionals in their professional codes of conduct and ethics.

Theory into practice

Research the following codes and summarise what each says about the relationship between service user, patient or client and the professional worker. This could be done as a group exercise and the information shared.

- Nursing and Midwifery Council (NMC) – Code of professional conduct, standards of conduct, performance and ethics – www.nmc-uk.org.uk
- British Association of Social Workers (BASW) – Code of Ethics – www.basw.co.uk
- General Medical Council (GMC) – Code of Good Medical Practice – www.gmc-uk.org.uk

Your research is likely to show that a relationship between a service user and a service provider should enable the service user to express their views or aims clearly and encourage their development. An example of this would be someone with learning disabilities expressing the view that they would like to go on holiday to Spain. A supportive relationship would endeavour to help the person achieve their wish. Such a relationship would also enable people to exercise their preferences. For example, Nancy, in the case study above, was not given the opportunity to express her preference as to whether she would prefer to stay at home, with help coming in, or choose to live in a particular care home in her community.

The person-centred or humanistic approach emphasises the importance of the individual making their own choices, once they have been given enough information on which to base an informed decision. This requires unbiased information being provided by key figures such as:

- GPs, for example, 'should I have an operation or not?'
- social workers, for example, providing information on a range of available care homes
- youth workers, for example, running a safe sex advisory campaign with information on different contraceptives and their effectiveness.

For this to happen, the service user needs to trust the source of the information.

Within a professional relationship, the emphasis on the support required can shift according to the individual's needs at any given time. While many individuals are able to express their preferences, some will not be able to do so for a range of different reasons.

Reflect

Spend a few moments identifying who might experience difficulty in expressing their preferences and why this might be the case. What degree of support would be required?

A person who has had a stroke, and is paralysed down one side of their body, could have difficulty making themselves understood. They would need someone to put across their views and preferences in a meeting that considered their care plan. An advocate, a person who was speaking on their behalf and representing their best interests, would do this.

The supportive professional relationship differs from the more informal relationship that exists between friends and family because of the framework within which it is set. Neil Moonie (2005) suggests that this difference is because:

- professionals must work within a framework of values
- professional work always involves a duty of care for the welfare of service users
- professional relationships involve establishing appropriate boundaries.

It is the responsibility of the professional to ensure such a relationship stays within the boundaries that have been laid down in legislation and by professional bodies. They are provided, through training and work-based experience, with clear guidelines whereas the service user does not necessarily have such a clear understanding of the boundaries. Although the relationship is seen as one of 'equals' in terms of being supportive, empowering and between two people, it is still a relationship between someone who is in need of help and a professional who has a helping role.

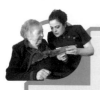
Mina is a student on placement in a care home. She has noticed that the care assistants talk to the residents in very loud voices even though most of them do not appear to have any hearing difficulties. They also talk to them as if they are children and stroke their hair, without first checking if the resident is happy with such behaviour, and often have a joke at their expense. For example, on Red Nose Day they coloured the end of Alice's nose without asking her. As soon as they left the room, Alice wiped it off.

1. **Which behaviour do you believe is patronising and which is belittling? Why?**

2. **What effect is this behaviour likely to have on the relationship between care-giver and care receiver?**

3. **Produce a ten-point Code of Conduct for care workers to ensure such behaviour does not happen again. How is such a code likely to affect relationships within the care home?**

In the past, many professionals believed that they knew what was best for people who needed help and did not involve them in the decision-making process. For example, in Canada, up until the early 1970s, women with learning disabilities were sterilised to stop them having unwanted babies. This was done without their permission and was passed off as a minor, but necessary, operation that was not fully explained to them.

This is an extreme, but not uncommon, example of professionals believing they knew what was best for their patients or clients. The services an individual received would not necessarily depend on their needs but on the decision of the professional. Equality in the relationship was replaced by power over subservience, with the service user accepting the decisions of the all-powerful professional without question.

Remember!

The person-centred approach emphasises the importance of unconditional positive regard, at all times.

Development of relationships

You choose to have a friendship, you do not necessarily choose to have a professional relationship – it is often thrust upon you! When you have toothache, you enter into a relationship with the dentist. The mutually agreed aim will be to repair whatever damage has caused the toothache and return you to pain-free oral health. During your time with the dentist, a relationship has been developing or an existing one rekindled. The type and quality of the relationship depends on a number of factors. What do you think these might be?

Initially, the first few seconds of contact with the dentist will produce an image on which your initial relationship will be based. You will decide whether you like the person or not and that will set the initial tone of the relationship. This will be based on the initial communication, facial expression, appearance, body language and behaviour or actions.

It is important that the professional projects an image of professional competence in order to put you at your ease and start to develop the trust which is essential in such a relationship.

This can be done through a person-centred approach that focuses on your needs. Your needs can be established through asking you how you are and what the problem is. This will be done while focusing on you, through eye

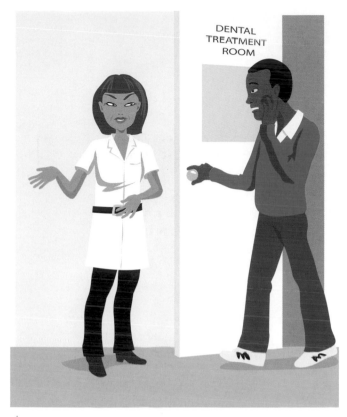

DENTAL TREATMENT ROOM

▲ Figure 11.3 You don't necessarily choose to enter into a professional relationship – sometimes it is thrust upon you!

contact and body language (facing you, not writing up the previous patient's notes) and listening to what you have to say. A welcoming action such as helping you onto the chair can also be seen as a factor in establishing a relationship. However, physical contact should first be checked with the recipient to ensure they are happy with it (for example, 'Can I help you on to the chair?') as the individual may have personal, cultural or religious reasons for not wishing to be touched. Why might this be?

Reflect

Think back to an occasion when you had to trust a stranger in a health and care situation. It might have been a visit to the A&E department at the local hospital for stitches, having a plaster cast put on a fracture or seeing a new dentist when you had toothache. How did you feel about trusting someone you had not met before with your health care?

The foundation on which a relationship is built is trust. It does not develop instantly although, in many circumstances, service users are forced to trust strangers.

The development of trust between two people is an indication of a developing relationship. To place yourself in the care of someone else can be scary and this is what many service users are experiencing on a daily basis. A young, physically disabled person living independently in their own home may have different agency carers coming in daily to prepare meals and help them with personal hygiene. An older person who has just moved into a care home might have four different carers, in 24 hours, helping them with their toileting. Service users may feel vulnerable until they reach the stage where they feel they can trust the care provider.

Trust can develop as a result of reliability and consistency of approach:

- A home carer says they will visit at 10 a.m. Monday to Friday and turns up on time.
- A patient in hospital has their dressing changed every four hours regardless of who is on duty.
- An older person attending the local day care centre is met with the same cheerful greeting every morning.

These actions enable trust to be built up between the service user and the professional as well as the service itself.

Being treated with fairness is another important factor in the development of a relationship and this relates to the care value: promoting equality and diversity. Equality is less about treating everyone equally but more about treating people fairly, without discrimination, and according to their needs. Service users who feel they are being treated unfairly will feel resentful. For example, if a patient is not offered a choice of appointment times for their next visit (when the person in front of them has) this is likely to have a negative effect on their relationship with the GP.

External factors can have a negative effect on relationships. Personal issues can distract a carer worker and affect their mood and reduce their effectiveness. This will be picked up on very quickly by service users who may feel they have done something wrong. It can detract from the quality of care being provided. Similarly, this can happen if one member of staff has an argument with another member of staff. They can carry the negative emotions from the argument with them, into their work. The professional, at all times, needs to focus on the individual with whom they are working and not be distracted by other focuses. This is a sign of true professionalism.

In context

Sasha, a care worker in a care home, has just split up with her boyfriend. She has started being snappy and bad tempered with some of the residents – so much so that her rough handling has accidentally bruised someone.

1   **What effect is this likely to have on her relationships within the home?**

2   **What should a professional do in such circumstances?**

3   **What action could the residents take?**

Individual rights

Since the introduction of the European Convention on Human Rights and Fundamental Freedoms 1950, the rights of the individual have been defined and enshrined in legislation and government policy. A person who turns to an organisation and its professionals for help does not lose their rights, unless they are believed to be a danger to themselves or other people, as a result of mental illness. Such restrictions are governed, at present, by the Mental Health Act 1983 but are likely to be changed under the 2006 Mental Health Bill and the subsequent act.

People's rights do not change because of a disability or because they use a health care service. It is the role of the professional to ensure that a supportive relationship develops for the benefit of the service user and that it is one that protects their rights.

Various legislation and policy over the years have identified the following as behaviour that should be expected as a right (see Table 11.2).

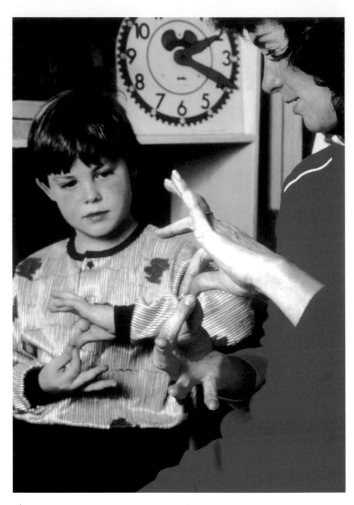

▲ It is important to use the service user's preferred means of communication.

Reflect

How would you want to be treated or cared for in a health or social care setting, for example, a hospital A&E department or a day centre for people with mental health conditions? List your expectations. Do you believe these are wishes that you would like to happen or are they rights that should happen, regardless of your need for help?

Rights	Example
To be respected	Being asked how you wish to be addressed, for example, by first name or family name – 'Jane' or 'Mrs Johnson'
To be treated equally and without discrimination	Being taken on the same trips as other people from the sheltered accommodation, regardless of wheelchair use
To be treated as an individual, taking into account one's diversity and differences	Being asked what you would like to eat and have cultural, religious, hygiene and eating habits taken into account, for example, having a meal served after sundown during Ramadan
To be treated in a dignified way	Having a GP actively listen to your description of the pain you are experiencing rather than dismissing it as 'something that you've got to get used to as you get older'
To have privacy	Being taken to a side room in hospital to discuss your diagnosis rather than in a busy corridor
To be protected from danger and harm	Setting up a password with a home care worker so that you can identify a relief worker
To have access to information about self	Being able to read, and check the accuracy of, the file that contains your personal information
To be communicated with in one's preferred manner	Staff at a day centre using Makaton sign language if this is someone's preferred means of communication
To be cared for in a way that meets one's needs and choices	Supporting an individual in the home they have lived in for the last 50 years, rather than in a care home (having first carried out a risk assessment and made the person aware of the potential risks)
To be able to practise one's own diversity and difference in terms of culture, religion, race, disability, sexuality, beliefs, behaviour, eating and hygiene habits	Continuing to practise your own diversity regardless of the setting, for example, having the privacy and space in which to pray at set times

Table 11.2 Behaviour that should be expected as a right.

Assessment activity 11.1

Annie is 18 and is a recovering drug user. She is living in a hostel for homeless people and attending a rehabilitation training course during the day. She has no friends and looks forward to chatting with Ian, her key worker at the hostel, each evening.

Joshua is 70 and is living in a care home for older people. He has difficulty dressing and taking care of his personal hygiene because of a recent stroke. He is a vegetarian and has little hearing, due to working all his life in the steel industry. His family moved back to the West Indies some years ago and he has a couple of visitors who drop in each week.

Kirin attends a day centre for people with physical disabilities. She is a Muslim and is fasting during the day, as it is Ramadan. She has mobility difficulties and needs to pray at various times during the day. She needs to be able to break her fast as soon as it gets dark. It is winter and daylight disappears an hour before she leaves the centre.

P1 Explain how individual rights can be respected in a supportive relationship.

1   Produce a guide for new care workers that explains the importance of developing supportive relationships with adult service users and how their rights can be respected. **P1**

Grading tip for P1

Remember – service users do not lose any of their rights because they need help. Use the given case studies to illustrate your points.

M1 Explain how supportive relationships can enhance the life experiences of individuals receiving health and social care services.

2   Using the case studies above, explain how such relationships can enhance the service users' life experiences.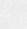

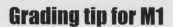
Grading tip for M1

The extent to which an individual is supported and empowered will enhance their experience. The relationship should be person-centred.

D1 Use examples to evaluate the role of supportive relationships in enhancing the life experiences of individuals receiving health and social care services.

3   Evaluate the strengths and weaknesses of the relationships.

Grading tip for D1

Consider how effective supporting relationships can be in improving service users' lives. What might the disadvantages be? Might people want to be told what to do rather than be involved in the decision-making process? Might there be confusion, in the service user's mind, about the difference between a friendship and a supportive professional relationship?

11.2 Types of abuse and indicators of abuse

If you find anything in the section that follows is disturbing or personal, it is important to talk with an appropriate adult with whom you feel confident.

Abuse is defined by the Department of Health as 'a violation of an individual's human and civil rights by any other person or persons'.

Historically, publicity relating to abuse tended to be linked with older people and, to a lesser extent, people with learning disabilities. Up until the late 1950s, older people who needed to be cared for often lived in large families or institutions. They tended to be invisible and, while abuse is likely to have existed, it went unreported as it happened behind closed doors.

In the 1960s and 1970s, families became more mobile, because of their jobs or having to move because of

divorce, and more older people started to live by themselves or in small residential homes or sheltered, supported accommodation. It was during the 1970s that the term 'granny bashing' first appeared in newspaper headlines as cases of physical abuse of older people became more widely reported. The term 'elder abuse' was first used in the late 1970s and early 1980s. In 1995 the charity Action on Elder Abuse defined elder abuse as 'a single or repeated act or lack of appropriate action, occurring within any relationship where there is an expectation of trust, which causes harm or distress to an elder person.'

The focus was later widened as abuse became more widely recognised in other vulnerable groups such as people with physical disabilities and sensory loss.

People who were seen to be 'at risk' were known as 'vulnerable adults'. These individuals were identified in the Department of Health white paper *No Secrets* (2000) as being a person:

- who is, or may be, in need of community care services by reason of mental or other disability, age or illness and
- who is, or may be, unable to take care of him or herself or unable to protect him or herself against significant harm or exploitation.

Theory into practice

Revisit the list of vulnerable people you made at the beginning of the unit (See p.81). Can you add other 'at risk' groups of service users to the list? Taking into account the previous definitions of abuse and people who are vulnerable to abuse, produce your own definition of abuse and a generic description of service users who may be vulnerable.

Types of abuse

The more common forms of abuse are:

- physical
- sexual
- psychological (previously known as emotional)
- financial
- neglect.

Reflect

Thinking about your own experiences and understanding of bullying (for example, from your school days) and knowledge of health and social care, identify and describe types of physical, sexual and psychological abuse that vulnerable adult users may experience.

Other forms of abuse include:

- discriminatory
- institutional
- self-harm
- domestic violence.

Physical abuse

Any physical contact has the potential to be seen as a form of physical abuse. It can depend on the degree of force, or the nature of the contact, used and the intention behind the action.

Clear cases of abuse would be classed as common assault and subject to criminal prosecution. This could include hitting, slapping, kicking and pushing – the sort of actions involved in bullying. These may be carried out by care workers who lose their temper with a service user because they are being difficult or it may be in retaliation for being hit with a walking stick by a confused patient. Possible scenarios could be:

- Jane often refuses to open her mouth when offered food on a spoon – she has had a stroke and is unable to feed herself. This time, when the care worker tries to feed her, she spits out a mouthful of food into the worker's face. The worker loses her temper and slaps Jane 'to teach her a lesson'.
- John is angry at having to move to a care home when his wife is no longer able to look after him. He is becoming confused and shows his anger by lashing out with his stick at anyone who comes near. An agency worker has come in to cover for sickness and hasn't been told about him. As she bends down to pick something up, he hits her across her back. He is surprisingly strong. The worker instinctively lashes out in pain and hits him back.

The more difficult to identify forms of physical abuse may occur within the context of 'caring'. Examples could be:

- A nurse might not take enough care and could roughly handle a patient when turning him over in bed to prevent bedsores. Another patient might be calling for her at the same time and she is rushing her work.
- A confused resident in a nursing home may be given extra medication to 'quieten her down' and make her

less demanding as there are staff shortages on the night shift.

- A boy in a children's home loses his temper and starts to attack other people. A staff member, who has not been trained in 'restraint', holds him down inappropriately and the boy ends up with a fractured arm.

In these situations physical abuse has taken place, although it is not necessarily done with intent to harm. It is sometimes the result of inappropriate actions by the staff when they are in difficult circumstances.

Sexual abuse

Such abuse may range from inappropriate touching to rape. Staff have a duty of care towards service users and it is inappropriate and against professional guidelines (and in some cases, illegal) for them to engage in a sexual relationship with someone who is in their care.

Reflect

Why do you think this is the case? In what situations could such activity be illegal?

There have been prosecutions in recent times of staff who have taken advantage of patients who have been paralysed or sedated. Other staff have had inappropriate relationships with service users in their care who have had learning disabilities. The individuals have not been able to give their full consent to such activities because of their limited understanding of the situation.

Psychological abuse

A service user who is being abused may also be threatened to keep quiet. They might be told that it is 'our little secret' or that they will lose their accommodation if they tell anyone what has happened.

Continuous put-downs and name calling in front of others humiliates people, causing them to lose self-

respect and pride. This can lead to a self-fulfilling prophecy. What has been predicted, for example, 'you are no good and a bad mother', may lead a woman to believe that she is a bad mother, and undermine her mothering skills.

Just as bullying at school can lead to the bullied being driven to take extreme action (for example, suicide) the same can happen to vulnerable adults. This can especially be the case if they have difficulty in getting away from the bully, for example, in a care home or closed psychiatric ward.

Although the focus so far has been on staff as the abuser, other service users can also carry out abuse. Examples have included:

- service users being assaulted by other residents in care homes
- patients in mixed psychiatric wards raping or sexually assaulting other patients
- groups of established tenants in sheltered accommodation picking on new tenants when they use communal lounges and facilities.

Financial abuse

Financial abuse might happen when a service user receives home care and support. They might be used to leaving their purse on the sideboard and then they think they are becoming forgetful because they don't seem to have as much money as they had originally thought. They might not be able to find a piece of jewellery they have not worn for some time and assume they have misplaced it or lent it to someone in their family. Sadly, it might be a support worker who is stealing from them.

An elderly person with restricted mobility may ask a neighbour to collect their weekly pension from the Post Office and do 'a bit of shopping' for them. The

Reflect

How would you feel if you found yourself in such a situation? What would be the effects on you of feeling you could not trust anyone?

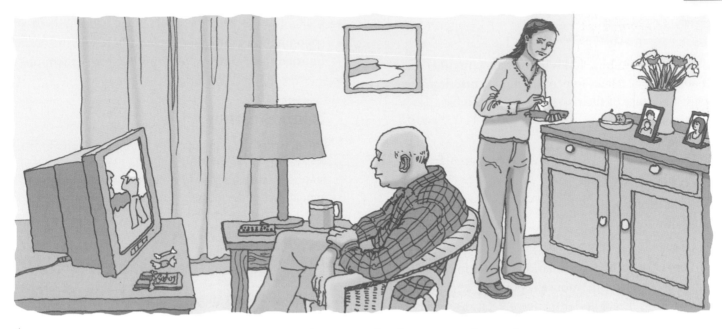

Figure 11.4 Financial abuse can happen when a service user receives home care and support.

neighbour might ask if they could buy a few items for themselves and promise to pay back the money when their giro comes through. This happens every week but the borrowed money is never forthcoming. The pensioner does not like to say anything because there is no one else available to collect her pension.

Neglect

Neglect can be said to take place when there is a failure to provide proper care and attention. In children, there is usually clear evidence of a failure to thrive and grow. They do not have regular meals or clean clothes that are appropriate for the time of year. Their personal hygiene can be poor.

For vulnerable adults, neglect may be self-imposed because of mental health problems. The individual may be suffering from depression and be unable to motivate themselves to prepare and eat food.

Neglect, as a form of abuse, would result from another person's inaction or failure to meet the individual's needs. Neglect has taken place in care homes and hospitals where individuals, who have not been able to feed themselves, have not been fed by carers. Meals have been taken away untouched on the assumption that the person did not feel hungry. As staff change three times

a day, and if accurate records are not kept, the patient's lack of food intake is overlooked. Patients have been admitted to hospital, from care homes, suffering from malnutrition.

Other needs can be neglected as shown in the table below.

Needs	Examples of neglect
Physical	Developing bedsores because of a lack of medical care and not being turned in bed often enough
Intellectual	Not having the opportunity to read your favourite books and newspapers because the staff keep forgetting to take your broken reading glasses for repair
Emotional	A lack of bonding and emotional care from staff because of their aloofness and 'must get the job done' attitude
Social	Living at home but being unable to get out and becoming socially isolated – not having your social needs taken into account in your care plan
Cultural	Not being provided with the opportunity to mix with people of your own culture
Spiritual	Being a devoted, disabled Catholic but not being helped to get to mass on Sunday

Table 11.3 Needs that can be neglected.

Discriminatory abuse

Discriminatory abuse tends to overlap with other forms of abuse but it relates to people who are discriminated against because of their:

- ethnicity
- gender
- age
- disability
- sexuality
- health status
- religion.

As a result of such discrimination, people may well be physically abused. Such abuse is not only a criminal assault but is illegal under the Race Relations Act 1976 (extended in 2000).

Institutional abuse

People's rights can be abused by the practices and procedures of the organisation that cares for them.

It was common practice in care homes and hospital wards to start waking service users from 5.30 a.m. onwards to enable the night staff to wash everyone and give them breakfast before the day staff came on duty. This was for the benefit of the organisation and not the service users.

Home-based service users who need help in going to bed and getting up in the morning may be put to bed at 8 p.m. and have to wait until 8 a.m. (or later) before the carer returns. Their choice of bedtime is overruled by the needs of the organisation to 'get around' a number of clients, using a limited number of staff.

In the past, care organisations have tied confused service users to chairs to stop them wandering and harming themselves. This form of abuse may even have been accepted as common practice across an organisation. New members of staff can be introduced to poor, and potentially abusive, care practices by staff telling them 'this is the way we do things here'. This can include:

- leaving toilet doors open so service users can be checked on
- having some residents as their 'favourites' and ignoring the quieter ones

- making fun of people's bodies when bathing them
- spooning food into people's mouths before they have finished their previous mouthful, to hurry them up.

Take it further

Produce a policy document for an organisation of your choice in which you identify, in general terms, how service users should be treated and what staff should do if they become aware of abusive practices.

Self-harm

Self-harm or self-abuse can take the form of self-inflicted wounds such as cuts to the arms and wrists, burns with lighters and cigarettes and the piercing of the skin with pins or sharp objects. These forms of abuse can be used to detract from, and replace, the psychological and emotional pain being felt by the individual. It can also be a reaction to feeling trapped in a situation from which there does not appear to be any escape. An example of this could be when a service user is being sexually abused by a member of staff in a care home and feels unable to complain or move. The fear and frustration can lead to self-harm as a cry for help.

Abuse through overuse of drugs, alcohol and prescribed medication can be another form of self-harm used to deaden psychological and emotional pain, as well as creating a sense of well-being. This applies to all age groups and care situations.

Theory into practice

Identify who might self-abuse using drugs, alcohol and prescribed medication and the reasons why.

Domestic violence/abuse

Recent legislation and policy relating to vulnerable adults, for example, *No Secrets* (2000) makes no reference to domestic violence as a form of abuse but it clearly fits in with the definitions of abuse.

If there has been domestic violence within a partnership or family before an individual became a service user, it may continue even after the service user moves into supported accommodation or a care home. Domestic violence covers physical, sexual and psychological abuse but other forms, such as financial abuse, may also exist.

In context

Mavis is 80 and lives in her own house. Her partner died some years ago and, when she started to have difficulty in moving around and looking after herself, her 50-year-old son offered to move in and help.

He has always had a short temper and shouts at her when she is slow to do things. He has been known to push her out of the way when he is in a rush. Once when this happened, she slipped and fractured her wrist. She told the hospital she had slipped on the stairs. He also 'charges' her for the care he provides. He has taken control of her pension book and gives her pocket money.

1   **What forms of abuse are taking place?**

2   **What difficulties might social services have in investigating suspected abuse?**

3   **Identify other situations in which domestic violence/abuse may take place. What forms might it take?**

As can be seen in the case study above, it is not always easy to identify when abuse is taking place. Vulnerable adults can be frail, afraid, prone to accidents, forgetful

Remember!

Abuse is not always inflicted with the intention of doing harm – it might be the result of bad practice. However, the result is still the same.

and not wanting to cause any 'bother'. It is therefore important for professionals to be alert for indications of abuse and self-harm so that early intervention can happen.

Indicators of abuse and self-harm

Medical opinion is often required to identify when an injury is non-accidental and even then it may not be clear cut. An injury resulting from a fall does not necessarily indicate if this is as a result of a push or an accidental trip. However, there are some clear indicators such as finger mark bruises on the upper arm that show the person has been grabbed and maybe shaken. Bruising around the mouth may be as a result of forced feeding. Burns from cigarettes and scalding, as a result of being placed in a bath with water that is too hot, are more obvious.

Malnourishment in an individual who has been in a 24-hour care environment, like a care home or hospital, shows itself in terms of unexplained weight loss and dehydration, and is a clear indicator of neglect.

Unexplained withdrawals from bank accounts (without any obvious benefit to the service user in terms of new clothes or furniture, etc.) can indicate that someone else is enjoying the financial benefits. It can be difficult to determine if the money was given or taken.

Reluctance to be touched or to undress for medical examination or be bathed by staff may indicate sexual

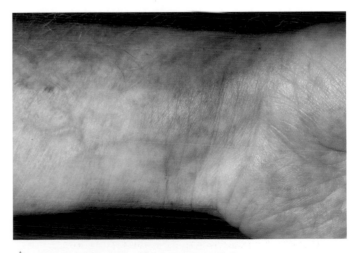

▲   Some injuries are clear indicators of abuse.

abuse, while physically flinching when a voice is raised may indicate psychological and/or physical abuse.

Service users who are bullied or threatened in any way are reluctant to admit they are experiencing abuse because of fear, embarrassment and/or low self-esteem. For some, they have come to accept abuse as 'normal', having experienced it for a lifetime in domestic or institutional settings. It can become a self-fulfilling prophecy in that they expect such behaviour to happen. For others, the answer is to withdraw into their own safe little world and shut out the painful external world. They may also find relief in self-abuse.

Assessment activity 11.2

P2 Describe different forms of abuse that may be experienced by vulnerable adults.

1 Produce a table that describes the different forms of abuse that vulnerable adults may be subject to.

Grading tip for P2

Identify the nine types of abuse and describe each. Use an example of your own for each one to demonstrate your understanding.

P3 Describe different indicators of abuse in vulnerable adults.

2 Describe the indicators of such abuse and give examples of each.

Grading tip for P3

The indicators fall under three main headings (physical, psychological and financial). Describe the signs, using examples, and link them to the types of abuse they could indicate.

11.3 The potential for abuse

The likelihood of abuse taking place can depend on a number of different factors. Some settings or contexts provide more opportunity than others for such behaviour.

Theory into practice

Identify settings and situations in which you feel service users are potentially at greater risk of being abused.

Contexts and the potential for abuse

Living alone, and depending on others, can be isolating for people who have limited social networks. They may find their main social contact is with their carers. Such isolation and dependency can increase the vulnerability of an individual who is confused, frail or has a learning disability.

Service users who live with their families may be subject to abuse by one or more family members. While not living in an isolated situation, they may be subject to a lack of privacy and financial abuse, for example, their mail might be opened and their benefits taken from them. They may suffer psychological abuse through name-calling and being the family scapegoat – being blamed whenever anything goes wrong.

Theory into practice

Identify the advantages and disadvantages, for vulnerable people, of living at home either by themselves or with their family.

In both situations, vulnerability is increased because the abuse takes place within the family and is more difficult to identify and resolve.

People with learning disabilities may live in the community in supported houses that are not staffed at night. They can become prey to local teenagers and young adults who take advantage of their open, trusting nature and use their accommodation as a drop in and a place to have drinking parties, etc. The service user finds they are swept up in the activities and are unable to control the situation. Neighbours may act as informal carers and develop an abusive relationship because of the imbalance of power in the relationship.

Residential care has the potential of abuse on various levels. In addition to abuse by carers and invasion of privacy, there is the possibility of abuse by other service users and by the organisation.

Bullying of new residents by cliques of long established residents is not uncommon, leading to psychological abuse and distress.

Residential care homes may have systems that deny the rights of service users. Residents may be put to bed early to allow night staff to get on with the laundry, ironing and cleaning. In theory, they may have a choice about bedtime but, in practice, they may be bullied into going early as staff start cleaning around them and ask

In context

Jonas has a mild learning disability and lives in a housing association flat. His next-door neighbours have suggested they will make his lunch and evening meal in return for half his money. He has agreed to this but finds the food is often cold and served in small portions. He is hungry most of the time and is having to spend his remaining money on snacks and chips. He feels unable to tackle them about this as he is afraid to lose their friendship. He does not know anyone else on the estate and he does not want any trouble.

1 As his social worker, what help could you offer?

2 Jonas is offered another flat, in a different area, for his own well-being and is happy to take it. He has a support worker, for two months, to help him settle in. What role and help could the support worker offer?

3 What longer-term plans could be discussed with Jonas to enhance his life experience?

Take it further

Social workers sometimes struggle to get the balance right. They have to balance protection of the vulnerable while enabling the development of autonomy and empowerment for the individual. In Jonas's case, what are some of the issues?

very pointedly 'Isn't it time you went to bed?' Service users are often over-compliant and accept whatever is happening to them. They have a lack of resistance because of their low self-esteem.

Reflect

Imagine you have just moved into a residential home. You walk into the TV lounge and sit down. Immediately, a resident comes in and tells you to move as that is her seat – she has sat there for the last five years. You go to move to a different seat and are told that this also 'belongs' to someone else. You finally find a seat at the back of the room where it is difficult to see the TV clearly. Everyone is glaring at you because you've interrupted their programme. An icy atmosphere continues for the next couple of days so you stop using the lounge. How would you feel?

However, it is not only service users who are vulnerable to abuse. Carers, both informal (relatives) and formal (professionals), are subject to abuse from service users. Relatives can be physically and psychologically abused by people they care for. This can happen when having close physical contact, for example, helping to dress and the person lashes out, or through verbal abuse, for example, name calling or negative comparison with siblings.

Professionals in institutions like hospitals are increasingly finding themselves on the receiving end of physical and verbal abuse. In some places, police have started to patrol A&E departments at weekends because of the level of threat. Staff in psychiatric units are also subjected to assault by patients, because of their illnesses.

Take it further

Research news items on the levels of abuse on NHS staff, especially in A&E departments. Produce a report on what you have found.

Predisposing factors

There are certain groups of service users who appear to be more vulnerable to abuse than others. These tend to be people with learning disabilities or mental health problems; older people suffering from dementia or in a state of confusion for some other reason; as well as those with a previous history of being abused.

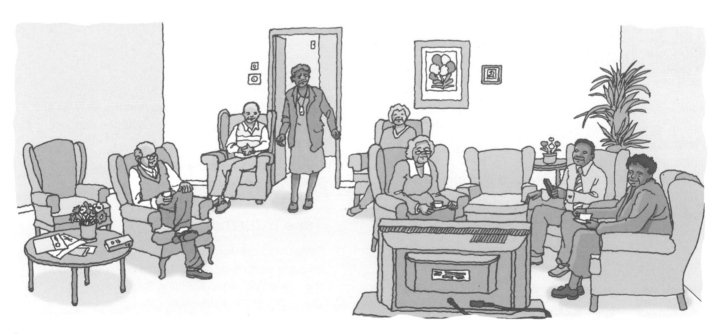

▲ Figure 11.5 Which seat would you use?

People in these groups tend to be over-compliant and to accept whatever happens to them. They have low expectations and low self-esteem. Their illness, condition or age tends to make them isolated and limit their social networks. As a result, they become dependent on their abusers, or potential abusers, for help, services and social interaction. Being vulnerable increases the fear of retaliation from the abuser. Service users can blame themselves for their abuse and believe they have deserved it. The abuser can reinforce this.

Individuals, such as those with learning or physical disabilities, may be naive and have limited sexual knowledge, which leaves them more open to being taken advantage of. There is evidence that adults can be groomed in the same way as children.

Service users who have a previous history of being abused can come to see it as a continuance, even in different circumstances and settings, of the norm. They feel disempowered and unable to resist.

The potential for abuse lies in the nature of the interaction and the powerlessness of the service users. The service user's need for help with personal care increases the opportunity for abuse and can make it harder to be sure it has actually taken place. It is an intimate and personal relationship that takes place behind closed doors privately and therefore it is difficult to monitor.

Vulnerable adults, who do not wish to make a complaint, or be involved in an investigation of alleged abuse, have the right of refusal. Even in cases where the adult is not considered capable of giving their informed consent or agreement (for example, in sexual relationships) their advocate might feel it is not in their best interests to have the matter pursued. Why do you think this may not be in their best interests?

Assessment activity 11.3

You are an inspector preparing to visit a small town. It has:

- a home that provides residential care for confused older people
- a long stay hostel for homeless men
- supported flats for people living in the community who have learning disabilities
- a home care service that provides home support for physically disabled people living in their own homes.

There have been a number of unconfirmed reports of abuse taking place and you have been asked to carry out an initial survey of the potential for abuse in these settings.

P4 Describe the potential for abuse in health and social care contexts.

1 Produce a short report that describes the potential for abuse in the care settings described above.

Grading tip for P4

Take a general view on the potential for abuse in care settings.

M2 Analyse the potential for abuse in four health and social care contexts.

2 Your report should go on to analyse the potential for abuse in each of these contexts.

Grading tip for M2

Consider the vulnerability of the service users in each of the settings before analysing the potential for abuse.

Having identified that adults can be vulnerable, a number of **strategies** have been put into place to minimise abuse. One of these strategies involves checking records to assess the suitability of people who wish to work as carers with vulnerable adults.

Key terms

Strategy A long-term plan, a way of working.

Protection of Vulnerable Adults Scheme (POVA)

This applies to:

- all care workers who wish to work in a care home and will have regular contact with residents
- those who would be providing personal care in an individual's own home
- those who would care for a service user in an adult placement (foster care for adults).

Since 24 July 2004, all care workers who apply to work with vulnerable adults:

- in care homes
- with domiciliary care agencies
- as adult placement carers

have to be checked against the POVA list. This list identifies professionals who have harmed service users and are banned from working with them. They may have intended to harm or caused harmed through poor practice. This requirement was set out in the Care Standards Act 2004 but does not cover other care settings such as hospitals.

Staff who were in post before this date are not subject to such a check but would have undergone a Criminal Records Bureau (CRB) check or **disclosure**.

Key terms

Disclosure Revealing information that is held about a person.

Care Homes Regulation 2001

This set out the requirements that providers and managers of care homes must meet in order to be registered as 'fit' or suitable for the job. It also sets out how care should be carried out within care homes. CRB checks are required for staff to assess their suitability to work with vulnerable adults. A fine (for example, for a minor traffic offence) would not normally preclude an individual from being employed but theft, or offences involving violence against a person, would preclude them.

National Service Framework

As well as protecting service users through the vetting of care workers, the government has:

- set national standards and defined service models, or ways of delivering services, to certain groups of people (for example, those with diabetes)
- introduced programmes that will support the introduction of such standards and ways of working, at a local level
- established performance measures or ways of measuring achievement of the standards.

These performance measures are known as the National Service Framework (NSF) and apply to health, social services and other organisations. By implementing good practice and high standards, the risk of abuse should be minimised.

The NSFs that set standards in the care of vulnerable adults are those covering mental health, older people and long-term conditions. The NSF for mental health aims to provide:

- safe services that protect and care for patients and service users
- sound services that provide access to a full range of different services
- supportive services that work with the patient, service user, families and carers for healthier communities.

Multi-agency working

A further strategy focuses on improving the ways in which agencies and professionals work together for the benefit of the service user. In the past, there has been rivalry over funding and arguments over 'who does what' that has obstructed closer professional working. This has been tackled in a number of ways.

- **Multi-agency working** – the **care planning** process and **single assessment** process has encouraged greater inter-agency working together, with the service user's needs being central to the process. Rather than working separately, and each agency providing their own service without reference to the others, joint working encourages a sharing of information, a co-ordination of approach and less duplication of services.

Key terms

Care planning The joint planning of an individual's treatment and/or care that involves all concerned.

Single assessment The assessment of an individual's needs carried out by one professional/co-ordinator on behalf of a multi-disciplinary/-agency team.

Multi-agency working produces a multi-disciplinary approach. This is where professionals from different agencies combine their skills and expertise to meet the holistic needs of the service user. For this to work well, good communication and an understanding of the way in which other agencies work is essential. It also requires a 'lead' or co-ordinating professional to ensure the needs of the service user are being met. This has not always happened in the past and agencies have assumed others were taking care of the service user, when they were not. This has led to the

death of a number of children and vulnerable adults through abuse or neglect.

The government guidance paper *No Secrets* (a separate guidance, *In Safe Hands*, applies to Wales) details how this should happen.

- **Working in partnership with service users** – this encourages greater trust and empowerment of service users. In turn, they are likely to feel more confident in talking about their worries, fears and possible abuse. The equality that is part of partnership working should encourage the growth of self-esteem, self-confidence and the strength to no longer accept abusive situations and behaviour as the norm. It also ensures an agreed approach that all involved are aware of and can monitor. Protection is provided by the clarity of the situation.

- **Closer working between professionals and within organisations** – this enables better communication and information sharing to take place. This may take the form of discussions amongst staff, team meetings, communication via emails and the use of written records such as a daily logbook. In a care home, or similar 24-hour caring context, there may be three shifts of different staff providing continual care. A daily log enables staff coming on shift to be aware of what has happened since they were last on duty. This could be a couple of weeks ago if they have been on holiday or off sick. A sharing of concerns can result in early preventive action being taken. Patterns of behaviour can also be identified, for example, if a resident's behaviour seems to change when a particular member of staff is on duty or when a certain relative visits.

Decision-making processes and forums

If decision-making is kept transparent and clear, everyone understands what is happening. There is also less likelihood that a culture of 'secret keeping' will develop in which abuse could take place. The use of forums (for example, a monthly meeting of residents in a care home) encourages a sharing of ideas, the exchange of opinions and provides the opportunity for service users to gain confidence in speaking out. They also have greater ownership of the decisions that affect their

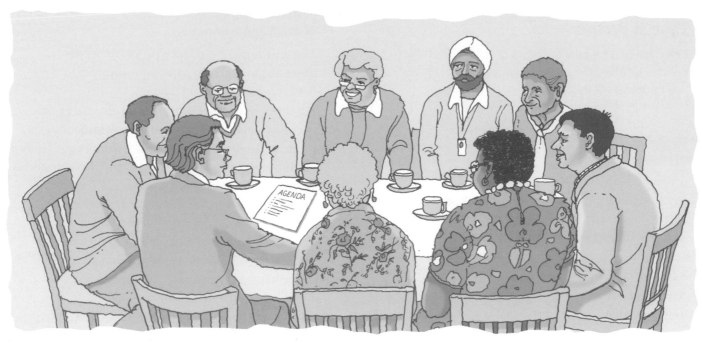

▲ Figure 11.6 Having the opportunity to speak out.

lives. This may include being involved in interviewing new care workers. It also provides the opportunity for procedures and guidelines to be explained, for rights to be emphasised and for service users to increase their expectations of the care they receive.

Organisational policies and training

Clear guidelines about expected behaviour from professionals are important, not only to guide the professionals, but also so that service users know what is acceptable and what is not. Complaints procedures need to be clearly understood and accessible to service users, together with independent support when making a complaint. This could take the form of an advocate from outside the organisation.

Training needs to be provided when new procedures and policies are put into place so that everyone understands what is required. New staff need a formal induction period during which all policies and procedures are explained.

Abuse is often the result of poor practice and a lack of understanding about the consequences of certain actions. Training is an important counter to this. The inclusion of role-play and service users talking about their experiences can give an insight into what it is like to be on the receiving end of care.

Reflect

If you were asked to take part in a training course for professionals (for example, for GPs, A&E nurses, dentists or doctor's receptionists) what improvements, based on your own experiences, would you recommend they make to the services you have received and the way in which they are delivered?

Working practices

The following are examples of good working practice which offer ways of minimising the risk of abuse.

Work practice	Purpose	Example
Needs assessment	Identifies service user's needs with their involvement and informs the care plan and professionals involved.	Josie is involved in identifying her needs and feels empowered by being included in the process rather than being ignored or marginalised.
Care planning cycle	A plan that sets out how needs are to be met, in detail, and by whom – all involved understand their responsibilities and the co-ordinator monitors its implementation and review.	Josie knows which professionals will be visiting her, and what they will be doing, and feels secure as she knows the co-ordinator will be checking that everything is working as planned.
Person-centred practices	The service user is central to the care process and services/professionals should be working to meet the person's needs – the individual should feel a partner in the process.	Josie feels her needs are being taken into account and she is part of a process that treats her with respect and dignity. She doesn't feel isolated or ignored – she is encouraged to speak out about her feelings.
Written and oral communications	Communication between services, professionals, service users and their families are clearly recorded so that everyone is aware of what is happening – the better the communication, the more those who are involved are kept informed.	By keeping up-to-date records, there is clarity in the process and individuals may check if they are unsure of what is happening – openness protects against abuse. Josie feels confident as all involved are kept fully informed.
Use of IT in sharing information between professionals	The rapid exchange of information between professionals is essential to ensure safe practice and a speedy reaction – early concerns over possible abuse can be investigated quickly.	A home visit by the district nurse finds Josie with a couple of bruises on her arm – she says it was an accident but this has happened once before following a visit from her son – other professionals can be quickly emailed and asked for their opinions/observations.
Anti-oppressive practice	Adopting the person-centred approach ensures the focus is on the needs of the service user and agencies or professionals are not forcing their ideas or agenda on the individual.	In the past, Josie had felt under pressure to move into a care home as it was a cheaper option to being provided with community-based care – an advocate argued against this as it was not in her best interests.
Anti-discriminatory practice	Services aim to meet the diverse needs of the individual and ensure they do not receive a lesser service than others who are in a similar position (which would be a form of abuse).	Whenever Josie sees her GP, she feels listened to and her pain is fully investigated – it is never dismissed as 'as you get older, you have to expect these things'.

Table 11.4 Good working practices.

Theory into practice

Using Table 11.4 as a guideline, what strategies would you introduce into a care home for people with physical disabilities, to minimise the possibility of abuse?

Procedures for protection

Each organisation involved in the delivery of care and the support of service users must have policies and procedures in place that will protect service users and investigate allegations of abuse.

All staff need to be aware of who to report any concerns to that they may have about possible abuse or poor practice. Depending on the size of the organisation, there may be a designated or named person who is likely to have received special training in dealing with any such concerns or complaints. In a small organisation, your line manager could well be the appropriate person although if the complaint relates to them, another manager would need to be involved.

Advocates, from an external body such as Age Concern or MIND, should be available to support service users with any complaint they may wish to make. The names and telephone numbers of advocates should be made easily and freely available, for example next to a public phone. This phone should be in a private zone to give the user some privacy. Service users should not feel they have to explain why they need to contact an advocate to members of staff first. It should be a confidential process.

From April 2007, the Independent Mental Capacity Advocates Service (IMCAS) has been available, under the Mental Capacity Act 2005. This aims to help vulnerable people who lack the capacity to make important decisions for themselves. The service focuses on such areas as health, welfare and finance. A new criminal offence of ill treatment or wilful neglect came into force at the same time, under the act.

While the rules of confidentiality normally apply, in situations where the service user, or others, are at risk of harm and abuse, confidentiality may be broken for their own protection. It is important that service users are aware of the circumstances when confidentiality is likely to be breached.

Reflect

At school, college and in the community, people are called names and are open to being abused if they are seen to 'grass', or tell, on someone. Young people grow up in a culture of not 'grassing'.

If you were working in a day centre and a person with learning disabilities told you that a member of staff had pushed them and helped themselves to their cigarettes, what would you do? If you told your line manager, would this be 'grassing'?

Care workers can find themselves in difficult situations when the service user confides in them about an abusive situation, on the understanding that it must be 'kept secret'. Organisations should have clear guidelines on such situations. It would be the role of the care worker to encourage the individual to allow disclosure so that appropriate action can be taken. This is more likely to happen where a trusting relationship has been developed. The fact that the individual has chosen to reveal such information is an indication that such a relationship exists.

While service users have the right to be protected, they also have the right to silence. Without their co-operation it will be difficult, if not impossible, to investigate suspected abuse. They may not wish to prosecute or have the case investigated because of fear, intimidation or misjudged loyalty to the abuser. They may not want to get involved because it is emotionally too painful or because they wish to put the memories behind them.

A study by Action on Elder Abuse in 2006, which looked into reported incidents of abuse, suggested that reporting of sexual abuse is lower that expected because of the shame and other negative feelings experienced by the victims. These feelings are similar to those experienced by rape victims but tend to be more so for older people. Why do you think this might be?

If abuse is suspected, it is important to follow the organisation's procedures to the letter. These should be clearly set out and the process should be overseen by the appropriate line manager or named person who is responsible for such investigations.

Information needs to be objective and carefully recorded. It could be used in a future disciplinary action against a member of staff and the correct procedures must be seen to have been followed. If a prosecution should follow, the records could be used as evidence in court.

The individual making the complaint or disclosure (revealing what happened) needs to write it up or have someone do it on his or her behalf. Great care needs to be taken at this stage, so that later accusations cannot be made about the complainant being 'led' into making certain statements by the type of questions being asked.

Legislation

The law exists to protect the individual. The vulnerable individual has the benefit of additional legislation and policies that apply to them specifically. This book's Appendix (see Resources and further reading) goes into this area in some depth and it is intended to provide a general overview of how protection is offered by the law.

The European Convention on Human Rights and Fundamental Freedoms 1950 and the Human Rights Act 1998 spelt out the basic rights of all humans, regardless of their condition or situation. This includes the right not to be abused and this is translated through various other acts. However, a 2007 House of Lords ruling on interpretation of the 1998 act has revealed that the rights of residents in private care homes are not protected in the same way as for those in local authority homes. For this to happen the contract between the home and the resident needs to include a clause requiring the home to observe the European Convention on Human Rights. It is thought that up to half of private homes include such a clause.

The anti-discrimination acts – Equal Pay Act, Sex Discrimination Act, Race Relations Act, Disability Discrimination Act and the Age Discrimination Act – all tackle abuse that occurs as a result of discrimination.

The Mental Health Act 1983 aims to balance the rights of the individual against the need to protect them and others because of their behaviour and illness. Their treatment, and restricted liberty, is under regular review to ensure it is appropriate and in the individual's best interests. This overview by professionals should also act as a deterrent against abuse taking place.

The Mental Health Act 1983 allows for the compulsory detention and treatment of people with mental illnesses such as schizophrenia. The illness can involve delusions of persecution – a belief that people are 'out to get you'.

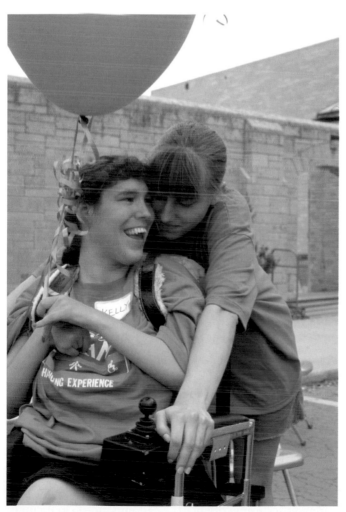

▲ The law exists to protect the individual.

In context

A patient, suffering from schizophrenia, has been detained in a psychiatric unit. He complains that a particular nurse is persecuting him – she takes cigarettes that are meant for him, has assaulted him and picks on him for no apparent reason. He says this has happened before. The nurse says she refused his request for a cigarette because he was drowsy from medication and in danger of burning himself. As a result, the patient became aggressive and she had to restrain him. She forgot to enter it in the appropriate log.

1   Do you investigate the allegation further or do you put it down as part of the patient's illness?

2   People with mental health problems or learning disabilities often find they are not believed when they have been assaulted. Why do you think that happens?

3   The police and the Crown Prosecution Service have, in the past, been reluctant to take up such cases because of the low success rates in court. Why do you think this happens?

The following legislation sets national standards for accommodation, services and good workplace practice in the care and protection of vulnerable people:

- The Nursing and Residential Care Homes Regulations 1984
- Care Standards Act 2000
- Care Homes for Older People: National Minimum Standards – Care Homes Regulations 2003

Part 7 of the Care Standards Act focuses on protection of vulnerable children and adults through screening care workers (it set up the POVA Scheme – see p. 100).

The Sexual Offences Act 1976 offers protection through the setting up of the Sex Offenders Register so that people can be identified and tracked, nationally. The same act protects those under the age of 16 from sexual abuse.

The NHS and Community Care Act 1990 places the service user at the centre of the care planning process. This empowers the individual, provides choice and sets standards of care by monitoring and reviewing needs that are being met. The more the service user is involved in decision making, the less isolated they become and the risk of abuse is reduced.

The Data Protection Act 1998 offers protection as it requires that personal details and information are kept secure and confidential.

The Special Educational Needs Act 2001 and Disability Act 2001 protect disabled students in further and higher education from being discriminated against because of their disability.

Policy documents such as *No Secrets* and *Speaking up for Justice* provide government guidance on the actual protection of vulnerable adults. *No Secrets* defines who is at risk and how this might be. It sets out a multi-agency framework, with the local social services authority having a lead role, to encourage greater working together and exchange of information between appropriate agencies. This can be achieved through the development of common policies, strategies and procedures, with each agency having a senior manager to lead the process.

Speaking up for Justice identifies the need to protect vulnerable adults when they appear as witnesses or the victims of abuse in the criminal justice system.

Theory into practice

If an investigation involves a vulnerable adult, as the alleged abuser, who should be present if the individual is to be questioned by the police, and why? (See *No Secrets* Section 6.21.)

Take it further

Research the policy and identify the steps that need to be followed by members of staff when investigating an allegation of abuse (see *No Secrets* Section 6.13).

Policies and procedures

In parliament, once a bill becomes an act, there is a need to implement it. The legislation sets out the legal requirements which need to be applied. How this is achieved is often set out in attached schedules, rules, regulations, directives or government guidelines. These explain the intentions of the act and suggest ways of carrying them out. These policies and procedures produce the strategies and working practice that aim to minimise abuse. The Mental Health Act, for example, included Mental Health Review Tribunal Rules. These set out the procedures for reviewing cases of individuals who had been compulsorily detained and who wished to appeal for discharge, or release.

As has been identified previously, the Care Standards Act 2000 Part 7 resulted in the establishment of the POVA Scheme. The associated Practical Guide for Placement of Adult Carers provided the detail of how this should be implemented.

Criminal Record Bureau (CRB) checks, under the 1997 Police Act, are now the norm for people who wish to work with vulnerable children and adults. This applies to anyone who is likely to come in contact with a vulnerable service user. A request for a standard (previous criminal offences) or an enhanced (to include other relevant information held by the police) disclosure or check is made before all new employees can take up their appointments. This applies to everyone including cooks, cleaners, teachers, care staff and managers. Once a check has been carried out, any previous criminal offences will be taken into account in terms of the risk the potential staff member may pose to the service users. A person with a recent record of theft, fraud or grievous bodily harm (GBH) is unlikely to be employed as a carer in a care home for vulnerable older people. However, if the theft was a minor, isolated incident which happened over 20 years ago, employment is more likely, depending on the organisation's policy towards previous offences.

All health and care employment opportunities are normally exempt from the Rehabilitation of Offenders Act 1974 and require the disclosure of previous offences. While 'enhanced disclosures' are valid for a period of three years, most employers prefer to have a new check carried out for each new employee, even though a current disclosure could be in force. This is because an offence could have taken place after the disclosure has been made.

The guidance in *No Secrets* identified the importance of having regional and local frameworks within which policies, strategies and procedures could be developed between agencies for the protection of vulnerable adults. These were along similar lines to those produced for child protection. It suggested a multi-agency management committee, which would oversee the development and implementation of such an approach, and set out procedures to be followed when investigating allegations of abuse. It also noted that abusers might be vulnerable adults who would need help, support and protection, in the form of an 'appropriate adult', throughout such an investigation.

Professional codes of practice require professionals to work to high standards, respect service users as individuals and minimise risk to them. Such codes are produced by the Nursing and Midwifery Council, the Department of Health (the Mental Health for Social Workers code of practice) and the British Association of Social Workers.

Theory into practice

Research two out of the three previously mentioned codes of practice and identify practices that are aimed at protecting vulnerable adults.

Assessment activity 11.4

P5 Describe strategies and working practices used to minimise abuse.

1   You work for a charity that is planning to open its first residential unit for people with learning disabilities. The aim is to prepare people for living independently in their own flats. Support workers will be employed to help residents develop the appropriate life skills, for example, cooking, budgeting, personal hygiene, leisure activities, etc.

Identify the various strategies, for example, POVA scheme and working practices (such as needs assessment) you need to put in place prior to opening the unit. Provide a summarised description of how they will be used to minimise the possibility of abuse.

Grading tip for P5

Demonstrate your understanding by taking an overview of appropriate strategies and working practices and describe the main points. Use examples based on your own work experience, or the various case studies used throughout the unit, to show your understanding and ability to apply it.

P6 Identify the legislation, policies and procedures that protect adults receiving health and social care services.

2   You are in charge of a charity that runs a small care home for people with mental health problems. The charity's work is overseen by a committee of volunteers. A new member has been elected to the committee and is meeting with you to find out more about the care home and how it is run. Produce a table that identifies legislation, policies and procedures that protect health and care service users at the centre. Briefly explain what each covers.   **P6**

Grading tip for P6

Focus on a generic approach of identifying and briefly explaining each policy, procedure and piece of legislation. (How each works comes under M3.)

M3 Explain how legislation, policies and procedures contribute to the protection of vulnerable adults.

3   Having identified the legislation, policies and procedures, you need to explain to the committee member how these contribute to the protection of the people living in the care home.   **M3**

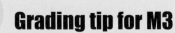

Grading tip for M3

Make sure you focus on *how* legislation, policies and procedures contribute to the protection of the people living in the care home. Use examples, based on your own experience, or from previous case studies, to demonstrate your understanding.

John lives in a supported house, run by a charity, for people with learning disabilities. He attends college for three days a week and a day centre for two days. He has a good relationship with a volunteer who visits him at weekends and takes him for trips.

A friend from college has started to turn up at the day centre and at home. John seems reluctant to see him at times but will not say why. He has started to spend more money than usual on CDs and electronic gadgets that he then gives to his friend as gifts, but is not his normal, cheerful self. The volunteer feels John is being taken advantage of and that financial and verbal abuse (threats) could be taking place.

D2 Analyse the role of multi-agency working in minimising the risks of abuse in health and social care contexts.

4   Analyse how multi-agency working could investigate and minimise the suspected abuse.   **D2**

Grading tip for D2

You need to first identify the agencies and individuals involved and then analyse how they could work together to minimise the suspected abuse. You also need to consider that John may not want to be involved in the process.

Remember!

Vulnerable adults, who do not wish to make a complaint, or be involved in an allegation of abuse, have the right of refusal. If they have an advocate, that person might decide it is not in the individual's best interests to pursue the matter, because of the trauma involved.

Knowledge check

Martin is 25 and lived with his father who recently died. He has a mild learning disability and is able to look after himself, with a little support. He has decided to stay in the family home and social services have assessed him as needing 10 hours a week social support. This will involve helping him with his shopping, budgeting, cooking and reminding him about such things as laundry, cleaning, etc. You have been appointed as his support worker.

1 Helping, enabling and empowering are important elements in developing a supportive professional relationship. How would you use them in developing a relationship with Martin?

2 What are the differences between a friendship and a supportive professional relationship?

3 Name four behaviours that service users, living in a care home, have the right to expect from professional workers.

4 In your own words, explain what is meant by the term 'vulnerable person'.

5 Give examples of physical abuse that might be experienced by adults receiving medical care.

6 Give examples of psychological abuse that could be experienced by a person receiving help in their own home.

7 Explain why an abused adult might self-harm.

8 What indicators of physical abuse should you be alert for?

9 Why might people with learning disabilities, who live independently in the community, be more vulnerable to abuse than others? Give examples of possible abuse.

10 What are the factors that increase the potential for abuse? Give examples.

11 In what way does the Protection of Vulnerable Adults Scheme (POVA) offer a way of minimising the likelihood of abuse?

12 What are the benefits for service users of 'multi-agency working'?

13 In what way can training for both staff and service users help tackle abuse?

14 Give a brief overview of the guidance offered in the policy document No Secrets.

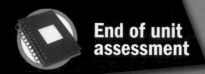
Preparation for assessment

Jane is 21 and led a busy life until 12 months ago when the car she was travelling in overturned and hit a wall.

After spending three months in hospital recovering from her injuries, and a further month on a rehabilitation ward, she was discharged home to her one-bedroom flat. She was paralysed from the waist down and became a wheel chair user. Her flat has been adapted so she can look after herself – widened doorways, lowered work tops, entry ramps and 'roll in' shower room – with the daily support of a care worker to help with personal hygiene and shopping.

Within two months of returning home, she became very depressed about her restricted lifestyle and was admitted to a psychiatric unit for treatment of her depression. This involved medication initially and then counselling to help her come to terms with her loss and change in lifestyle. She was an inpatient for one month before returning home, with her medication balanced. She now attends a day centre, run by MIND for people who are recovering from mental ill health. She still receives counselling once a week and home support daily.

There have been some concerns expressed that she is vulnerable to possible abuse because of her current mental frailty and tendency to become involved with anyone who shows her some interest. She also tends to buy friendship by being over generous with the large amount of money she received in compensation after the accident.

1   Explain how Jane's individual rights have been, and will continue to be, respected in the various supportive relationships she has been in over the last two years (nurses, rehabilitation workers, home support staff, mental health workers in hospital and at the day centre). **P1**

2   Explain the ways that these relationships have enhanced her life experience and evaluate their benefits. **M1**, **D1**

3   To guard against possible abuse, it is important to carry out a risk assessment of her home and day centre as potential arenas for abuse from care workers. Identify the different forms of abuse that could take place, and describe the signs or indicators that need to be looked for. **P2**, **P3**

4   Describe and analyse the potential for abuse in four of the settings, or contexts, she has been in. **P4**, **M2**

5   Describe strategies and working practices that could be used to minimise the likelihood of abuse taking place. **P5**

6   Identify the legislation, policies and procedures that are there to protect Jane and explain how they work. **P6**, **M3**

7   Analyse how a multi-agency approach to minimising abuse could continue to minimise the potential for abuse in Jane's case. **D2**

Resources and further reading

See this book's Legislation Appendix at www.harcourt.co.uk/btechsc

Brown, K. (ed) (2006) *Vulnerable Adults and Community Care* Exeter: Learning Matters

Crawford, K., Walker, J. (2004) *Social Work with Older People* Exeter: Learning Matters

Criminal Justice Performance, Justice, Victims & Witnesses Unit (2003) *Speaking up for Justice* Home Office

Department of Health and Home Office (2000) *No Secrets: Guidance on Developing and Implementing Multi-agency Policies and Procedures to Protect Vulnerable Adults from Abuse*

Fisher, A. (2006) *OCR National Level 3 Health, Social Care & Early Years* Oxford: Heinemann

Fisher, A. et al (2006) *Applied AS Health and Social Care* Dunstable: Folens

Johns, R. (2005) *Using the Law in Social Work,* second edn. Exeter: Learning Matters

Moonie, N. (ed) (2005) *GCE AS Level Health & Social Care* Oxford: Heinemann

Pritchard, J. (ed) (2001) *Good Practice with Vulnerable Adults* London: Kingsley

Criminal Justice Performance, Justice, Victims & Witnesses Unit (2003) *Speaking up for Justice* Home Office

Useful websites

Action on Elder Abuse
www.elderabuse.org

Age Concern
www.ageconcern.org.uk

Better Government for Older People
www.bgop.org.uk

British Association of Social Workers
www.basw.co.uk

Commission for Social Care Inspection
www.csci.gov

Department of Health
www.doh.gov.uk

Department of Health social care bulletin
www.careandhealth.co.uk

General Medical Council
www.gmc-uk.org

Home Office
www.homeoffice.gov.uk

Information on the Court of Protection
www.lcd.gov.uk/family/mi

International Network for the Prevention of Elder Abuse
www.inpea.net

Legislation and explanatory notes
www.legislation.hmso.gov.uk/acts

Legislation and policies
www.direct.gov.uk

MIND
www.mind.org.uk

The NHS Plan
www.nhsia.nhs/uk/nhsplan/summary.htm

Nursing and Midwifery Council
www.nmc-uk.org

Office of Public Sector Information
www.opsi.gov

Valuing People White Paper
www.valuing people.gov.uk

GRADING CRITERIA

To achieve a pass grade the evidence must show that the learner is able to:	To achieve a merit grade the evidence must show that, in addition to the pass criteria, the learner is able to:	To achieve a distinction grade the evidence must show that, in addition to the pass and merit criteria, the learner is able to:
P1 explain how individual rights can be respected in a supportive relationship **Assessment activity 11.1 page 89**	**M1** explain how supportive relationships can enhance the life experiences of individuals receiving health and social care services **Assessment activity 11.1 page 90**	**D1** use examples to evaluate the role of supportive relationships in enhancing the life experiences of individuals receiving health and social care services **Assessment activity 11.1 page 90**
P2 describe different forms of abuse that may be experienced by vulnerable adults **Assessment activity 11.2 page 96**		
P3 describe different indicators of abuse in vulnerable adults **Assessment activity 11.2 page 96**		
P4 describe the potential for abuse in health and social care contexts **Assessment activity 11.3 page 99**	**M2** analyse the potential for abuse in four health and social care contexts **Assessment activity 11.3 page 99**	
P5 describe strategies and working practices used to minimise abuse **Assessment activity 11.4 page 107**		
P6 identify the legislation, policies and procedures that protect adults receiving health and social care services. **Assessment activity 11.4 page 108**	**M3** explain how legislation, policies and procedures contribute to the protection of vulnerable adults. **Assessment activity 11.4 page 108**	**D2** analyse the role of multi-agency working in minimising the risks of abuse in health and social care contexts. **Assessment activity 11.4 page 108**

12 Public health

Introduction

Public health is concerned with improving the health of the population, as opposed to treating the diseases of individual patients. Public health professionals work in partnership with many other agencies to monitor the health status of the community, identify health needs, develop programmes to reduce risk, screen for early disease, control communicable disease, foster policies which promote health, plan and evaluate the provision of health care and manage and implement change.

This unit aims to develop your understanding of the role of public health systems, their origin and development and the range of key groups in influencing public health policy. You will also identify current patterns in ill health and consider factors which contribute to those patterns. The unit closes by looking at the different methods of promoting and protecting public health in terms of health education, health protection and environmental measures. You will find more about the principles and practice of health education in Unit 20: *Health education*.

How you will be assessed

This unit will be internally assessed by your tutor. A variety of exercises and activities has been provided to help you understand all aspects of public health and prepare for the assessment. You will also have the opportunity to work on some case studies to further your understanding.

After completing this unit you should be able to achieve the following outcomes:

- Understand public health strategies in the UK and their origins
- Understand patterns of ill health and factors affecting health in the UK
- Understand methods of promoting and protecting public health.

Thinking points

If you were asked to name the most important medical advance in the past 150 years, what would you suggest?

If the biggest threats to public health in the nineteenth century were communicable diseases such as cholera and typhoid, what do you think might be the biggest threats today?

Think about the issues which are covered in print and broadcast media everyday. What do you see as possible future threats to the health of the UK?

If public health is about safeguarding the population's health, how does this differ from promoting the health of individuals (discussed in Unit 20: *Health education*)?

Key aspects of public health

The official definition of public health is 'the science and art of preventing disease, prolonging life, and promoting health through the organised efforts of society'.

This definition, coined in 1988 in a report by Sir Donald Acheson (*Public Health in England*), reflects the essential focus of modern public health – an emphasis on collective responsibility for health and on prevention.

It relies on a multi-disciplinary approach which emphasises partnership with the people who are being served. The table below sets out key aspects of public health practice in more detail with examples:

Key terms

Obesity A Body Mass Index in excess of 30 (BMI is explained on p. 132).

Role	Explanation	Example
• **Monitoring the health status of the population**	Tracking changes in the health of the population and alerting people to potential problems.	For example, the rising levels of **obesity** within the population.
• **Identifying the health needs of the population**	Once trends and patterns are established, the likely implications for services can be identified.	In relation to obesity, this means assessing the likely increase in the need for diabetes support services.
• **Developing programmes to reduce risk and screen for disease early on**	Attempting to reduce the levels of ill health by introducing new programmes which identify people as being 'at risk' of a condition and engaging them with preventative programmes.	For example, a doctor identifying that someone is at risk of developing diabetes because of their obesity and referring them to a weight management programme for support to lose weight.
• **Controlling communicable disease**	Reducing the impact of infectious diseases through immunisation and other control measures.	While there are obvious examples such as measles, mumps and rubella, this might also include food hygiene measures in restaurants and takeaways to control the spread of food poisoning.
• **Promoting the health of the population**	Health-promoting activities to reduce ill health in the population.	For example, for **obesity**, this might include campaigns which encourage people to be more active or eat more fruit and vegetables.
• **Planning and evaluating the provision of health and social care**	Assessing the provision of relevant health services and whether or not they are having sufficient impact on the problem.	In the case of obesity this might include assessing whether or not: • local services can meet the demand for weight management advice • there is sufficient 'capacity', i.e. service provision to meet the rising demand for obesity-related services • the existing model of services is managing to help people to reduce their weight and sustain that change.

Table 12.1 The key roles within public health practice.

Sources of information for studying patterns of ill health

The study of **epidemiology** is the study of diseases in human populations. It is particularly important in helping us to understand the spread of infectious diseases and how they can lead to epidemics. It attempts to understand the factors that influence the number of cases of a disease at any one time, its distribution and how to control it. This most clearly applies to infectious diseases such as influenza or HIV but is equally applicable to the diseases of the Western world such as coronary heart disease and cancer. Epidemiological data is essential for identifying what health problems are occurring in a population and targeting the relevant health promotion activity to address those problems. Ill health data, i.e. that which deals with illness and death, is routinely collected and interpreted by a range of organisations including:

- **World Health Organisation** which collects information about national and international health and can make comparisons between countries
- **the government** which collects information to inform policies, for example, information about substance use can inform national drugs policy, as information about rising rates of obesity can influence policy on nutrition
- **regional statistics and reports** – this is a key role for public health observatories which produce regional information about aspects of population health
- **local reports and statistics** – we will see later how the report from the local director of public health should inform local health planning
- **epidemiological studies** – occasionally specific studies are necessary to highlight topics, for example, trends in cancers were highlighted in the Cancer Atlas published by the **National Statistics Office** in 2005
- **Public health observatories** whose role is to provide regional data about health for local planners to use. For example, profiles of alcohol-related harm which compare local authority areas against national rates can be found on the North West Observatory site
- **Health Protection Agency** which routinely produces

reports about communicable disease rates and reports which focus on specific outbreaks or events.

Key terms

Epidemiology The study of diseases in human populations.

World Health Organisation (WHO) Established on 7 April 1948, in response to an international desire for a world free from disease, and since then 7 April has been celebrated each year as World Health Day.

National Statistics Office (NSO) The national body which compiles information on the UK population and which is responsible for carrying out the census every 10 years.

Health Protection Agency (HPA) An independent organisation dedicated to protecting people's health in the UK.

One example of information which can be collected and used at all these levels is demographic data or information about the population. For example, the numbers of people by age band 0–4, 5–9, 10–14, etc., numbers from minority ethnic communities, etc. This is important information which helps people to plan services. For example, one current challenge is to deal with an ageing population.

Historical perspectives of the public health system

Public health, as we know it today, originated from the nineteenth century Poor Law system and the Victorian sanitary reform movement. The Poor Law ensured that the poor were housed in workhouses, clothed and fed. Children who entered the workhouse would receive some schooling. In return for this care, all workhouse paupers would have to work for several hours a day.

Industrialisation and the rapid growth of cities during this period led to concerns about environmental problems such as poor housing, unclean water supplies, 'bad air' and the impact that these had on the health of the working population.

■ The first national Public Health Act 1848

Edwin Chadwick was an active campaigner on a number of public health issues including poor housing and working conditions and sanitary reform. Chadwick's *Report on an inquiry into the sanitary conditions of the labouring population of Great Britain, 1842* contained a mass of evidence supporting the relationship between environmental factors, poverty and ill health. It recommended the establishment of a single local authority, supported by expert medical and civil engineering advice, to administer all sanitary matters. Six years later, the national Public Health Act was passed and the first Board of Health was established.

■ John Snow and the Broad Street pump

In 1854, John Snow was interested in the role of drinking water in the spread of cholera and had observed that people who had drunk water provided by one water company were more likely to contract the disease than those who had not. By plotting the cases of cholera on a map, Snow was able to establish that all those falling ill were getting their water from a single pump, which drew its supplies from the sewage-contaminated River Thames. People using nearby wells to obtain their water had escaped infection. The connection between cholera and contaminated water was therefore established, before bacteriology was able to identify the causative organism.

Having identified the source of the infection as polluted water, he went on to remove the handle of the Broad Street water pump and halted the outbreak of cholera in Soho, London.

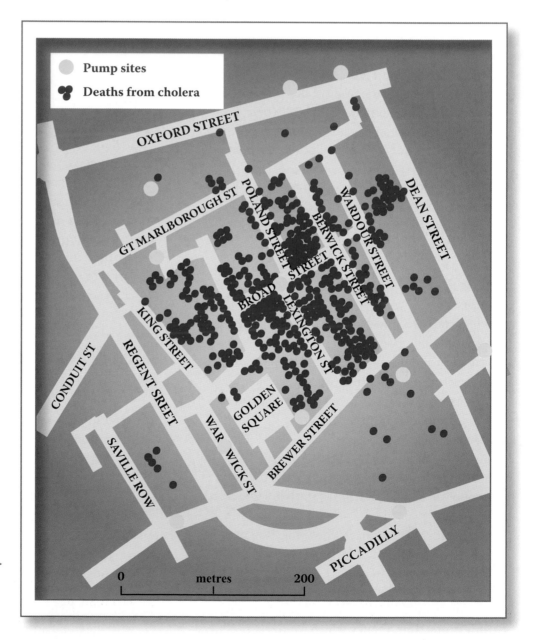

Figure 12.1 Snow's map showed the cholera cases plotted around the Broad Street pump.

John Simon and the 1866 Sanitary Act

John Simon was the third 'founding father' of public health. He succeeded Edwin Chadwick in his role in public health administration. John Simon was a physician by profession and became medical officer to the Board of Health in 1855. Advised by a team of scientists and engineers, Simon was instrumental in helping a number of towns to install their first sewage systems throughout the 1850s and 1860s. In 1866 the Sanitary Act placed a duty of inspection on local authorities and extended their range of sanitary powers.

Even today the work of these three public health campaigners is held in the highest regard. In a recent poll by the *British Medical Journal* (January 2007) sanitation, and the efforts of Snow and Chadwick in particular, were rated the greatest medical advances of the last 150 years.

The twentieth century

The Beveridge Report, 1942

Following the Second World War there was a strong feeling that the British people should be rewarded for their sacrifice and resolution. The government promised reforms that would create a more equal society, asking Sir William Beveridge to write a report on the best ways of helping people on low incomes. In December 1942, Beveridge published a report that proposed that all people of working age should pay a weekly contribution. In return, benefits would be paid to people who were sick, unemployed, retired or widowed.

The National Health Service (NHS)

In the aftermath of the Second World War, Clement Attlee's Labour government created the NHS, based on the proposals of the Beveridge Report. A white paper was published in 1943 which was followed by considerable debate with resistance organised by the **British Medical Association (BMA)**. The structure of the NHS in England and Wales was established by the National Health Service Act 1946 and the new arrangements were launched on 5 July 1948. This was under health and

Key terms

British Medical Association (BMA) This is the professional body for the medical profession. It represents their interests at a national level, for example in negotiations with the government over changes in management of the medical profession.

housing minister Aneurin Bevan. Contrary to popular belief, the founding principles of the NHS called for its funding out of general taxation, not through national insurance. Services in the NHS were provided by the same doctors and the same hospitals but:

- services were provided free at the point of use
- services were financed from central taxation
- everyone was eligible for care (even people temporarily resident or visiting the country).

The original structure of the NHS had three arms:

1 **hospital services**
2 **primary care** (i.e. family doctor services)
3 **community services** such as maternity and child welfare clinics, health visitors, midwives, health education, vaccination and immunisation and ambulance services.

Acheson Report into inequalities in health, 1998

In July 1997, Donald Acheson was invited by the Secretary of State for Health to review and summarise inequalities in health in England and to identify priority areas for the development of policies to reduce them. This followed in the wake of two famous reports in this field that had been carried out earlier – the report of Sir Douglas Black in 1977 and the updated version from 1987, *The Health Divide*. Both these reports were kept quiet to some degree at the time of their release because of the bleak picture of widening health inequality in such a developed country and the implications for the government of the day.

Donald Acheson concluded his report with a list of 39 recommendations for addressing health inequality, 'judged on the scale of their potential impact on health inequalities and the weight of evidence'. The three areas identified as crucial to this process are:

- All policies likely to have an impact on health should be evaluated in terms of their impact on health inequality.
- A high priority should be given to the health of families with children.
- Further steps should be taken to reduce income inequalities and improve the living standards of poor households.

In context

John is the estates officer for a local Primary Care Trust (PCT). His role is to manage the construction of new buildings. The PCT has agreed to construct a new health centre in the middle of the most deprived estate in the district. On paper this seems like an excellent opportunity for the PCT to improve the health of this community. However, John has been asked to carry out a simple health impact assessment to help the PCT senior managers consider what the likely changes are that the new building might bring. When you answer the questions below, don't just think of this in terms of health care provision. What about the impact on local employment, the environment, crime and other aspects of local life?

1 What improvements might a health centre bring for the locality?

2 What problems might it create for people who live nearby?

3 What measures would you suggest to overcome these potential problems?

■ *Saving Lives: Our Healthier Nation, 1999*

This was the health strategy released by the Labour government shortly after it came to power in 1997. It made clear links to the Acheson Report, proposing to tackle the root causes of ill health including air pollution, unemployment, low wages, crime and disorder and poor housing. It focuses on prevention of the main killers which include cancer, coronary heart disease and stroke, accidents and mental illness. It also includes a wide range of service providers such as local councils, the NHS and local voluntary bodies and businesses. Included within the strategy were specific health targets in key disease areas:

- cancer – to reduce the death rate in under-75s by at least 20 per cent
- coronary heart disease and stroke – to reduce the death rate in under-75s by at least 40 per cent
- accidents – to reduce the death rate by at least 20 per cent and serious injury by at least 10 per cent
- mental illness – to reduce the death rate from suicide and undetermined injury by at least 20 per cent.

Twenty-first century

■ The public health White Paper – *Choosing Health: Making Healthy Choices Easier*, 2004

The White Paper of 2004 recognised that interest in health was increasing and recommended a new approach to public health reflecting the rapidly changing and increasingly technological society we live in. The document acknowledged the role for government in promoting social justice and tackling the wider causes of ill health and inequality as well as recognising the need to support and empower individuals to make changes in their own lives.

The strategy set out in the document had three underpinning principles:

1 informed choice: although with two important qualifications:
   - protect children and
   - do not allow one person's choice to adversely affect another, for example passive smoking
2 personalisation: support tailored to the needs of individuals
3 working together: real progress depends on effective partnerships across communities.

Its main priorities were to:
- reduce the number of people who smoke

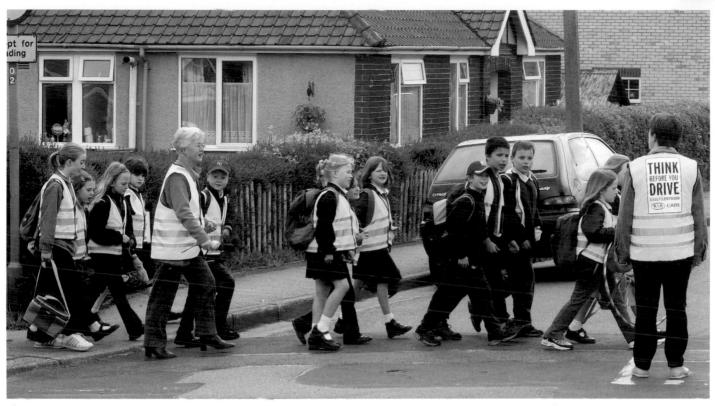

▲ By 2010, all schools in England should have active travel plans.

- reduce obesity and improve diet and nutrition
- increase exercise
- encourage and support sensible drinking
- improve sexual health
- improve mental health.

The public health paper set out the following areas for action:

- **Children and young people** – by 2010, all schools in England should have active travel plans.
- **Communities leading for health** – local authorities, working with the national transport charity Sustrans, are to build over 7000 miles of new cycle lanes and tracks.
- **Health as a way of life** – NHS health trainers will help people to make healthy choices and stick to them. This will be a new kind of personal health resource.
- **A health-promoting NHS** – all NHS staff will be trained to help them deliver key health messages effectively as part of their day-to-day work with patients.

- **Work and health** – the NHS will become a model employer.

Take it further

Look at the difference between the types of actions in the most recent public health white paper *Choosing Health* and *Our Healthier Nation* (OHN). *Choosing Health* is built around programmes of work as opposed to disease reduction targets.

- Which type of targets are more meaningful for the public and why?
- Both documents include actions which may take many years to produce improvements in health. Do you think it likely that the same government will be in power at the end of the ten-year time span set for achieving the targets?
- How does this influence campaigning at election times when the health agenda tends to focus on ill health services?

Your tutor has asked you to present a report which outlines both what current public health practice looks like today and how this has evolved from its early roots in the late nineteenth and early twentieth centuries.

P1 Describe key aspects of public health practice in the UK.

1   What are the key aspects of public health practice in the UK? How might each aspect of the public health approach be applied to reducing the rising rates of the sexually transmitted infection syphilis?   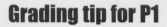 **P1**

Grading tip for P1

The task requires you to describe the key aspects of practice, i.e. you don't need to cover everything but you do need to identify the most important aspects of practice.

P2 Describe the origins of public health in the UK.

2   Who are the three key founding fathers of public health practice and what was their contribution to the development of modern-day public health practice?

3   What are the main policy documents from the twentieth century which have framed current public health practice?

4   Draw up a timeline showing the key dates for the evolution of modern day public health practice starting in 1840.   **P2**

Grading tip for P2

This question asks you to focus on the origins so it is not asking you to list everything that has contributed, i.e. to simply restate the contents of your timeline, but it is asking you to focus on the early developments on which current practice is based.

■ The Health Protection Agency (HPA)

The Health Protection Agency is an independent organisation dedicated to protecting people's health in the UK. It does this by providing impartial advice and authoritative information on **health protection** issues to the public, professionals and the government. It combines public health and scientific expertise, research and emergency planning within one organisation. It works at international, national, regional and local levels and has links with many other organisations around the world.

Key terms

Health protection The measures taken to safeguard a population's health, for example, through legislation, financial or social means. This might include legislation to govern health and safety at work, or food hygiene, and using taxation policy to reduce smoking levels or car use by raising the price of cigarettes or petrol.

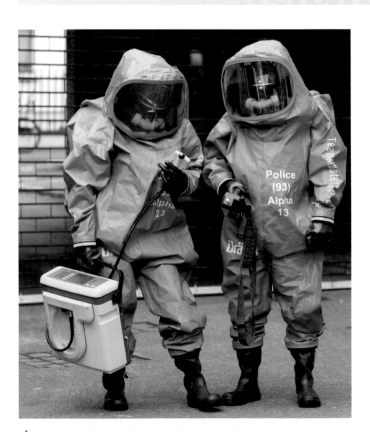

▲ The role of the HPA is to prevent and reduce the impact of infectious diseases, chemical and radiation hazards and major emergencies.

The role of the HPA includes:

- providing impartial expert advice on health protection and providing specialist health protection services
- identifying and responding to health hazards and emergencies caused by infectious disease, hazardous chemicals, poisons or radiation
- anticipating and preparing for emerging or future threats
- supporting and advising other organisations with a health protection role
- improving knowledge about health protection through research and development, education and training.

In context

Ahmed is a public health nurse from the local health protection unit. His role is mainly involved with identifying and understanding local outbreaks of infectious diseases, specifically those which are termed 'notifiable', i.e. they have to be reported to the relevant authorities because they are important to control (for example salmonella, tuberculosis and other diseases which you will read more about later in this section). In each case he visits the patients infected by the disease and takes a detailed case history to understand what might have led to them being infected and who else might have caught the disease. If there are several cases of one type of disease then this might be identified as an 'outbreak'. In this case, a team of people drawn from the PCT public health department, the HPA and the local environmental health department might be convened to manage the outbreak, identify the source and control its spread.

1 **Have you seen or heard about local outbreaks of infectious diseases?**

2 **How are they usually reported in the media?**

3 **What problems might this present for Ahmed if he is dealing with an outbreak of a potentially fatal disease such as meningitis?**

■ The National Institute for Health and Clinical Excellence (NICE)

NICE is the independent organisation responsible for providing national guidance on the promotion of good health and the prevention and treatment of ill health. The Department of Health commissions NICE to develop guidance to inform practice in:

- public health – the promotion of good health and the prevention of ill health for those working in the NHS, local authorities and the wider public and **voluntary sector**
- health technologies – the use of new and existing medicines, treatments and procedures within the NHS
- clinical practice – the appropriate treatment and care of people with specific diseases and conditions within the NHS.

Key terms

National Institute for Health and Clinical Excellence (NICE) The independent organisation responsible for providing national guidance on the promotion of good health and the prevention and treatment of ill health.

Voluntary sector Agencies which obtain their funding from charitable giving, specific funding from public sector organisations such as PCTs or through the National Lottery.

Target setting

National and international targets for health

The European Observatory for Health describes health targets as follows:

Health targets express a commitment to achieve a specified outcome in a defined time period and enable monitoring of progress towards the achievement of broader goals and objectives. They may be quantitative (for example the immunisation rate) or qualitative (for example the introduction of a national screening programme).

International targets for health don't fall easily into this model because to set a SMART (see Unit 20) target would require all the countries involved to agree to a single course of action and often this is not possible. Therefore international targets are more usually loosely framed as goals or frameworks which describe broad objectives or common approaches. A good example would be the UN Millennium Declaration, agreed in September 2000. The declaration, endorsed by 189 countries, set out goals to be reached by 2015. The eight Millennium Development Goals represent commitments to reduce poverty and hunger and to tackle ill health, gender inequality, lack of education, lack of access to clean water and environmental degradation.

Theory into practice

More detailed information can be found about the millennium goals and the convention on tobacco control on the Internet. What specific targets underpin the broad goals outlined in the Millennium Development Goals? What actions does the framework commit signatories such as the UK to undertake?

It is perhaps surprising that, until quite recently, this country had few targets for improving health. In fact it wasn't until the 1992 White Paper *The Health of the Nation* that the UK had a first-ever health (as opposed to health services) strategy. It set for the first time 27 specific targets within five key areas:

- coronary heart disease (CHD) and stroke
- cancers (breast, lung, cervical and skin cancers)
- mental Illness
- HIV/AIDS and sexual health
- accidents.

These areas were selected because they were major causes of premature death or avoidable ill health, as they are today. This fact provides the health policy of following administrations with consistency, as we can see in the targets in *Saving Lives: Our Healthier Nation*.

Regional/local targets for health

Local health strategy should be driven by the annual report of the local primary care trusts' director of public health. This provides a summary of local health trends and makes key recommendations about future local policy to improve health.

Theory into practice

Find your local director of public health's (DPH) most recent annual public health report. It is a public document which should inform your local community about the health problems it faces. This is likely to be available on the PCT website.

What does it identify as local priorities for improving public health? What recommendations does it make? This report is not a report of the PCT but of the DPH in their role as public health advocate – find out what is meant by 'public health advocate'.

The PCT's main business is to invest in treatment services such as those provided by local hospitals but the DPH's role might be to encourage greater investment in more preventative activity – which might mean in services outside the NHS. Can you foresee any situations where the view of the DPH and the PCT might be at odds? What tensions might this bring for the DPH in writing and agreeing their report?

Local health targets to improve health are likely to be found in many planning documents, for example, the Local Development Plan of the PCT which might include investment in health promotion programmes or improving local services.

Targets can also be found in the Local Area Agreement (LAA) – a partnership plan with high-level targets which might include reducing teenage conceptions, poverty, alcohol-related harm and a wide range of other potentially health-promoting initiatives.

An example of a local target from the Lancashire LAA includes:

- Reduce health inequalities across Lancashire by improving lifestyles and addressing the wider determinants of health by:
  - halting the year-on-year rise in obesity in children under 11 by 2010
  - reducing smoking prevalence across Lancashire
  - reducing the percentage of retailers who sell tobacco to under-age young people as measured by test purchases.

Key groups in influencing public health policy

Pressure groups

Pressure groups are collections of individuals who hold a similar set of values and beliefs based on ethnicity, religion, political philosophy or a common goal. Based on these beliefs, they take action to promote change and further their goals. Pressure groups often represent the viewpoints of people who are dissatisfied with the current conditions in society and which are not well represented in the mainstream population. By forming a pressure group, people seek to express their shared beliefs and values and influence change. The roles of some major pressure groups are outlined below.

■ Greenpeace

Greenpeace is a non-profit organisation with a presence in 40 countries across Europe, the Americas, Asia and the Pacific. Greenpeace relies on contributions from individual supporters and foundation grants to maintain its activities and in this way ensures its independence from government. Greenpeace has been campaigning against environmental degradation since 1971 when a small boat of volunteers and journalists sailed into Amchitka, an area north of Alaska, where the US government was conducting underground nuclear tests. As a global organisation, Greenpeace focuses on the most crucial worldwide threats to the planet's biodiversity and environment. It campaigns to:

- stop climate change
- protect ancient forests
- save the oceans
- stop whaling
- stop genetic engineering
- stop the nuclear threat
- eliminate toxic chemicals
- encourage sustainable trade.

■ Friends of the Earth

Friends of the Earth is another environmental pressure group which seeks to influence policy and practice. Their work is underpinned by three beliefs:

1 There is a need to look after our planet, i.e. to live within the limits of the natural world, which means polluting and using less.

2 People's needs should be met but, at the same time, the environment must be kept safe both now and in the future. This is termed 'environmental justice' – implying that everyone has a fair share of the earth's resources.

3 Realistic alternatives are possible and countries' economies should only grow and develop using ways that focus on quality of life and protection of the planet.

Friends of the Earth operate campaigns in a range of areas including:

- fighting climate change
- challenging the influence of the global free trade system
- exposing poor business practice
- working towards greener farming and seeking a ban on genetically modified (GM) food
- campaigning for increased recycling
- working to reduce the impact on the environment of the movement of people and goods
- campaigning to protect the world's wildlife habitats.

International agencies

Organisations operating at this level include a range of charities such as Christian Aid, Oxfam and Save the Children, as well as pressure groups such as Greenpeace and key statutory organisations like the United Nations, European Commission, World Health Organisation and UNICEF.

The World Health Organisation

In 1945, meeting in San Francisco, the United Nations Conference on International Organisations unanimously approved a proposal by Brazil and China to establish a new and autonomous international health organisation. In 1946, at a meeting in New York, the International Health Conference approved its constitution, and finally the WHO came into being on 7 April 1948. The WHO's constitution defines it as 'a directing and co-ordinating authority on international health work,' its aim being 'the attainment by all peoples of the highest possible level of health'. The following are listed among its responsibilities:

- strengthening health services
- information, advice and assistance in the field of health
- improved nutrition, housing, sanitation, working conditions and other aspects of environmental hygiene
- international conventions and agreements on health matters
- research in the field of health
- international standards for food, biological and pharmaceutical products.

The United Nations (UN)

The United Nations is central to global efforts to solve problems that challenge humanity. Co-operating in this effort are more than 30 affiliated organisations, known together as the UN system. The UN and its family of organisations work constantly to promote respect for human rights, protect the environment, fight disease and reduce poverty. UN agencies define the standards for safe and efficient air travel and help improve telecommunications and enhance consumer protection. The UN leads the international campaigns against drug trafficking and terrorism. Throughout the world, the UN and its agencies assist refugees, set up programmes to clear landmines, help expand food production and lead the fight against AIDS.

Health Protection Agency

We have already heard about the role the HPA plays in the UK in managing communicable disease and preparing for emergency situations. Here are a few of the areas where the HPA provided national information and guidance in 2005/6, to illustrate their role in determining national policy:

- the first report on the burden of hepatitis C in the UK which estimated that 4500 people in the UK were living with severe liver disease
- the annual report on HIV and sexually transmitted infections published by the HPA showed that 58,300 people were living with HIV in the UK
- the HPA reported an increase in cases of listeria over the past five years which showed that the trend was continuing
- the publication of guidance on spa pools, advising commercial and domestic owners about the risks of infections if they are not maintained properly.

NICE

NICE guidance provides recommendations on the promotion of good health and the prevention of ill health. The guidance is for people working in the NHS, local authorities and the wider public, and private and voluntary sectors.

There are two types of NIHCE public health guidance:

1 public health intervention guidance – this provides recommendations on clear types of activity ('interventions') that are provided by local organisations and which help to reduce people's risk of developing a disease or condition, or help to promote or maintain a healthy lifestyle

2 public health programme guidance – this deals with broader action for promotion of good health and the prevention of ill health. This guidance may focus on a topic, such as smoking, or on a particular population, such as young people, or on a particular setting, for example, the workplace.

In context

An example of guidance from the recent NICE obesity intervention review states that local authorities should work with local partners, such as industry and voluntary organisations, to create safe spaces for physical activity. They need to address as a priority any concerns about safety, crime and inclusion by:

- providing facilities and schemes such as cycling and walking routes, cycle parking, area maps and safe play areas
- making streets cleaner and safer, through measures such as traffic calming, congestion charging, pedestrian crossings, cycle routes, lighting and walking schemes
- ensuring buildings and spaces are designed to encourage people to be more physically active (for example, through positioning and signing of stairs, entrances and walkways).

1 Why do you think people are less and less active?

2 How might the recommendations from NICE change this situation?

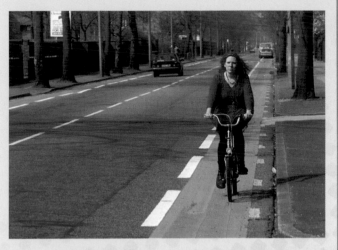

▲ Increasing the number of cycle routes is a measure suggested by NICE for reducing obesity levels.

3 If the town where you live had been improved in this way, would you be more active? For example, would you walk and cycle instead of using the car or bus? If not why not?

■ Cancer Research UK

Cancer Research UK is the world's leading independent organisation dedicated to cancer research. It was launched in February 2002 following the merger of the Cancer Research Campaign and Imperial Cancer Research Fund.

- It is the world's leading independent organisation dedicated to cancer research.

- The charity supports research into all aspects of cancer through the work of more than 3000 scientists, doctors and nurses.
- Cancer Research UK is the European leader in the development of novel anti-cancer treatments.
- They are an important training agency for cancer scientists and doctors.

Patterns of ill health and inequalities

Generally people are living longer than ever before. Boys born in 2004 can expect to live to the age of 76, compared with a life expectancy of 45 in 1900, and girls can expect to live to 80, compared with 50 in 1900. A child born today is likely to live nine and a half years longer than a child born when the NHS was established in 1948. While the threat of childhood death from illness is falling and the infectious diseases of the last century have been eradicated or largely controlled, the relative proportion of deaths from cancers, coronary heart disease and stroke has risen. They now account for around two-thirds of all deaths. Cancer, stroke and heart disease not only kill but are also major causes of ill health.

Although on average we are living healthier and longer lives, health and life expectancy are not shared equally across the population. In the early 1970s death rates among men of working age were almost twice as high for unskilled groups as they were for professional groups. By the early 1990s, death rates were almost three times higher among unskilled groups. There are regional differences too. In 1999/2001, the difference between areas with the highest (North Dorset) and lowest (Manchester) life expectancy at birth was 9.5 years for boys and 6.9 years for girls. The highest life expectancy for girls was in West Somerset and the lowest was in Manchester. We are going to explore some of the landmark reports which document these differences and the factors contributing to these inequalities.

The Black Report, 1980

At the end of the 1970s, the outgoing Labour government appointed Sir Douglas Black to review the evidence on inequalities in health and to suggest policy recommendations that should follow. The report was published under the incoming Conservative government in 1980 with no press release and only 260 copies were initially printed. The major finding of the Black Report was that there were large differentials in **mortality** and **morbidity** that favoured the higher social classes and that these were not being adequately addressed by health or social services. The report presented a number of costed policy suggestions and concluded: 'Above all, we consider that the abolition of child poverty should be adopted as a national goal for the 1980s.'

Key terms

Mortality Deaths due to a particular condition.

Morbidity This refers to the number of people who have a particular illness during a given period, normally a year.

The Acheson Report, 1998

We have already touched on the background and findings from the Acheson Report but below are some of the specific recommendations the report called for (many of which informed later government policy):

- **Benefits** – an increase in benefit levels for women of childbearing age, expectant mothers, young children and older people. The report stated that poverty has a disproportionate effect on children. In the mid 1990s, around a quarter of people in the UK were living below the poverty level.
- **Education** – more funding for schools in deprived areas, better nutrition at schools and 'health promoting schools' promoting health through the curriculum, for example, by teaching children not just about cooking but also about budgeting for food.
- **Smoking and drinking** – restrictions on smoking in public places, a ban on tobacco advertising and promotion, mass educational initiatives, increases in the price of tobacco and the prescribing of nicotine replacement therapy on the NHS.

'Tackling Health Inequalities: A Programme for Action', 2003

In 2003 the Labour government released the health White Paper *A Programme for Action* which set out plans to tackle health inequalities over the following three years. It established the foundations required to achieve the two national health inequalities targets, one relating to infant mortality and the other to life expectancy. They complemented a range of other
targets that had been set with an inequalities focus, in the areas of smoking and teenage pregnancy. The targets were:

- starting with children under one year, by 2010 to reduce by at least 10 per cent the gap in mortality between manual groups and the population as a whole
- starting with health authorities, by 2010 to reduce by at least 10 per cent the gap between the quintile (fifth or 20 per cent) of areas with the lowest life expectancy at birth and the population as a whole.

The strategy set out the following key priorities for delivering the targets:

- supporting families, mothers and children – to ensure the best possible start in life and break the inter-generational cycle of health
- engaging communities and individuals – to ensure relevance, responsiveness and sustainability
- preventing illness and providing effective treatment and care – making certain that the NHS provides leadership and makes the contribution to reducing inequalities that is expected of it
- addressing the underlying determinants of health – dealing with the long-term underlying causes of health inequalities.

'Choosing Health: Making Healthy Choices Easier', 2004

As we saw earlier, this White Paper of 2004 recognised that interest in health was increasing and recommended a new approach to public health.

Socio-economic factors affecting health

By now you will have begun to recognise the range of factors which together impact on someone's health. We will explore some of these in more detail below.

Social class

Social class has long been used as the method of measuring and monitoring health inequalities. Since the Black Report of 1988, it has been clearly identified and acknowledged that those from the lowest social groupings experience the poorest health in society. Current research suggests the countries with the smallest income *differences* have the best health status (rather than the richest countries). Where income differences remain great, as in this country, health inequalities will persist. For example:

- children in the lowest social class are five times more likely to die from an accident than those in the top social class
- someone in social class five is three times more likely to experience a stroke than someone in class one
- infant mortality rates are highest among the lowest social groups
- the difference in life expectancy between a man from one of the most affluent areas in this country and a man living in Manchester is six years.

Age

As one might expect, as people get older they are more likely to experience a wide range of illnesses. The health inequalities recorded above remain in the older generations but are often compounded by the loss of income that comes with retirement. This significantly increases the proportion of the population who are living on benefits as compared to other age groups in the population. Another factor is the longer lifespan of women which means that, because women make up a higher proportion of the older population, there are often higher rates of illnesses specifically associated with women.

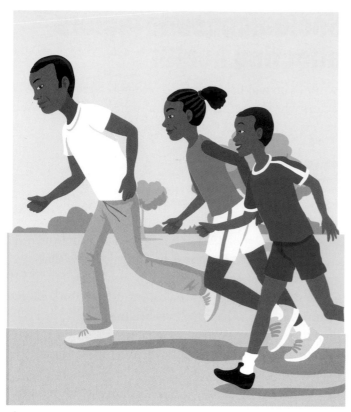

▲ **Figure 12.2 We are all raised to accept different types of health behaviours.**

Culture

One of the most powerful influences on our health is the culture we are raised in. Culture can mean many things including our ethnicity, the region we live in, religious beliefs, etc. but probably the most important cultural influence is our family, which can play a significant part in determining our health status through its key role in our socialisation, i.e. the types of behaviours we are raised to accept as normal. The health behaviours of adults in key positions in the family can have a major impact on the health of young people.

Gender

Men and women have widely differing patterns of ill health. In the main this can be best summarised by saying that men suffer a higher rate of early mortality (deaths) while women experience higher rates of morbidity (illness). There are many specific examples which illustrate these points and they are linked to

physiological, psychological and other aspects of gender characteristics influenced by the differing roles that the two genders are expected to adopt by society at large. Typically men are less likely to access routine **screening** and other forms of health service, while women who are viewed as the carer in the family are more able to do so and therefore they could identify potential health problems earlier. The results can be seen in the following patterns:

- Under the age of 65, men are 3.5 times more likely to die of coronary heart disease.
- Suicide is twice as common in men as in women.
- Women experience more accidents in the home or garden while men experience more accidents in the workplace or sports activities.

Key terms

Screening The identification of unrecognised disease or defect by the application of tests, examinations and other procedures which can be applied rapidly. Screening tests sort out apparently well people who may have a disease from those who do not.

Sexuality

Sexuality is a central aspect of being human and encompasses sex, gender identities and roles, sexual orientation, eroticism, pleasure, intimacy and reproduction. Sexuality is experienced and expressed in thoughts, fantasies, desires, beliefs, attitudes, values, behaviours, roles and relationships. While sexuality can include all of these dimensions, not all of them are always experienced or expressed. A person's sexuality can be influenced by including biological, psychological, social, economic, political, religious and many other factors. With such a range of facets it is inevitable that sexuality has a major part to play in influencing health. For example:

- Young gay men have the highest rate of suicide of all groups, a situation which is directly related to the prejudice and discrimination about their sexuality.

- Some faith-based schools will not allow discussion of contraception and sex outside of marriage because it breaches their faith-based guidelines.
- Sexuality has strong political ties, for example, the introduction of section 28 of the Local Government Act 1988 that prohibits local authorities 'promoting homosexuality by publishing material, or by promoting the teaching in state schools of the acceptability of homosexuality as a pretended family relationship'. This prevents any discussion of the health needs of gay and lesbian young people in schools.

Reflect

What examples of homophobia do you see in your college? These might be aimed at someone in particular or at gay people generally. What negative comments or 'put downs' do people use that are about sexuality? If a gay person hears these comments, how do you think it might make them feel about themselves and the people around them?

In context

John is employed by the local PCT as an outreach worker for the local gay community. His work specifically focuses on the needs of young gay men, because of their high risk of suicide, but his work also encompasses other aspects of health such as substance use, smoking and sexual health. His work includes direct support of young gay men through a local community group, one-to-one client support and the creation of a local helpline which volunteers now help to staff.

There is another aspect to his role which is to challenge organisational homophobia. For example, he encourages schools to challenge homophobic bullying through the development of appropriate policies coupled with training for staff on how to recognise homophobic bullying and how to challenge it appropriately. National research demonstrates that experience of homophobia and bullying at school is a significant contributor to the high rate of suicides in young gay men.

1   Does your college have an anti-bullying policy? If it does, get a copy and read it.

2   Is homophobic bullying mentioned specifically in the policy?

3   What would you suggest as being appropriate action to take for students who regularly breach this aspect of a policy?

Income and expenditure

Disposable income has a clear link to health status. The poorest people in England are over 10 times more likely to die in their 50s than richer people despite receiving similar healthcare. Obesity and smoking, two of the leading causes of preventable death, are more common in lower socio-economic groups. A person is more likely to smoke if:

- they have no educational qualifications
- they live in rented accommodation
- they do not having a car and/or phone
- the adults in the household are traditionally involved in manual labour
- they live off means-tested benefits.

In a recent survey, two-thirds of respondents agreed that tackling poverty would be the most effective means of preventing disease and improving health. Not surprisingly, people in the lowest socio-economic groups (67 per cent) and the socially excluded (71 per cent) are more likely to agree than people in the higher socio-economic groups.

Employment status

For the vast majority of people, being unemployed leads to significantly poorer health. The unemployed have higher levels of depression, suicide and self-harm and a significantly increased risk of morbidity and mortality across all causes of death and illness. Men unemployed at both census dates in 1971 and 1981 had mortality rates twice those of other men in the same age range and those men who were unemployed at one census date had an excess mortality of 27 per cent.

Housing

It is true to say that public health campaigners have been advocating improvements in housing to better the public's health since the middle of the nineteenth century. As we have seen, Edwin Chadwick's *Report on an inquiry into the sanitary conditions of the labouring population of Great Britain* (1842) resulted in the first national Public Health Act in1848.

The link between housing and health remains true to this day: the Office for National Statistics Longitudinal Study shows that, between 1971 and 1981, age-standardised mortality rates for social tenants (those in rented accommodation) were 25 per cent higher than for owner-occupiers. Although death rates have declined since that time, the gap between these groups has widened. Owner-occupiers see greater reductions in death rates than those living in rented accommodation.

Diet

Nutrition has recently become a high-profile health issue, not least because obesity has risen up the health agenda (as illustrated by its prominence in *Choosing Health*). This is particularly because of startling recent trends in young children which show a 60 per cent increase in the prevalence of being overweight among 3–4-year-olds and a 70 per cent increase in rates of obesity, while most adults in England are now overweight and one in five (around 8 million) are obese (with a **Body Mass Index** in excess of 30). Some 30,000 deaths a year are linked to obesity at an estimated cost to the NHS of £500 million.

Obesity is a major public health concern contributing substantially to:

- type 2 diabetes
- coronary heart disease
- hypertension
- depression
- cancers
- high blood pressure
- stroke.

Key terms

Body Mass Index (BMI) A reliable indicator of total body fat which is related to the risk of disease and death. Body Mass Index can be calculated using weight and height with this equation:

$$BMI = \frac{\text{weight in kilograms}}{\text{(height in metres)} \times \text{(height in metres)}}$$

The score is valid for both men and women but it does have limits. It may overestimate body fat in athletes and others who have a muscular build and it may underestimate body fat in older persons and others who have lost muscle mass.

	BMI
Underweight	Below 18.5
Normal	18.5 – 24.9
Overweight	25.0 – 29.9
Obese	30.0 and above

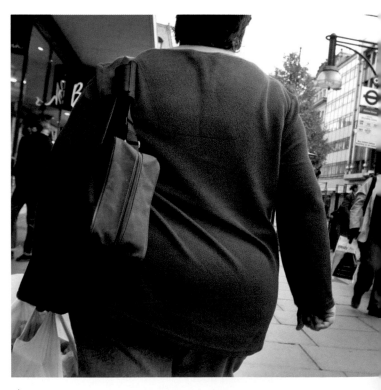

▲ **Obesity is a major public health concern today.**

As well as its role in relation to obesity, diet also has a major part to play in managing the current trends in cancers. Over the past 25 years the **incidence** of all cancers has risen by 8 per cent in men and 17 per cent in women. Up to 80 per cent of bowel and breast cancer may be preventable by dietary change.

Key terms

Incidence The rate of a disease at a given point in time.

Peer pressure

You will read more about peer pressure in Unit 20 which deals with health promotion but it is important to recognise that peer pressure (and peer preference) has an important role to play in influencing people's health.

Mass media

The role of the media in influencing health patterns has been most graphically illustrated through coverage of concerns about the safety of the measles, mumps and rubella (MMR) vaccine. A research paper by Andrew Wakefield, suggesting that the MMR vaccination in young children might be linked to autism, sparked a media frenzy which gave considerable coverage to his viewpoint, despite findings from many other researchers which provided no support for the MMR-associated form of autism. In spite of this, findings from a tracking survey of mothers with children aged 0–2 years old found that 8 per cent considered the **MMR vaccine** a greater risk than the diseases it protects against and that 20 per cent considered the vaccine to have a moderate or high risk of

Key terms

MMR vaccine A vaccination against measles, mumps and rubella.

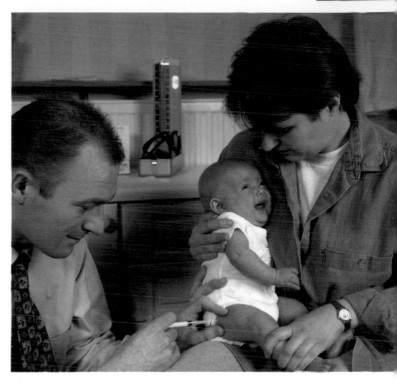

▲ **Who can parents trust to give them the right information to help them make the right choice for their child?**

Theory into practice

What examples of health information/campaigning can you find in the printed media? Collect any examples in your own newspaper and magazines from a seven-day period. This exercise will be more effective if you work with others to maximise the number of different papers and magazines you can cover.

What examples did you find which were:

- advertising (i.e. they were paid for)
- unpaid coverage of new information
- news coverage of new services/health-related projects?

What are the messages being conveyed in these pieces? Did you find any examples of the same information presented differently in various papers and magazines? What problems do you think this might present for the health promoter seeking media coverage?

side effects. Worryingly, the survey also showed that 67 per cent of people knew that some scientists had linked the MMR vaccine with autism and they also thought that the evidence in favour of such a link was evenly balanced, or that the evidence even favoured a link. The long-term media coverage of controversy over the vaccine appears to have led the public to associate MMR and autism, despite the overwhelming evidence to the contrary.

The impact of the media story continues today with MMR coverage still only at 86 per cent in June 2006 and as low as 73 per cent in London, some way short of the 95 per cent coverage required to prevent an outbreak.

Race and discrimination

We have already seen how prejudice and discrimination can lead to higher rates of suicide in young gay men, but black and minority ethnic (BME) groups also experience poorer health due to prejudice and discrimination. BME groups experience higher mortality from a range of diseases such as diabetes, liver cancer, tuberculosis, stroke and heart disease. Establishing the cause of these variations has proved difficult: while interventions have tended to concentrate on cultural practices, this has ignored the compounding factors of poverty and low employment levels in these groups. Sixty seven per cent of people from ethnic minority backgrounds live in 88 deprived areas which receive targeted neighbourhood renewal funding compared with 40 per cent of the total population, i.e. people from ethnic minorities are more likely to live in poor/disadvantaged communities. The only possible explanation for this situation is one which acknowledges that **racism** must also be a factor which leads to a higher than average experience of poverty and unemployment in these groups and hence contributes to their poorer health status.

Key terms

Racism Discrimination against a person on the basis of their race background, usually based on the belief that some races are inherently superior to others.

Education

It is now well-established that educational success is associated with better health. There are a number of possible explanations for this linkage:

- Educational success is linked to higher earnings, higher socio-economic status and lower rates of unemployment. Higher income tends to allow for a healthier lifestyle through being able to afford more nutritious but more expensive food, as well as better housing and holidays, etc.
- Studies suggest that people with more years of education and higher level qualifications tend to exercise more, eat more nutritious and healthy diets and smoke less, etc.
- Education enables individuals to learn problem-solving skills. It gives them a sense of purpose and this, together with social competence, instils in individuals a greater sense of belief in their ability to cope with adversity.

In general, children from low-income households go on to leave full-time education much earlier and with fewer formal qualifications than their more affluent counterparts. Of all children born in 1970, for example, some 24 per cent failed to achieve any O levels or equivalent by the age of 30, while 23 per cent went on to get a degree. Among children from low-income households, however, 38 per cent achieved no formal qualifications, and only 11 per cent went on to get a degree.

Access to services

An understanding of the health care professional/patient relationship can help explain the way in which people engage with local health services. It is suggested that this relationship is often at its least effective in the most disadvantaged communities. In 1994, Baldock and Ungerson attempted to summarise people's attitudes to community care services using a simple model which described four roles people can adopt when services are made available to them in a free market format:

- **Consumers** – people who expect nothing from the state and who set out to arrange the necessary care by buying it themselves. They believe that using the market in this way gives them control and autonomy, much like buying a car or any other kind of consumer goods. These people know about services but prefer to purchase their own care for a variety of reasons including convenience, perceived quality, etc.

- **Privatists** – people who have learnt to manage alone. Adapting to being cared for in later life can mean leaving the family home and increased dependency which they find hard to come to terms with because it means having to ask for help. They can become isolated and fail to access the necessary health care. Generally they do least well of the four in accessing services.
- **Welfarists** – people who believe in the welfare state and their right to use it; they expect and demand their rights to the relevant services. They have both the understanding and the know-how to make sure they get the most from the system and use it effectively to access both public and voluntary provision.
- **Clientists** – they accept passively what they are offered without demanding or expecting more. They don't expect services to be flexible in being able to respond to their specific needs. This is commonly seen in older people and low-income groups, explaining how people in disadvantaged communities will often accept the poor state of their local health services and not challenge and demand better provision.

This model is just that – a model – a means of helping us to understand how real world systems operate. It doesn't mean that people have to rigidly fit one role: they may move between roles dependent upon their circumstances. However, it can explain why people will have different experiences of using the same health services and how this can contribute to local health inequalities.

Environmental factors affecting health

The impact of the environment on health can be seen from two perspectives:

- its capacity to provide benefits to health, for example, parks and recreational spaces can encourage us to participate in regular exercise or even just allow us the opportunity to experience time away from the stresses and strains of everyday life
- its capacity to do harm, for example, through pollution or poor housing.

Urban

It is almost a universal truth that people living in the major urban centres experience the poorest health.

In context

Mary is 76 and a lifetime smoker since the age of 16. She has recently developed a recurrent chest problem which she just can't seem to shake off. She has been to her GP, who has examined her but who thought this infection was probably just a result of her poor physical health due to a recent hip operation. He has prescribed her two treatments of antibiotics recently but hasn't seen her for a couple of weeks.

Mary is a classic clientist. She has accepted faithfully the GP's prescription and diagnosis without question, having been brought up to respect professionals like the GP and not question them. Martin is Mary's son.

He is less confident and is worried that the GP might have missed something, particularly in light of her long-term smoking habit.

1   **What problems might Martin face in challenging the GP's diagnosis?**

2   **If the GP is Martin's doctor, how might this affect their relationship in the longer term?**

3   **What does this tell you about the power balance between doctor and patient and how prepared people might be to challenge decisions about their treatment?**

There can be no better illustration of this than Manchester which has on balance possibly the worst health profile in England and Wales:

- Men can expect to live 72.3 years in Manchester and women 77.9 years. This is the lowest life expectancy for men and the second lowest for women in England.
- Deaths from heart disease and stroke, smoking and cancer are the second highest in England.

The likely explanations of these trends should be no surprise to you now – they strongly correlate to income deprivation and the other markers we have already considered earlier in this unit. In Manchester, deprivation is significantly high with 73 per cent of the population living in the most deprived areas and 46.4 per cent of children under 16 living in 'low income households'.

Rural

By contrast, rural areas appear idyllic with their wide open green spaces – an environment which by definition should be beneficial to health. However, they also have a very specific set of their own health problems. For example:

- Road traffic accident (RTA) rates are higher in rural areas. The Eden Valley area has the second highest RTA rate nationally.
- Isolation, occupational stress, economic crises and unforeseen events (such as crop failure due to bad weather) can all contribute to mental health problems.
- Suicides are higher in rural areas, as in particular are farm suicides. People in rural communities (farmers and vets in particular) have ready access to firearms and drugs if they are seeking to take their own lives.

In rural communities, the stigma attached to certain illnesses can be more of an issue because it is so hard to keep secrets. Families, patients and carers can 'soldier on' with mental health problems masked to the outside world. In these areas, community psychiatric nurses have been known to leave their cars some distance from a patient's home to maintain confidentiality and avoid stigmatising the patient.

Water supply

As we saw earlier, the link between contaminated water and disease was clearly established in the nineteenth century by John Snow. Contaminants that may be in untreated water include microorganisms such as viruses and bacteria; inorganic contaminants such as salts and metals; pesticides and herbicides; organic chemical contaminants from industrial processes and petroleum use; and radioactive contaminants. In the developing world today, poor access to safe water and adequate sanitation continues to be a threat to human health. In 2003, 1.6 million deaths were estimated to be attributable to unsafe water and sanitation, including lack of hygiene; 90 per cent of this burden is concentrated on children under five, mostly in developing countries. In spite of the considerable investment in the provision of water supply and sanitation in the 1980s and 1990s, in 2000 an estimated 1.1 billion people were without access to improved water sources and 2.4 billion people lacked access to improved sanitation.

Waste management

Consumerism is a major contributor to the growth of household waste through rising income, increasing household numbers, more small households and a growing acceptance of discarding products in order to upgrade to newer ones. In the UK, an increasingly urban environment, municipal waste is growing at a rate of 3 per cent a year, one of the fastest growing rates in Europe. In the UK we have a very high level of unsustainable waste disposal, specifically in landfill where nearly 80 per cent of the 28 million tonnes of municipal waste is disposed of each year. This is significantly higher than France (49 per cent), Austria (35 per cent) and the Netherlands (12 per cent). Historically this has been a cheap option economically but it is environmentally costly. It contributes:

- 25 per cent of the UK's methane production (a powerful greenhouse gas)
- nothing to sustainable development (all waste disposed of in this way is simply lost)
- significantly to our individual ecological footprint.

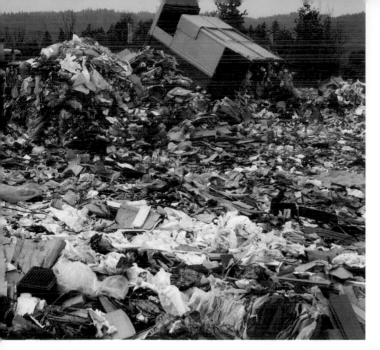

▲ In the UK we have a very high level of waste disposal in landfill.

Housing

The link between housing and health status is probably best explained as housing being an indicator for income deprivation, or social class. Those on low incomes are more likely to be living in poor housing conditions experiencing overcrowding, poor washing and cooking facilities, damp and disrepair. Children who live in such houses with damp are known to have higher than usual rates of respiratory conditions like asthma and other communicable infections which are transmitted more easily in overcrowded conditions. Childhood accident rates are also highest in areas of high density housing where play facilities are limited and it is difficult for parents to supervise children at play outside.

Pollution

Pollution can be said to have occurred when the environment is negatively affected in some way. Pollution comes in many forms including pollution to land, air, water and aesthetic pollution (visual). Many of these forms of pollution have the potential to bring about long-term damage to both the environment and human health and well-being on a global and national scale. It is argued that pollution should be monitored and measured to allow action to be taken to reduce the amount of all kinds of pollution.

We can also include indoor air pollution in an exploration of the home environment. For example, inhaling other people's tobacco smoke (passive smoking) is clearly a risk to health.

Access to health and social care services

We have already considered how the ways in which people engage with services may influence their treatment outcomes but the physical location of services is just as important. If we return to the issue of rurality, we have already seen that these areas have higher rates of RTAs. This problem is then compounded by having to wait longer before receiving initial medical care. This is because the response times are usually slower as ambulances must travel longer distance to reach the casualty. There are also access issues for community-based services such as the GP who is the first point of contact in health care. He or she also controls access to other services such as secondary hospital care. Problems in accessing a GP are reflected in the fact that urban residents with a car and telephone use their GP three times more than remote rural residents who do not have a car or phone.

Access to leisure and recreational facilities

How we use our spare time in terms of recreation can have a significant influence on our health. Recreational pursuits can contribute to a wide range of health benefits such as physically active lifestyles, weight management, stress release and a sense of well-being which leads to improved mental health status. In 2004, the **Health Development Agency (HDA)** published a

Key terms

Health Development Agency (HDA) A national health agency set up in 2000 to provide information about what works in terms of health promotion activity. This in turn enables evidence-based practice in health promotion. Its role has subsequently been taken up by NICE.

review of how people use their leisure time. It found that:

- those who participate in sporting activities are also more likely to participate in cultural activities, and vice versa
- for both sport and culture, the majority of people tended to do very little of anything
- higher levels of household income, education and social class usually predicted higher rates of participation in most cultural and sporting activities
- after accounting for household income and social class, not having access to a vehicle was important in determining the amount of sporting and cultural activity that individuals are able to participate in
- there were no especially marked regional differences in participation in culture and sport.

Men were found to be more likely to participate in sports activities than women (either including or excluding walking). Active forms of recreation were found to be in decline – in 1996, 54 per cent of men and 38 per cent of women had participated in at least one activity, excluding walking, but by 2002 participation had fallen to just over half (51 per cent) of men and 36 per cent of women. Participation rates also decreased with age. In 2002, 72 per cent of young adults (aged 16 to 19) compared with 54 per cent of adults aged 30 to 44 and 14 per cent of adults aged 70 and over had participated in at least one activity (excluding walking) in the four weeks before the interview.

Genetic factors affecting health

For some conditions, the key influencing factor is the presence or absence of a specific gene or gene combination. Specific examples are explored below.

Sickle-cell anaemia

This disorder affects haemoglobin in red blood cells (which carries oxygen from the lungs to all parts of the body). People with sickle-cell anaemia have sickle haemoglobin (HbS) which is different from the normal haemoglobin (HbA). While normal red blood cells can bend and flex easily, when sickle haemoglobin gives up its oxygen to the tissues, it sticks together to form long rods inside the red blood cells making these cells rigid and sickle-shaped. Because of their shape, sickled red blood cells can't squeeze through small blood vessels as easily as the normal cells. This can lead to the small blood vessels getting blocked which then stops the oxygen from getting through to where it is needed. This in turn can lead to severe pain (called crises) and damage to organs.

Everyone has two copies of the gene for haemoglobin – one from their mother and one from their father. If one of these genes carries the instructions to make sickle haemoglobin (HbS) and the other carries the instructions to make normal haemoglobin (HbA) then the person has sickle-cell trait and is a carrier of the sickle haemoglobin gene. This means that this person has enough normal haemoglobin in their red blood cells to keep the cells flexible and they don't have the symptoms of the sickle cell disorders.

If both copies of the haemoglobin gene carry instructions to make sickle haemoglobin then this will be the only type of haemoglobin they can make and sickled cells can occur. Over time, people with such sickle-cell anaemia can experience damage to organs such as liver, kidney, lungs, heart and spleen. Another problem is that red blood cells containing sickle haemoglobin do not live as long as the normal 120 days and this results in a chronic state of anaemia. A special blood test (haemoglobin electrophoresis) can tell whether a person has a sickle cell disorder or is a healthy carrier, for example for sickle cell trait.

Thalassaemia

Beta thalassaemia is a genetic blood disorder. A person who carries the beta thalassaemia gene can appear perfectly healthy. However, where both partners carry the gene there is a 1 in 4 chance that their child could inherit both their genes and develop beta thalassaemia major. This condition requires intensive medical care including monthly blood transfusions and a continuous injection for 8 to12 hours each night at home. Beta thalassaemia major has a serious impact, not just on the quality of life of the sufferers and their family, but also on the NHS as treatment for one person up to the age of 30 costs about £1 million.

- Up to 23 births of babies with beta thalassaemia major occur each year in the UK. Of these births, 79 per cent are to Asian parents who originate from India, Pakistan and Bangladesh. Up to 1 in 7 Asians may be carriers of the thalassaemia gene.

- Beta thalassaemia major can be prevented by diagnosing and screening potential at-risk couples and offering them counselling both before and during pregnancy.

- A survey carried out in 1995 by the UK Thalassaemia Society found that only 25 per cent of South Asians living in England were aware of thalassaemia, and only 4 per cent had had the blood test to find out if they carry the gene.

Cystic fibrosis

Cystic fibrosis (CF) is the UK's most common life-threatening inherited disease. It affects over 7500 people in the UK and over 2 million people in the UK carry the gene that causes it (around 1 in 25 of the population). If two carriers have a child, the baby has a 1 in 4 chance of having cystic fibrosis.

Cystic fibrosis affects the internal organs, especially the lungs and digestive system, by clogging them with thick sticky mucus. This makes it hard to breathe and digest food. Average life expectancy is around 31 years, although improvements in treatments mean a baby born today could expect to live for longer. Cystic fibrosis is increasingly being diagnosed through screening but some babies and older children (and even adults) are diagnosed following unexplained illness. There are three types of screening for cystic fibrosis:

- **newborn testing** – a heel-prick to sample blood as part of the normal test carried out on all children

- **carrier testing** – a simple mouthwash test can be taken to tell if a person is a carrier

- **antenatal testing** – this test is used early in pregnancy to show whether a baby has cystic fibrosis.

Disease susceptibility

In many cases, a single defective gene is not sufficient to cause a disorder. However, many of the common diseases of adult life, such as diabetes mellitus, hypertension, schizophrenia and most common congenital malformations (such as cleft lip, cleft palate and neural tube defects) have a strong genetic component to their occurrence. In these examples it is thought that a large number of genes each act in a small but significant manner to predispose an individual to the genetic condition. This can result in a disease caused by the interaction between multiple genes and environmental factors.

Scientists have been able to separate the random from the genetic by inspecting the occurrence of disorders in identical *and* non-identical twins because identical twins are genetically identical and non identical twins are not.

Disease	Chances of both twins being affected (% age)	
	Identical twins	Non-identical twins
Diabetes (mellitus)	50	10
Hypertension	30	10
Manic depression	80	10
Multiple sclerosis	20	5

Table 12.2 Genetic influence in common disorders.

As the table shows, in many conditions, the chance of both identical twins being affected by the same disorder is much higher than non-identical, inferring that a strong 'non random' or genetic component is influencing the chance of having these conditions.

Assessment activity 12.2

Imagine you are the Director of Public Health for your area. Each year you must produce a report which describes the local health patterns and explains what might be contributing to those patterns. Draw up a local report for your area. It should include two main sections:

- a first section which describes local patterns of health
- a second section which explains possible contributory factors to the pattern of ill health.

A starting point for this task would be to look for examples of local public health reports which will not only show you how to set out this information but also give you the necessary public health information for your report. You will probably find these on your local Primary Care Trust website. Use these reports to answer the following questions.

P3 Identify current patterns of ill health and inequality in the UK.

1   Collate data that identifies current patterns of ill health and inequality on a wall chart to present to a local pressure group.

P4 In a written report, describe six factors that potentially affect health status.

In your second section you need to address some of the major contributors to ill health in more detail. Do this by describing two socio-economic, two environmental and two genetic factors which potentially affect health status in the UK. Be sure to acknowledge your sources.

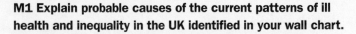

Grading tip for P3

You need to identify at least *three* key patterns of ill health and inequality in your locality, using major national reports to help you. Include graphs and charts where possible and add explanatory notes.

Grading tip for P4

For this first stage you simply need to describe each, explaining the contribution to ill health it makes.

M1 Explain probable causes of the current patterns of ill health and inequality in the UK identified in your wall chart.

What are identified as the main causes which are contributing to these patterns of death and disease? Evaluate the extent to which these contribute to patterns of ill health and inequality, referring to your sources.

D1 Evaluate the role of factors that contribute to the current patterns of ill health and inequality in the UK.

Summarise your report by assessing which factors make the greatest contribution to ill health and therefore are the priorities for action to reduce ill health locally.

Grading tip for M1

To gain a merit grade you would need to identify at least *four* probable causes and explain how they might contribute to these patterns of ill health and inequality.

Grading tip for D1

Always make sure any claims you make in your evaluation are supported by evidence in your report. Draw conclusions as to which factors are most important, both locally and nationally.

Aims of promoting and protecting public health

To improve health

Perhaps the best summary of governmental aspirations in this area can be found in the introduction to the White Paper *Choosing Health: Making Healthy Choices Easier*:

> *There have been big improvements in health and life expectancy over the last century. On the most basic measure, people are living longer than ever before. Boys born in 2004 can expect to live to the age of 76, compared with a life expectancy of 45 in 1900, and girls to 80, compared with 50 in 1900. A child born today is likely to live nine and a half years longer than a child born when the NHS was established in 1948. Future progress on this dramatic scale cannot be taken for granted … the relative proportion of deaths from cancers, coronary heart disease (CHD) and stroke has risen. They now account for around two-thirds of all deaths.*

Clearly the government has recognised that while we now live longer, and the major causes of premature death of the last century are largely under control, the same cannot be said for today's main killers.

To reduce health inequalities

The government's *Tackling Health Inequalities: a Programme for Action* set, for the first time, national targets for reducing the levels of health inequalities by 2010. It suggested that there were a number of specific interventions among disadvantaged groups that were most likely to help in achieving the targets including:

- reducing smoking in manual social groups
- preventing and managing other risks for coronary heart disease and cancer such as poor diet and obesity, physical inactivity and hypertension through effective primary care and public health interventions – especially targeting the over-50s

- improving housing quality by tackling cold and dampness and reducing accidents at home and on the road
- improving the quality and accessibility of antenatal care and early years support in disadvantaged areas
- reducing smoking and improving nutrition in pregnancy and early years
- preventing teenage pregnancy and supporting teenage parents
- improving housing conditions for children in disadvantaged areas.

Health promoting activities/health education

Healthy eating campaigns

As we have already seen, improving nutrition has a key role to play in reducing obesity and its associated disorders as well as reducing cancers. Current recommendations are that everyone should eat at least five portions of a variety of fruit and vegetables each day, to reduce the risks of cancer and coronary heart disease and many other chronic diseases. Yet average fruit and vegetable consumption among the population in England is less than three portions a day.

The government-led 5 A DAY programme aims to increase fruit and vegetable consumption by:

- raising awareness of the health benefits
- improving access to fruit and vegetables through targeted action.

The 5 A DAY programme has five strands which are underpinned by an evaluation and monitoring programme:

- National School Fruit Scheme
- local 5 A DAY initiatives

- national/local partners – government health consumer groups
- communications programme including 5 A DAY logo
- work with industry including producers, caterers and retailers.

Standards for school lunches

The School Food Trust (SFT) was commissioned in 2005 to advise ministers on standards for food in schools. These standards will apply to school lunches and other food provided in all local authority maintained schools in England. There are two sets of standards for school lunches:

- food-based, which will define the types of food that children and young people should be offered in a school lunch and the frequency with which they are offered
- nutrient-based, which will set out the proportion of nutrients that children and young people should receive from a school lunch.

The government has also decided that similar standards should apply to all school food other than lunches, as recommended by the SFT, which will mean:

- no confectionery will be sold in schools
- no bagged savoury snacks other than nuts and seeds (without added salt or sugar) will be sold in schools
- a variety of fruit and vegetables should be available in all school food outlets (this could include fresh, dried, frozen, canned or juiced varieties)
- children and young people must have easy access at all times to free, fresh drinking water in schools.

National No Smoking Day

No Smoking Day was established as a national event on Ash Wednesday in 1984. The campaign has always been aimed at encouraging and helping smokers who want to stop smoking and has helped over 1.2 million to do so since then. The success of the day is largely due to the commitment of local organisers throughout the UK. There are now over 5000 registered campaigners for No Smoking Day and around 30,000 campaign packs are distributed to organisers each year. The No Smoking Day campaign has become one of the best-known awareness days in the UK. Each year around 70 per cent of the population are aware that it is No Smoking Day. Smokers are using the day more than ever as their day to try to stop smoking. Considering that the percentage of adults who smoke has dropped nearly 10 per cent since the campaign began, the proportion of smokers who use the day has actually risen over the last 24 years.

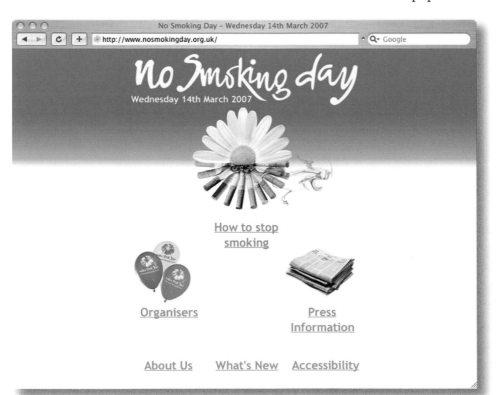

Figure 12.3 You can find out more at www.nosmokingday.org.uk

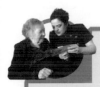

In context

Janet is the manager of the local stop smoking service (SSS) which offers people one-to-one and group support in their efforts to quit smoking. National No Smoking Day is a key point on the calendar for the service because it is one of two peaks in the year when people attempt to quit smoking.

Each year the service invests heavily to encourage as many people as possible to engage with the service and quit smoking. The success of the SSS is based on '12-week quitters', i.e. the number of people who manage to stay stopped for three months – this is known to be the length of time it takes for someone to have a high chance of succeeding in staying stopped for life. The annual performance of Janet's service is measured from 1 April to 31 March.

1 **When is No Smoking Day each year?**

2 **About what date will the service know how many 12-week quitters they have gained from the focus at national No Smoking Day?**

3 **What problems might this present for Janet when submitting her annual returns?**

Specific protection

Immunisation

It is possible to make people immune to certain diseases. This is done by challenging their immune system with a weak or inactivated version of the disease organism which then stimulates the person to create antibodies to the disease. This will enable their immune system to respond quickly should they contract the disease later on, resulting in no more than mild symptoms instead of experiencing the worst aspects of the disease. Children are routinely immunised for diphtheria, typhoid, polio, measles, mumps, rubella, etc.

The immunisation programme creates what is known as 'herd immunity'. That is, if enough people within the population are immunised, the likelihood of any epidemic is greatly reduced. For this reason the government sets immunisation targets for local health services to meet. Any regular fall below these levels signals a potential epidemic and becomes a serious cause for concern.

Disease surveillance

Key infections are under constant surveillance in order to detect significant trends, to evaluate prevention and control measures and to alert appropriate professionals and organisations to infectious disease threats. As part of this programme, certain diseases have to be reported to the HPA to enable these trends to be monitored. Examples include some classes of food poisoning, sexually transmitted infections such as syphilis and other communicable diseases such as TB. Samples from the infected people are checked at key laboratories which are able to identify new or virulent strains of specific organisms that may be causing higher levels of illness. This information can then be used to put together appropriate responses to possible outbreaks.

Screening

Screening can be defined as 'the identification of unrecognised disease or defect by the application of tests, examinations and other procedures which can be applied rapidly. Screening tests sort out apparently well people who may have a disease from those who do not.' However, screening a well population can be a contentious issue: in almost all cases the majority of people screened will not be ill with the condition screened for. This begs the question, are we right to be treating a well population in this way?

Environmental

Waste disposal/treatment

We explored earlier how waste poses a serious threat to health and the concerns over the quantities of waste we currently produce as a nation. However, there are some significant improvements being seen due to government recycling targets for local authorities. These have changed the nature of kerbside collections to include collections for glass, paper, plastics, etc. for recycling. This has resulted in:

- the proportion of recycled household waste rising steadily from 7 per cent in 1996/7 to 11 per cent in 2001/02
- the proportion of households served by kerbside recycling schemes increasing from 48 per cent in 1999/00 to 51 per cent in 2000/01
- the amount of waste disposed of in landfill falling from 80 per cent in 1999/00 to 78 per cent 2000/01
- in 2000/01 around 60,000 tonnes of metal was collected for recycling
- the amount of material collected through civic amenity sites rose by 9 per cent from1999/00 to 2000/01.

Supply of safe water

Drinking water quality in England and Wales is regulated by the government through the Drinking Water Inspectorate (DWI). The DWI was set up in 1990 after the water industry was privatised to operate as an independent body with staff experienced in all aspects of water supply.

The DWI's main task is to check that the water companies in England and Wales supply water that is safe to drink and meets the standards set in Water Quality (Water Supply) Regulations. To achieve this, DWI staff carry out technical audits of each water company.

The legal standards for drinking water quality in England and Wales are set down in the Water Quality Regulations. Most of these standards come directly from European law and are based on World Health Organisation guidelines. The UK regulations include additional standards to safeguard the already high quality of water in England and Wales. The standards are strict and generally include wide safety margins.

Pollution control

Pollution from industrial installations in England and Wales has been controlled to some extent for over 150 years. The Pollution Prevention and Control (England and Wales) Regulations 2000 (the PPC Regulations) are a regime for controlling pollution from certain industrial activities. The regime introduces the concept of Best Available Techniques (BAT) to environmental regulations.

Operators must demonstrate the use of BAT to control pollution from their industrial activities if they are to gain a permit. The aim of BAT is to prevent, and where that is not practicable, to reduce to acceptable levels, pollution to air, land and water from industrial activities. BAT also aim to balance the cost to the operator against benefits to the environment.

The system requires the operators of certain industrial and other installations (for example landfill sites, bleachworks, chemical plants, etc.) to obtain a permit to operate. Once an operator has submitted a permit application, the regulator (usually the Environment Agency) then decides whether to issue a permit. If one is issued, it will include conditions aimed at reducing and preventing pollution to acceptable levels.

Assessment activity 12.3

You have been asked to make a PowerPoint presentation to your group to explain the role that the following key interventions make to promoting and protecting health:

- the 5 A DAY programme
- National No Smoking Day
- immunisation
- recycling targets
- the PPC regulations.

P5 Describe ways to promote and protect public health.

1 Describe each intervention. Take one slide for each and summarise what the nature of the activity is, and what aspect of ill health it protects us against, using the notes pages to provide extra detail.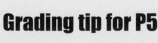

Grading tip for P5

The question asks you to 'describe' the intervention, so to attain this grade you simply need to explain what the activity is and what the aspect of ill health is that it is working to protect us against.

M2 Explain methods of promoting and protecting public health.

2   Use a second slide for each activity which explains how each intervention promotes and protects our health. **M2**

Grading tip for M2

To help you achieve a merit grade you need to explain how each of these methods contributes to promoting and protecting public health.

Communicable diseases

As previously explored, some communicable diseases are of specific interest and are routinely monitored to observe trends. This statutory requirement came into being in 1891. Some of these key diseases are discussed in more detail below.

Tuberculosis (TB)

Tuberculosis (TB) is an infection caused by the bacterium *Mycobacterium tuberculosis*. It is most commonly spread in droplets which are coughed or sneezed into the air but frequent or close prolonged contact with an infected person is necessary to catch the disease. TB most commonly affects the lungs but it can affect other parts of the body such as the lymph nodes, bones, joints and kidneys and can cause meningitis. With effective treatment, it is possible to make a full recovery from tuberculosis. Treatment involves a combination of 3–4 antibiotics for a period of six months or more. However, sometimes longer courses of treatment are needed, for example for TB meningitis, or if the bacteria are resistant to one or more antibiotics.

Prevention of TB is through the use of the BCG vaccine developed using a strain of *Mycobacterium bovis,* the organism that causes TB in cattle. This organism has been modified in the vaccine so that it produces immunity against TB without causing the disease. Studies in the UK have shown the vaccine gives about 70 to 80 per cent protection. Vaccination is recommended for people such as health care workers who may be exposed to TB at work, and immigrants from, or people going to live in, countries with a high prevalence of TB (if they have not previously been immunised). In the UK, BCG is also offered to babies who are more likely than the general population to come into contact with someone with TB.

Sexually transmitted infections (STIs)

The government first set targets for improving the sexual health of the population in *The Health of the Nation* (1992), where it focused on a reduction in rates of gonorrhoea and in the rate of conceptions among the under-16s by 50 per cent by 2000.

The government recognised a steady rise in rates of both gonorrhoea and chlamydia. Between 1995 and 1997 there was a 53 per cent rise in rates of gonorrhoea and a 47 per cent rise in rates of chlamydia among the 16–19 year age group. These are both areas of considerable concern with chlamydia being the single most preventable cause of infertility in women.

As a result, the government invested heavily in a national chlamydia screening programme which aims to screen and treat where necessary at least 15 per cent of under-25s (this being the most sexually active and promiscuous age group). One likely spin-off from the programme will be an increase in diagnoses and treatment of other sexually transmitted infections as services actively seek out young people to test.

Meningitis

Meningococcal disease results from a bacterial infection caused by the organism *Neisseria meningitides*, which causes an inflammation of the lining of the brain (the same organism can also cause septicaemia). The disease is usually spread in droplets being coughed or sneezed into the air, or more directly through kissing. Levels of the disease tend to peak during the winter months, and drop to their lowest rate by late summer. The highest risk group for meningococcal disease is the under-1s, with the 1–5 age group following closely. The next highest risk group is young people aged 15–19 years. Immunisation with MenC vaccine became part of the routine childhood immunisation programme in the UK in November 1999. All babies should receive three doses of MenC vaccine by injection as part of their primary immunisation course at 2, 3 and 4 months of age. Children and young people from 1 to 24-years-and-364-days-old who have not previously been vaccinated should receive a single dose of MenC. While the risk of the disease is generally low in adults, there is a greater risk for people aged between 20–24. People in this age group who have already had the new MenC vaccine will not need to have it again.

Salmonella

Salmonella is a common type of food poisoning caused by bacteria which can be caught by eating food contaminated with the bacterium, for example, unpasteurised milk, raw meat, undercooked poultry and eggs, etc. It is also possible to catch salmonella from someone else who is infected and from pets and farm animals. Salmonella usually causes diarrhoea, stomach ache, sickness, tiredness and fever. The incubation period is usually 12 to 36 hours but can be as short as 6 hours or as long as 10 days. Infection is mainly caused by poor kitchen hygiene. The following advice is routinely given to commercial food premises by environmental health officers to prevent its spread:

- Uncooked food and cooked food must not be kept together in a fridge or on work surfaces.
- Always ensure raw food is never stored above cooked food in the fridge.
- All food should be well cooked, especially eggs and chicken.
- Wash hands after handling raw chicken.
- If you have an illness with diarrhoea and sickness, you must stay away from work

Methicillin-resistant Staphylococcus aureus (MRSA)

Staphylococcus aureus is a very common bacterium that around 30 per cent of the population carry on their skin or in their nose without knowing it. It is a very common cause of bacterial infections such as boils, carbuncles and infected wounds. Some strains of the *Staphylococcus aureus* bacterium have developed a degree of resistance to the more commonly used antibiotics (for example penicillin) and are called MRSA. It is this resistance to certain (not all) antibiotics that makes MRSA different, as it may not be as easy to treat if it does cause an infection. People can carry MRSA in the same way as the usual *Staphylococcus aureus* without causing harm to themselves or others. Although it was first identified in hospitals, it is now found in the general community and care homes. MRSA can be spread by hands so handwashing is the most important way to stop it spreading particularly:

- between caring for clients/patients
- after using the toilet
- before eating/preparing food
- after handling soiled linen/bedding/nappies
- after touching animals
- when hands appear dirty.

Healthcare workers can use an alcohol handrub to help to ensure that their hands are properly clean.

Poliomyelitis

Poliomyelitis is an infectious disease that used to be the most common cause of paralysis in young people. For this reason, it was known as infantile paralysis. Myelitis means an inflammation of the spinal cord which can lead to lasting damage to the nervous supply and hence paralysis. Polio was once a common cause of death but widespread vaccination has greatly reduced it. Better hygiene and sanitation have also helped, but vaccination is the most important reason why this disease is now so rare in the UK. There now seems a real prospect that, like smallpox, polio may be eradicated entirely from the world. Polio is prevented by the Hib vaccine (five-in-one) which is given during childhood. It provides immunity to polio, as well as diphtheria, tetanus, pertussis and Hib. The vaccine was introduced in the UK in 2004 and has been used in Canada since 1997. Before the five-in-one vaccine, children were immunised against polio with an oral (taken by mouth) vaccine called Sabin. Although this is still available, the five-in-one vaccine provides a similar or better level of protection and is the preferred form of immunisation.

Measles

Measles is a highly infectious viral disease that causes a range of symptoms including fever and distinctive red-brown spots. Most people recover within 7 to10 days but there can be serious complications, some of which can be fatal. Although the rash is the most well-known and obvious sign of measles, it is just an outward symptom of what is mainly a respiratory infection. Measles mainly affects young children but can be caught at any age. The virus is spread by droplets in the air from coughs and sneezes, contact with the skin or via objects with the live virus on them.

The mumps, measles and rubella vaccination (MMR) has made measles quite rare in the UK but there have been recent outbreaks in children who have not been immunised. The first MMR vaccination should be given to all children at around 13 months old, with a booster dose given before they start school (3–5 years old). Between 5 to10 per cent of children are not fully immune after the first dose, so the booster jab helps to increase protection, with the result that less than 1 per cent remain at risk.

Non-communicable diseases

Skin cancer

The major cause of ill health associated with skin care is malignant melanoma or skin cancer. Skin cancer is distributed in the reverse pattern to other forms of cancer both regionally and by social class. That is, it is most common in the south west and east and in social classes 1 and 2. The incidence of malignant melanoma among men in class 1 is nearly five times that for men in class 5 and this is repeated for women, where the incidence is approximately twice in class 5 what it is in class 1.

The major cause of malignant melanoma (skin cancer) is exposure to the sun, which explains both the regional and social variations. In the northern areas of the country the number of days where lengthy exposure to the sun is likely is far fewer than in the south. The variations by social class are most usually explained by the use of tanning facilities and holidaying abroad, which those with greater disposable income can afford. Since the advent of the cheap package holiday this gap has narrowed as more and more people have greater access to holidays in hotter countries with stronger sunlight levels. Countries such as Australia have led the way in addressing this problem, with campaigns such as Slip, Slap, Slop which have been adopted in many other areas worldwide.

SunSmart is the national skin cancer prevention campaign run by Cancer Research UK. The campaign is funded mainly by the UK health departments and is supported and guided by the UV Health Promotion Group.

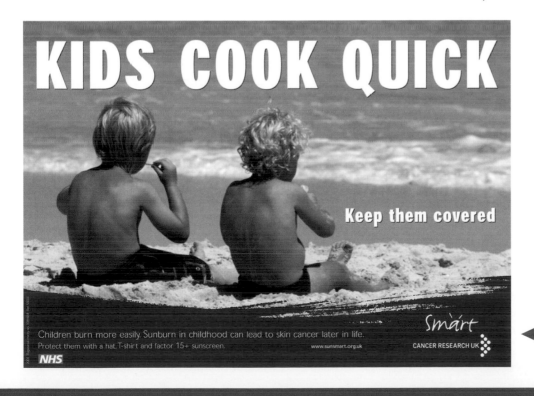

KIDS COOK QUICK
Keep them covered

Children burn more easily. Sunburn in childhood can lead to skin cancer later in life. Protect them with a hat, T-shirt and factor 15+ sunscreen. www.sunsmart.org.uk

Figure 12. 4
For more information, go to www.info.cancerresearchuk.org

Reflect

The current sun safety messages are:

- **S**eek the shade – especially at midday
- **H**ats on – use a wide-brimmed hat
- **A**pply sunscreen of at least spf 15
- **D**on't burn – it won't improve your tan
- **E**xercise care – always protect the very young

How often do you see people following this advice? Why might people choose not to follow this advice? What wider principle does this illustrate?

Lung cancer

The link between smoking and ill health is now well-documented.

Smoking is the single most important modifiable risk factor for coronary heart disease (CHD) in young and old.
Our Healthier Nation, section 6.5

A lifetime non-smoker is 60 per cent less likely to have CHD and 30 per cent less likely to have a stroke than a smoker. Smoking mirrors other patterns of ill health in that the highest levels are in the lowest social groups. Although the proportion of young people who smoke is similar across all social groups, by their mid-30s, 50 per cent of young people from higher social classes have stopped as opposed to only 25 per cent from the lowest income groups. The result is that about one third of the smokers in the population are concentrated in only the lowest 10 per cent of earners in the country.

Remember!

- Tobacco smoking causes most lung cancers.
- It is implicated in a wide range of other cancers including those of the nose and throat but also cervical cancer.
- Overall about one third of cancer deaths can be attributed to smoking.
- Smoking also contributes to coronary heart disease and stroke deaths.

In context

Following on from the commitment to reduce smoking-related deaths in the NHS plan, the government set up a comprehensive NHS 'stop smoking' service. Services are now available across the NHS in England, providing counselling and support to smokers who wanting to quit. This complements the use of the 'stop smoking' aids Nicotine Replacement Therapy (NRT) and bupropion (Zyban).

Services are provided in group sessions or on a one-to-one basis, depending on the local circumstances and service user's preferences. Most 'stop smoking' advisers are nurses or pharmacists and all have received training for their role.

The Department of Health funded an evaluation of the NHS 'stop smoking' services programme, which was carried out by a team led by Glasgow University. The main findings were that:

- the services can contribute to a reduction in health inequalities
- long-term quit rates for the services show about 15 per cent of people are still not smoking at 52 weeks, which is comparable with earlier clinical trials.

The services are cost-effective in helping smokers to quit. The evaluation showed that a smoker who tries to quit with the NHS 'stop smoking' service and NRT/Zyban is up to four times as likely to succeed as by willpower alone.

1 **Find out how to access your local 'stop smoking' service.**

2 **What range of support does it offer for people who are trying to quit smoking?**

3 **How many people did they help to quit last financial year (i.e. April to March)?**

Bowel cancer

About one in 20 people in the UK will develop bowel cancer during their lifetime. It is the third most common cancer in the UK and the second leading cause of cancer deaths, with over 16,000 people dying from it each year. Regular bowel cancer screening has been shown to reduce the risk of dying from bowel cancer by 16 per cent. Bowel cancer screening aims to detect bowel cancer at an early stage (in people with no symptoms), when treatment is more likely to be effective.

Bowel cancers sometimes bleed and the faecal occult blood (FOB) test works by detecting tiny amounts of blood which cannot normally be seen in faecal matter (occult means hidden). The FOB test does not diagnose bowel cancer but the results will indicate whether further investigation (usually a colonoscopy) is needed. The NHS Bowel Cancer Screening Programme offers screening every two years to all men and women aged 60 to 69 while people over 70 can request a screening kit. People eligible for screening receive an invitation letter explaining the programme and an information leaflet. About a week later, an FOB test kit is sent out along with step-by-step instructions for completing the test at home and sending the samples to the laboratory.

Coronary heart disease

In most advanced industrial societies the death rates from coronary heart disease (CHD) have fallen by 30 to 70 per cent over the last two decades. The risk factors for CHD have been well known for many years and we can now also say that changing these risk factors has a clear effect on the incidence of CHD. Some of these risk factors can be affected by primary prevention activity, for example, changing behaviours such as smoking, diet and exercise. However, they can also be reduced by drug therapy for people with raised blood lipids using a class of drug called statins. In a recent briefing, the Health Development Agency suggested that if the prescription of statins was increased so that 80 per cent of eligible patients received them in line with existing guidance, this would result in approximately 20,000 fewer deaths each year.

However, by the same token, modestly reducing average cholesterol levels in the UK to levels similar to those in Sweden, Finland, the US and Australia would prevent approximately 25,000 deaths each year and reducing smoking prevalence to American levels would result in 17,000 fewer deaths annually. Together with a small reduction in population blood pressure, over 50,000 CHD deaths could be prevented annually, halving current mortality rates in England and Wales. This emphasises the potential impact of health promotion activity (which you will read more about in Unit 20).

Stroke

Stroke (also known as cerebrovascular accident or CVA) is when the blood supply to a part of the brain is interrupted. The part of the brain with disturbed blood supply no longer receives adequate oxygen and brain cell death or damage can result, impairing local brain function. Stroke is a medical emergency and can cause permanent damage or even death if not promptly diagnosed and treated. Strokes are the third leading cause of death and adult disability. They affect around 200 per 100,000 population in the UK each year. It tends to be thought of as a disease of the elderly and incidence certainly rises with age but about 30 per cent occurs under the age of 65. Strokes account for 11 per cent of all deaths in England and Wales. The incidence doubles for every decade after 45 years.

The risk factors are very similar to CHD and include advanced age, hypertension (high blood pressure), diabetes, high cholesterol and cigarette smoking. Therefore many of the same interventions work for both.

Diabetes

In 2006, according to the World Health Organisation, at least 171 million people worldwide suffered from diabetes. Its incidence is increasing rapidly and it is estimated that by the year 2030 this number will double. Diabetes mellitus occurs throughout the world but is more common (especially type 2) in the more developed countries. The greatest increase in prevalence is, however, expected to occur in Asia and Africa, where most patients will likely be found by 2030. The increase in the incidence of diabetes in developing countries follows the trend of urbanisation and lifestyle changes, perhaps most importantly a 'Western-style' diet. Type 2 diabetes can be prevented in many cases by making changes in diet and increasing physical activity. Again, this emphasises the overlapping nature of many of the risk factors for CHD, obesity, CVA and other conditions and therefore the potential for relatively simple interventions such as increasing exercise, changing diet and quitting smoking to make major impacts on public health.

Assessment activity 12.4

A key role for public health practitioners is to argue for resources for public health programmes which control diseases or protect us against them. Imagine you are a member of your local public health team and have to prepare a short report explaining why you want funding for a public health programme to protect or control:

- either MRSA or TB and
- diabetes or coronary heart disease.

Your report should have clear three sections.

P6 Identify appropriate methods of prevention/control for a named communicable disease and a named non-communicable disease.

1   Identify the best methods of prevention/control for your chosen diseases.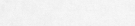

Grading tip for P6

For each disease you must describe the activities which can be put in place to control its spread or to protect people from contracting it. To do this you will need to describe how the disease is spread and then identify what the control measures are that relate to this method of spread.

M3 Explain appropriate methods of prevention/control for a named communicable disease and a named non-communicable disease.

2   Explain how these methods work in protecting or preventing the spread of these diseases.

Grading tip for M3

To help you achieve a merit grade you need to *explain* how these methods of prevention/control protect the public. This means you must show what the control method does to stop the disease from being spread, i.e. it is not enough to simply say what the measure is, you must describe *why* it stops the spread of the disease.

D2 Evaluate the effectiveness of methods of protecting public health for the two named diseases.

3   Evaluate how successful these methods are for promoting and protecting public health for the two named diseases.

Grading tip for D2

To do this you will need to check whether the current rates of the diseases are rising or falling, and to what extent the method has contributed to that trend.

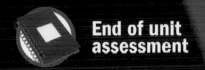
Preparation for assessment

You may be assessed in a variety of ways including reports, presentations, group discussion or the production of leaflets and posters. Whatever the mix of methods used by your tutor(s) you will need to explain the key aspects of public health in the UK **P1** and its origins giving an historical perspective which draws on the Beveridge Report and other key milestones as discussed at the beginning of this unit **P2**.

You will also need to explore current patterns of ill health **P3** explaining the ways in which health is unequally distributed within the UK, i.e. the current patterns of health inequality. This will require the use of health statistics drawn from local and national reports and websites. You should look for information on the Department of Health website and the National Statistics site, both of which can provide suitable information.

It is important to be able not just to describe the patterns of health inequality but also to suggest probable causes of the current patterns of ill health and inequality in the UK **M1**. You should also be able to describe six factors that potentially affect health status in the UK **P4** and assess the contribution to ill health and health inequalities in the UK that they make **D1**. The text will give you some of this information but again you will find more on key health sites such as those listed above and on page 152.

The final grading criteria deal with the subject of health protection, requiring you to both describe **P5** and explain **M2** methods of promoting and protecting public health. These methods are described in the text above but you can find additional information on the Health Protection Agency site as well as the sites for the NHS and the Department of Health. You will need to look at methods of promoting and protecting public health with particular reference to two named diseases, one communicable and one non-communicable. For each disease you must be able to identify appropriate methods of prevention/control **P6**, describe how these methods work **M3** and evaluate how effective they have been **D2** in promoting and protecting public health.

Resources and further reading

Baldock, J., Ungerson, C. (1994) *Becoming Consumers of Community Care* York: Joseph Rowntree Foundation

Benzeval, M., Judge, K., Whitehead, M. (1995) *Tackling Inequalities in Health: An Agenda for Action* London: Kings Fund Publishing

Downie, R.S., Tannahill, C., Tannahill, A. (1996) *Health Promotion Models and Values* Oxford: Oxford University Press

Draper, P. (1991) *Health Through Public Policy* London: Green Print

Ewles, L., Simnett, I. (1999) *Promoting Health: A Practical Guide* Edinburgh: Baillière Tindall

Hall, D. (1996) *Health for all Children* Oxford: Oxford University Press

HM Government (2004) *At Least Five a Week: Evidence on the Impact of Physical Activity and its Relationship to Health* London: HMSO

HM Government (2004) *Choosing Health: Making Healthy Choices Easier* London: HMSO

HM Government (1992) *The Health Of the Nation* London: HMSO

HM Government (1992) *Immunisation Against Infectious Disease* London: HMSO

HM Government (1998) *The Independent Inquiry into Inequalities in Health* London: HMSO

HM Government (2001) *The National Strategy for HIV and Sexual Health* London: HMSO

HM Government (1997) *The New NHS: Modern, Dependable* London: HMSO

HM Government (1997) *Saving Lives: Our Healthier Nation* London: HMSO

HM Government (2003) *Tackling Health Inequalities: A Programme for Action* London: HMSO

Jones, L., Sidell, M. (1997) *The Challenge of Promoting Health: Exploration and Action* Buckingham: The Open University

Katz, J., Peberdy, A. (1997) *Promoting Health: Knowledge and Practice* Buckingham: Macmillan/OU Press

Naidoo, J., Wills, J. (1996) *Health Promotion: Foundations for Practice* Edingurgh: Baillière Tindall

Whitehead, M., Townsend, P., Davidson, N., Davidsen, N. (1998) *Inequalities in Health: The Black Report and the Health Divide* Harmondsworth: Penguin Books

Useful websites

British Heart Foundation
www.bhf.org.uk/

Calculate your Body Mass Index
www.nhlbisupport.com/bmi/bmicalc.htm

Cancer Research UK
www.info.cancerresearchuk.org

Department of Health
www.doh.gov.uk

Drinking Water Inspectorate
www.dwi.gov.uk

European Observatory on Health Systems and Policies
www.euro.who.int/observatory

Gateway for Our Healthier Nation
www.ohn.gov.uk

Give up smoking
www.givingup-smoking.co.uk

Health Protection Agency
www.hpa.org.uk

Information about immunisation programmes
www.immunisation.org.uk

Mind, Body & Soul
www.mindbodysoul.gov.uk

NHS cancer screening programmes
www.cancerscreening.nhs.uk/

NHS in England
www.nhs.uk/england/

NHS immunisation information
www.mmrthefacts.nhs.uk

National Institute for Health and Clinical Excellence (NICE)
www.nice.org.uk

No Smoking Day
www.nosmokingday.org.uk

Office for National Statistics
www.statistics.gov.uk

Quick guide to checking information quality on the Internet
www.quick.org.uk

Wired for Health
www.wiredforhealth.gov.uk

World Health Organisation
www.who.int/en/

GRADING CRITERIA

To achieve a pass grade the evidence must show that the learner is able to:	To achieve a merit grade the evidence must show that, in addition to the pass criteria, the learner is able to:	To achieve a distinction grade the evidence must show that, in addition to the pass and merit criteria, the learner is able to:
P1 describe key aspects of public health practice in the UK **Assessment activity 12.1 page 122**		
P2 describe the origins of public health in the UK **Assessment activity 12.1 page 122**		
P3 identify current patterns of ill health and inequality in the UK **Assessment activity 12.2 page 140**	**M1** explain probable causes of the current patterns of ill health and inequality in the UK **Assessment activity 12.2 page 140**	**D1** evaluate the role of factors that contribute to the current patterns of ill health and inequality in the UK **Assessment activity 12.2 page 140**
P4 describe six factors that potentially affect health status in the UK **Assessment activity 12.2 page 140**		
P5 describe methods of promoting and protecting public health **Assessment activity 12.3 page 144**	**M2** explain methods of promoting and protecting public health **Assessment activity 12.3 page 145**	
P6 identify appropriate methods of prevention/control for a named communicable disease and a named non-communicable disease. **Assessment activity 12.4 page 150**	**M3** explain appropriate methods of prevention/control for a named communicable disease and a named non-communicable disease. **Assessment activity 12.4 page 150**	**D2** evaluate the effectiveness of methods of protecting public health for the two named diseases. **Assessment activity 12.4 page 150**

Knowledge check

1 What are the main roles within public health practice? How might each of these apply to a specific situation like an outbreak of E. coli food poisoning?

2 Name three founding fathers of public health. What did they contribute to improving public health?

3 Define *pressure group*. Give an example to explain how they influence public policy.

4 Give three examples of socio-economic factors which influence health and explain how each impacts on health.

5 Briefly compare and contrast the differences in health issues in rural and urban communities.

6 What influences whether or not a person has sickle-cell anaemia? What are its effects and how can it be prevented?

7 Select three health-promoting activities and explain how each contributes to improvement of health.

8 Whose role is it to monitor the supply of safe water and how do they ensure the water we drink is safe?

9 Identify three communicable diseases. Explain how they are spread and how best to control them.

10 What is the impact of lung cancer on the nation's health? What steps is the government taking to reduce it?

Physiology of fluid balance

Introduction

Water is essential for the maintenance of life. Therefore, the maintenance of fluid balance in the human body is of primary importance when caring for individuals. This unit aims to provide you with an understanding of a number of fundamental scientific principles that will underpin further studies in health-related science, as well as an overview of physiology in relation to the homeostatic control of water.

The unit builds on the basic knowledge of the cells introduced in Book 1, Unit 5: *Fundamentals of anatomy and physiology*, in which the microstructure of cells and the contribution made by cell organelles to the overall functioning of cells was explored. The movement of materials into and out of cells is then considered, followed by the distribution of fluids and the role of water and dissolved substances in the body.

You will then go on to examine the renal system and its role in homeostasis, in particular in relation to water balance.

The unit will be useful to those of you intending to work in the health or social care sectors, or to anyone progressing to further or higher studies. The scientific principles gained through the study of this unit link with several other science units within the programme.

How you will be assessed

After completing this unit you should be able to achieve the following outcomes:

- Understand the microstructure of a typical animal cell
- Understand the movement of materials into and out of cells
- Understand the distribution and constituents of fluids in the human body
- Understand homeostatic processes in relation to water balance.

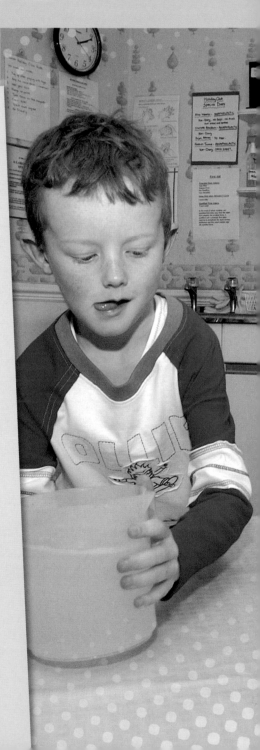

Thinking points

Have you ever considered how the millions of cells in a human body, which all have the same genetic 'footprint', are able to manufacture different materials to carry out their functions? How does a cell in the pancreas know that its job is to produce the hormone insulin, when cells in other places such as skin and muscle cannot make insulin? They all have the same DNA.

Skin, muscle and pancreatic cells all possess the same basic cell organelles but do entirely different jobs.

Have you thought how old cells are removed to make way for new cells as our bodies move on through the different life stages? The old cells must go somewhere! The body cannot just keep on making new cells and cell parts forever or we would get bigger and bigger.

We take water into our bodies in enormously varied amounts every day, yet our bodies don't swell up when we take in a lot or shrink on days when we don't take in much. Clearly, this vitally important substance is closely monitored.

This unit will provide some answers to questions, and give you a further insight into the fascinating and complex processes at work in the human body.

Despite the title of this section, you must understand that there is no such thing as a typical animal cell. This is a theoretical concept to help you learn about cell structure and physiology and apply this knowledge and understanding to particular cells such as liver or hepatic cells, white blood cells, red blood cells, etc. All these different cell types will have different roles to play in the body as well as having different shapes, sizes, functions and sometimes cell parts.

Cell structure

Human body cells are so small that they are invisible to the naked eye and for approximately 300 years they were viewed under light microscopes. Early light microscopes consisted of crude lenses used with daylight and really very little was seen.

As seen under the light and the electron microscope

The light microscopes gradually became more sophisticated, lenses became stronger and bright electric lamps were incorporated – but still, knowledge of cell structure advanced very little. This was mainly due to limits to the **resolution** of light with optical lenses. Special dyes were invented to stain particular structures to make them stand out more easily. A central **nucleus** (or several nuclei) readily took up stains and sometimes darker spots inside the nucleus were visible – the

Key terms

Resolution The capability of making individual parts or closely adjacent images distinguishable (in the absence of good resolution, stronger lenses make images blurred).

Nucleus Membrane-surrounded organelle, containing genetic material.

Nucleoli Dark spots inside the nucleus, probably the site of ribosome synthesis.

nucleoli. This was surrounded by a shapeless type of jelly called the **cytoplasm**, (or **cytosol**) bounded by a cell or plasma membrane. The cytoplasm showed dark granules and fluid-filled 'cysts' scattered around. This was generally thought to be some kind of organic jelly.

In the 1950s, another type of microscope was developed which avoided the use of light. It substituted a beam of electrons to produce an enormously enlarged image of a very small object.

This eventually opened up a whole new 'world' of the interior of a cell. The organic jelly of the cytoplasm was seen to be complex and structured. A new branch of science was born – **cytology**, or the study of cells.

Key terms

Cytoplasm Jelly-like material found between the cell membrane and the nucleus (also: **cytosol**).

Cytology The study of cell structure.

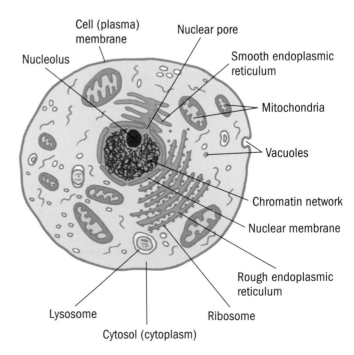

▲ Figure 13.1 The structure of a cell as seen under an electron microscope.

You learned some of the difficult terms in cytology in Unit 5: *Fundamentals of anatomy and physiology* in Book 1. You will now take this basic understanding further.

Nuclear and cell membranes (as a phospholipid bilayer)

Cells are bounded by their cell or plasma membranes and nuclei are bound by nuclear membranes. These membranes have the same biochemical structure. The membranes are composed of a double layer of **phospholipid** molecules, cholesterol and, sometimes, sugars and proteins (see Figure 13.3).

The double layer (which has a sandwich-like appearance) is often called a bilayer as the molecules are arranged in a special way. A phospholipid molecule looks rather like an old-fashioned clothes peg (see Figure 13.2). The head is made of **glycerol** and a group of phosphorus and nitrogen atoms; the 'legs' are made of chains of fatty acids.

The head is electrically charged and is often referred to as the **polar** head. It is said to be **hydrophilic** because it is able to exist against water molecules. The fatty acid chains do not carry charges and (like most fats or lipids) dislike water and are called **hydrophobic**.

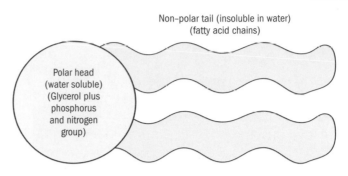

Non-polar tail (insoluble in water) (fatty acid chains)

Polar head (water soluble) (Glycerol plus phosphorus and nitrogen group)

▲ Figure 13.2 **The structure of a phospholipid.**

In the cell membrane the polar heads face both outwards and inwards, while the fatty acids face each other, like the meat in a sandwich (see Figure 13.3).

Cholesterol molecules are inserted into the bilayer at intervals and these tend to act as a stabiliser of the freely moving bilayer, which acts rather like a fluid itself. The original model of the cell membrane was called *the Fluid Mosaic model*. The phospholipid bilayer is dynamic but also flexible; its action is rather like when you place a spoon into a cup to stir it and lift it out – there isn't a 'hole' or space left behind with either action.

Also present are protein molecules: some lie only on the inner surface, others only on the outer surface and yet more others pass all the way through the membranes and act as pores or channels for substances moving into and out of the cell. Various sugar chains may add to phospholipids (**glycolipids**) or proteins (**glycoproteins**) and seem to form a 'sugar coating' to the outside of a cell. Proteins, glycolipids and glycoproteins may enable cells to stick together to form tissues and act as identity markers or receptor sites for hormones, enzymes, etc.

Key terms

Phospholipid A molecule consisting of glycerol, phosphate and lipid chains.

Glycerol A sugary alcohol.

Polar Carrying an electric charge, positive or negative.

Hydrophilic Having an affinity for water.

Hydrophobic Lacking an affinity for water.

Remember!

Tissue fluid bathes the outside of cells and is mainly water. Cytoplasm (inside the cell) is also a watery gel.

Key terms

Cholesterol A type of fatty steroid present in cells.

Glycolipid Phospholipid with a sugar chain attached.

Glycoprotein Cell protein with a sugar chain attached.

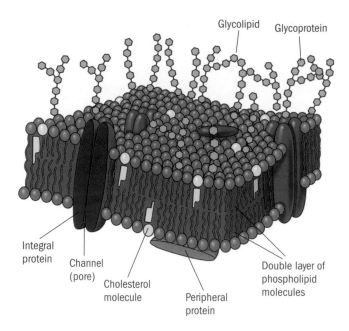

Glycolipid Glycoprotein

Integral protein
Channel (pore)
Cholesterol molecule
Peripheral protein
Double layer of phospholipid molecules

▲ Figure 13.3 The structure of the cell membrane.

Nucleus and chromosomes

The nucleus is limited by the nuclear membrane, which is a phospholipid bilayer interrupted at intervals known as **nuclear pores**. These 'gaps' provide direct communication between the cytoplasm and the nucleus. The soft material inside the nucleus is called **nucleoplasm** and it has no particular features. Embedded in the nucleoplasm is the **chromatin** network composed of **DNA** and proteins. When a cell is dividing, the chromatin network condenses to form distinct

Key terms

Nuclear pore Gap in the nuclear membrane.

Nucleoplasm Soft featureless material contained in the nucleus.

Chromatin A complex of DNA and protein that forms chromosomes during cell division.

DNA Short for deoxyribose nucleic acid, responsible for transmitting inherited characteristics.

Chromosomes Thread-like structures seen during cell division composed of DNA and proteins.

chromosomes carrying genetic units. There are 23 pairs of chromosomes in humans. Other species have different numbers of chromosomes.

Another type of nucleic acid is also found in the nucleus and this is **RNA**. It is linked with controlling certain chemical activities taking place inside the cell. Lastly, there is the nucleolus or several nucleoli and these are believed to be the site for the production of RNA.

Key terms

RNA Ribose nucleic acid, associated with controlling the chemical activities within the cell.

DNA

DNA is made up of units called **nucleotide**s and these repeat along the length of the molecule. A nucleotide consists of a **base**, sugar and phosphate grouping. There are four different bases in DNA: adenine, guanine,

Key terms

Nucleotide Structural unit of DNA and RNA consisting of a base, sugar and phosphate grouping.

Base Chemically a purine or pyrimidine structure such as adenine, guanine, thymine, cytosine and uracil.

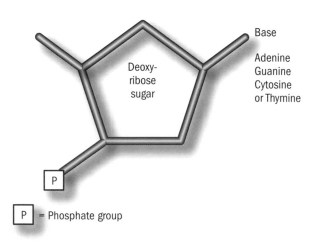

Deoxy-ribose sugar

Base

Adenine Guanine Cytosine or Thymine

P

P = Phosphate group

▲ Figure 13.4 A nucleotide.

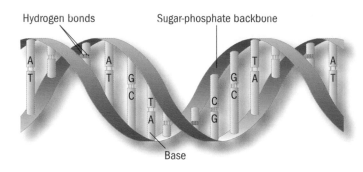

Hydrogen bonds   Sugar-phosphate backbone

Base

▲ Figure 13.5 The structure of DNA.

Theory into practice

The only difference between one strand of DNA and another is the sequence of the bases but if we know the bases on one strand of DNA we can work out the sequence of the other strand.

1 When the sequence is TAGGCAATC, what will the sequence on the other strand be?

2 If the sequence is TGGACTAAGT, what will it be?

3 What do you think needs to happen for DNA to repeat or replicate itself during cell division?

cytosine and thymine, often referred to by their initial letters for simplicity. Using a sophisticated form of X-rays and chemical analyses, teams of scientists were able to propose a model for DNA and later work has proved this to be true.

The bases always combine in the same way, adenine and thymine together and guanine and cytosine. So A and T and G and C form chemical 'rungs' with the sugar and phosphate molecules forming the sides of the ladder. The pairs of bases are held together by hydrogen bonds. However, the ladder looks as if it has been in a tornado as it is twisted in to a spiral shape known as a double helix (a helix is a spiral shape).

The DNA must unwind and split at the hydrogen bonds so that each strand can form a new strand using raw materials in the cytoplasm. Enzymes assist in the process.

Thus two new DNA strands are formed, still in the nucleus, using the 'old' one as a pattern or template. Each has one 'old' strand and one new strand made from raw materials and is an exact copy of the original.

If the DNA is in the nucleus and the raw materials are in the cytoplasm, how do you think they get together? The answer is that the nuclear membrane contains pores and the

raw materials enter the nucleus through the pores.

A sequence of bases on a section of DNA forms a code, or set of instructions, for cell metabolism. A particular pattern of bases will form a gene or unit of inheritance.

Metabolism is governed by enzymes which catalyse all reactions. Enzymes are proteins and the sequence of bases on a particular stretch of DNA forms the code for production of enzymes and other proteins. Proteins are made up of amino acids and the bases control which amino acids are linked together to form the specific protein.

DNA never leaves the nucleus under normal circumstances and proteins are made in ribosomes on the rough endoplasmic reticulum in the cell, so clearly an intermediary must carry this code of bases from DNA

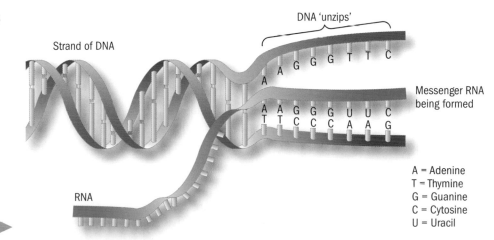

Strand of DNA

DNA 'unzips'

Messenger RNA being formed

RNA

A = Adenine
T = Thymine
G = Guanine
C = Cytosine
U = Uracil

Figure 13.6 Transcription of messenger ▶ RNA (mRNA) from a section of DNA.

in the nucleus to the ribosomes in the cell. This is the function of a type of RNA called messenger RNA and written briefly as **mRNA**.

Theory into practice

When DNA is not faithfully copied, this is called a mutation and so cell metabolism is affected.

1 Name two inherited conditions produced by mutations.

2 Explain why cell metabolism would be affected.

3 Explain why inherited diseases are currently difficult to treat.

4 What may happen if an individual with an inherited condition has children?

Key terms

mRNA Messenger RNA; carries the code for the synthesis of a protein and acts as a template for its formation.

In RNA, which exists mainly as a single strand, the sugar structure is slightly different (ribose instead of deoxyribose) and thymine is replaced by another base called uracil (U).

This type of RNA is made when a particular protein is needed, rather like a special order, but it is made in exactly the same way as DNA replicates itself. A section of DNA unwinds and splits and this time only one strand acts as the template and using enzymes and raw materials, the mRNA is made up on the template strand, sometimes called the coding strand.

The section of mRNA formed detaches itself from the DNA, which 'zips' back up into its double helix. Newly-formed mRNA moves through the nuclear pores to the

Theory into practice

The mRNA is made opposite the coding strand.

1 What would be the sequence of bases for a section of DNA as TCCGAGT?

2 Try another one – CCTCAAGAG.

3 What do you think happens next?

Don't forget to substitute uracil for thymine.

ribosomes. The process of making mRNA on the DNA template is called **transcription.**

There are special gene regulatory proteins that tailor the number of transcripted copies to be made according to cell needs.

Genes can code for similar proteins and the mRNA can be cut and spliced to make different proteins. The parts of the mRNA that have been copied and removed from the gene are called introns and those that have been kept are called exons.

Ribosomes are made of another type of RNA called ribosomal RNA or **rRNA** in short. Ribosomes become attached to the mRNA strand and the process of converting the code into a sequence of amino acids begins. This process is known as **translation.**

Three bases on the mRNA correspond to one amino acid and this is known as a **codon**. There are

Key terms

Transcription The process of forming mRNA from a template of DNA.

Ribosome A tiny cell organelle responsible for protein synthesis.

rRNA Ribosomal RNA, the type of RNA found in the ribosomes.

Translation The process of forming a protein molecule at ribosomes from an mRNA template.

Codon A sequence of bases on mRNA which correspond to a particular amino acid.

many more codons than amino acids, so several codons can form one particular amino acid. There are 20 known amino acids. The sequence of bases for all amino acids has long been known. Three amino acids and their codons are given below as an example:

Phenylalanine   UUC and UUU
Glutamine   CAA and CAG
Valine   GUA, GUC, GUG and GUU.

A small molecule of yet another different type of RNA carries the amino acids to the ribosome to be formed into a protein chain – this is known as transfer RNA or **tRNA** in short.

tRNA

Two tRNA molecules with their amino acids can attach to a ribosome at the same time and a **peptide bond** will form between them; the ribosome then rolls on the mRNA and third and fourth amino acids are added, each forming a peptide bond with the next in the chain and so on.

All types of RNA are made by transcription of a relevant section (gene) of DNA in the nucleus.

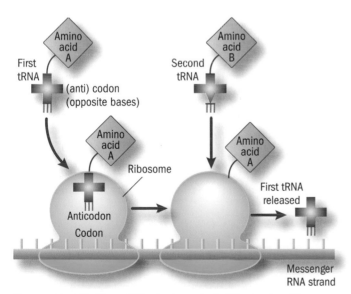

There are at least 20 different tRNA molecules coding for different amino acids

▲ **Figure 13.7 How mRNA translates into protein synthesis at a ribosome.**

Theory into practice

In Book 1, Unit 5: *Fundamentals of anatomy and physiology*, you learned about the digestion of proteins in the diet and that the end products of protease digestion were amino acids.

1 What is the composition of both dietary and metabolic proteins?

2 Which substances are needed to make proteins and to break them down?

3 What are the chemical bonds called that link units together in a protein?

Endoplasmic reticulum (ER)

This is a system of flattened membranous sacs which fills the cytoplasmic part of the cell. It is continuous with the plasma membrane and the nuclear pores. Much of the ER has a rough appearance because it is studded with tiny black bodies known as the ribosomes – this is known as **rough ER**. Some parts of the membranous sacs do not carry ribosomes and this is known as **smooth ER**.

Key terms

tRNA A small molecule of RNA which carries amino acids to the ribosome to be made into protein.

Peptide bond A chemical bond formed between the amine and carboxyl groups of two amino acids by the removal of the elements of water.

Rough ER Endoplasmic reticulum studded with ribosomes.

Smooth ER Endoplasmic reticulum without ribosomes.

Ribosomes

You have already learned the location of most ribosomes as small spherical bodies on the ER. However, some also exist freely in the cytoplasm. They consist of 65 per cent rRNA and 35 per cent protein and exist in very large numbers, particularly in cells producing proteins for export (for example, certain cells in the pancreas which manufacture insulin, a protein hormone). rRNA is closely associated with the nucleoli, which are believed to be the site of synthesis. Structurally, ribosomes consist of two sub units, one large and one small, each composed of protein and rRNA.

Golgi body

This has also been called the Golgi complex or apparatus. It appears as a stack of flattened membranes with numerous **vesicles** pinched off the ends. These are termed Golgi vesicles. Some scientists believe that it is a specialised part of the smooth ER.

Key terms

Golgi body A series or pile of flattened membranes which lie close to the nucleus.

Vesicles These can also be called cysts, vacuoles, etc., which usually mean fluid-filled sacs or pouches.

Mitochondria

Mitochondria (the singular is mitochondrion) are round or sausage-shaped bodies found in large numbers (1000 plus) in the cytoplasm. Each is double-layered and the inner layer is folded to form internal 'shelves' called **cristae**. Enzymes which catalyse the breakdown of glucose are dissolved in the internal fluid while enzymes associated with the formation of **ATP** lie in order on the cristae. Strangely, mitochondria have their own ribosomes and some believe that they are the remnants of simple bacteria which became trapped inside cells millions of years ago.

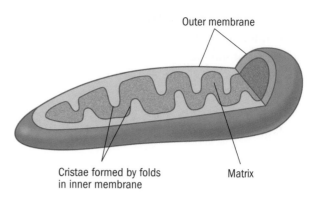

Outer membrane

Cristae formed by folds in inner membrane

Matrix

▲ Figure 13.8 The structure of a single mitochondrion.

Key terms

Cristae Internal folds or shelves of mitochondria holding an orderly arrangement of enzymes for ATP production.

ATP Adenosine triphosphate; a chemical whose role in the cell is to store energy and release it for use when necessary.

Lysosomes

Scattered throughout the cell are vesicles of digestive enzymes known as **lysosomes**. They are the 'cleaners' or recyclers of the cell, clearing up debris, digesting old unwanted organelles and infectious agents like bacteria. Unwanted material, usually membrane-bound, fuses with one or more lysosomes and the digestive enzymes break the material down to raw materials. Whole, damaged or old cells can also be destroyed in this way, a process called **autolysis**. Some believe that cancer-causing agents, infectious organisms and poisons may act by damaging the membranes of lysosomes,

Key terms

Lysosomes Membranous vesicles filled with digestive enzymes.

Autolysis Self-destruction of the cell by lysosomes.

thus causing cell damage or even mutations of genetic material.

Other microstructures

Certain other microscopic structures, including centrioles and cilia, exist in some cells or in most cells at particular times.

■ Centrioles

These are two tiny hollow cylinders that exist in a darkly-staining part of the cytoplasm called the centrosome, close to the nucleus. Each contains a complex system of microtubules (nine groups of three called triplets) that are capable of replicating themselves. They do this at the beginning of cell division, migrating to opposite ends of a cell. A spindle of microtubules is formed between them and these control the separation of the chromosomes to form two new cells.

■ Cilia

These are microscopic filaments that protrude from the free surface of a cell and in humans they are usually found adjacent to mucus-secreting cells. They 'beat' rhythmically to effect transport of mucus and other materials such as debris in the respiratory passages and ova in the reproductive tract. The base of a cilium has the same microtubular structure of the centrioles and is believed to be formed from them.

Functions

You have already learned many functions of the parts of the cell (organelles) as you explored their structure and also when you studied them in Book 1, Unit 5: *Fundamentals of anatomy and physiology*. The following table will serve as both revision and supplementary information.

Organelle	Functions
Cell membrane	• Acts as a selective barrier to substances entering and leaving the cell. • Holds certain receptor sites to which other molecules, such as hormones, can attach. • Contributes to the immunological identity of the cell. • Interacts with the surrounding environment. • Interacts with adjacent cells. • Due to the fluid-like behaviour of the membrane, 'holes' or damage can be repaired almost instantaneously.
Nuclear membrane	• Acts as a selective barrier to substances entering and leaving the nucleus. • Nuclear pores allow communication between the ER (see below) and the nucleus. • Defines the boundary of genetic material such as DNA.
Nucleus	• Controls cellular activities. • Contains chromosomes and thus genetic information. • Site of transcription of mRNA from DNA. • Ultimately responsible for protein production in the ribosomes. • Nuclear division precedes cell division.
Chromosome	• Carries theoretical units of inheritance called genes. • Contains DNA responsible for controlling the protein production. • Capable of replication prior to cell division.
Endoplasmic reticulum (ER)	• Forms an internal cellular transport system. • Enables communication between the cell membrane, the nucleus and the environment. • Carries ribosomes responsible for the production of proteins (rough ER). • Synthesises lipids from fatty acids and glycerol and transports these to the Golgi body (smooth ER).
Ribosomes	• Bind to rough ER. • Bind to mRNA. • Enable translation of mRNA to produce proteins.

(Continued overleaf)

Organelle	Functions
Golgi body	• Receives proteins from the ribosomes via the ER and chemically modifies them for export (particularly in secreting cells). • Produces vesicles to transport the modified proteins to the cell membrane for release. • Receives and modifies lipids from the smooth ER for transport to the cell membrane. • Produces lysosomes containing digestive enzymes.
Mitochondria	• Complete the oxidation of glucose (initially this begins in the cytoplasm) to release energy. • Trap the energy released to form ATP which is used to power the metabolic functions of the cells.
Cilia	• Transport mucus and other materials that may be stuck in them to the exterior by continuous rhythmic beating.

Table 13.1 Organelle functions.

Cell types

You have learned about the types of cells in Unit 5 and understand that there are basic categories of epithelia, connective, muscle and nervous tissues with many subdivisions. You may like to revisit this section of Unit 5. In this unit, you will learn how some of these types of cells are specifically associated with the ultrastructure of the cell you have just studied.

Epithelia

Remember!

Epithelia line internal and external surfaces and body cavities. Cuboidal epithelia are often associated with glandular activity, while columnar cells bearing cilia line, for example, the trachea and bronchi.

The basement membrane on which epithelial cells lie is a **mucopolysaccharide**, a complex mix of protein and long sugar chains; mucopolysaccharides are started at the ribosomes and the polysaccharide or sugar chains are then added in the Golgi body.

Simple squamous epithelia are much flattened cells which have a large surface-area-to-volume ratio, allowing rapid passage of substances through the cell membrane.

Goblet cells which secrete mucus have prominent Golgi bodies which package the mucopolysaccharide for export from the cell. The protein component of mucus is made in the ribosomes on the rough ER.

Ciliated columnar epithelia, lining the trachea and bronchi for example, have prominent centrioles, always associated with cilia, and large numbers of mitochondria to release energy for the rhythmic movement.

Cuboidal epithelia are associated with the inner lining of glands, such as in the breast, thyroid and sweat glands.

They contain large numbers of mitochondria, ribosomes and prominent Golgi bodies.

Key terms

Mucopolysaccharide A molecule made from protein and long sugar chains; it is one of the most important biological molecules.

Connective tissues

Theory into practice

Blood is a loose connective tissue that you have already learned about.

1 Which blood cell is usually portrayed as spherical but is rarely that shape in life?

2 This type of blood cell is often said to be granular. Under the electron microscope, these granules were found to be a particular type of cell organelle. Which organelle is more abundant in this blood cell?

3 Explain the function of these organelles in relation to the role of these blood cells.

4 Which cell organelle is conspicuously absent in red blood cells?

Key terms

Myofibrils Bundles of parallel myofibrils are contained in a muscle fibre.

Filaments Protein filaments of two types, actin and myosin, are contained in a myofibril. Contraction is achieved when these slide between each other.

Sarcolemma The special name given to the cell membrane of a muscle fibre.

Sarcoplasm The name given to the cytoplasm of a muscle fibre.

Take it further

The theory of muscle contraction is known as the sliding filament hypothesis. You can research this further in advanced science or biology texts.

Calcium is also required for muscle contraction and is supplied through vesicles from the Golgi body.

All connective tissues consist of a matrix (background material) in which particular cells are found. The matrix is secreted by these connective tissue cells.

Muscle

Muscle is composed of multinucleate muscle fibres which are in fact very long cells. Embryonic cells fuse together to make the multinucleate fibres. Muscle cells and nerve cells (neurones) are called excitable cells because they are capable of responding to stimuli. Each fibre is composed of **myofibrils**, long elements lying parallel to the fibre. Each myofibril is made of protein **filaments** which in some muscle gives a characteristic banding appearance. The cell membrane is known as a **sarcolemma** and the cytoplasm is **sarcoplasm** ('sarco' means flesh). Muscle contraction occurs by filaments sliding between each other with great amounts of energy from ATP. It is not surprising, therefore, to find huge numbers of mitochondria sandwiched between muscle fibres.

Nervous tissue

Nerve cells or neurones are highly specialised excitable cells with long processes called **axons** and **dendrons**. Neurones have lost their ability to divide as a result of specialism so there is very little chromatin in the nucleus although nucleoli are prominent. Distinctive granules in the cytoplasm (called **Nissl granules**) are concentrations of rough ER and mitochondria, lysosomes and Golgi bodies can be found. At the swollen

Key terms

Axons These are processes leading nerve impulses away from the cell body.

Dendrons These are processes taking impulses towards the cell body.

Nissl granules Characteristic dark granules found in the cytoplasm of neurones.

end of the axon is the **synaptic knob** containing vesicles of **neurotransmitter,** commonly acetylcholine. These are Golgi vesicles and ATP is required for their discharge and recycling. The cell membrane has special sites for receptors.

Assessment activity 13.1

P1 Describe the microstructure of a typical animal cell and the functions of the main parts.

1   What do the cell organelles look like and what do they do?

M1 Use four examples to explain how the functions of the main cell components relate to overall cell function.

2   How do the functions of the cell organelles play their parts in the role of each of four named types of cells?

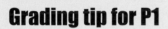

Grading tip for P1

In order to display this without writing up lots of material, you could produce a large diagram of a cell (similar to the one for Book 1, Unit 5, or use the same one) to show the detailed structures of the organelles and use annotations to describe the structure and functions. This could be drawn by you or cut and pasted from downloaded images of organelles. It must be a display of your own work and not a downloaded cell and description from the Internet. If you want to show transcription and translation, for example, you could add extra strips of paper that unfold to display the activities.

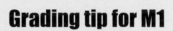

Grading tip for M1

You could choose a ciliated columnar cell or goblet cell, a motor or effector neurone, a white blood cell and a muscle fibre.

The examples listed show one cell from each different type of tissue. However, you could choose two cells from the same type if you wish. You should illustrate your answer to display the various features. If you wish to avoid long descriptions, you could again annotate your diagrams of the cell types with structures related to functions.

You are fully aware that cells are separated from the tissue fluid which bathes them by the cell membrane and that most of the cell organelles have membrane boundaries. Cells are continuously requiring materials from the surroundings and conversely exporting or eliminating materials from the cell to the surroundings. This section will examine the methods by which materials are moved in this two-way process.

States of matter

Matter is material that has substance and occupies space. There are three states of matter that must be distinguished:

- solids
- liquids
- gases.

All these types of matter are made of atoms and molecules. Atoms are the smallest 'bits' of matter that can take part in chemical reactions whereas molecules are composed of one or more atoms and are the smallest amount of a substance that can exist independently and keep its characteristic features. Even an atom is composed of smaller particles known as protons and neutrons in a positively charged nucleus and has negatively charged electrons present in a shell which orbits the nucleus. All atoms exhibit random motion and this is important in the state of matter.

Solid

Theory into practice

There are many solids in the human body.

1   Name three solids in the body.

2   How do you know these are solids?

3   Can you suggest what is happening to their atoms or molecules to make them solids?

You might have mentioned bone, cartilage and skin and thought that they were solids because they were firm to the touch or because you know that they are not liquids or gases. These responses would be acceptable, but did you know that they are solids because the atoms/molecules are packed so tightly together that the motion is reduced to a very tiny vibration, so tiny that you could not perceive it? These features define a solid – they cannot flow!

Liquid

Theory into practice

Similarly there are several liquids in the human body.

1   Can you name three liquids in the human body?

2   How do you know that these are liquids?

3   Using the same sort of information that you had with solids, state the features of a liquid.

You probably chose blood, tissue fluid, lymph or urine and said that they were liquids because they could flow. The atoms/molecules are further apart than in a solid and so the atoms have more movement, resulting in flowing. Liquids take up the shape of their 'container' whether this is a vessel (as in blood and lymph), tiny spaces between cells or a hollow organ, like the bladder.

Gas

Gases also occur in the human body – oxygen, carbon dioxide and nitrogen are common constituents of the air that we breathe in. The atoms/molecules of gases are much further apart from each other and are able to move about quite freely. Gases also flow.

Materials

In this section, you will learn about different types of material that you will meet in the body.

Particulate material

Particles such as dust from coal, asbestos, silica, etc., and carbon particles in polluted air can reach even the finest air passages, causing scarring and disease. Such particles are very fine and as small as 0.005 mm in diameter. Particulate material can enter any open wound and rest in deeper tissues where the macrophages will attempt to engulf and digest them. Invading bacteria digested by lysosomes will leave some debris behind such as particulate matter. Images of the lungs of smokers or workers in 'dust' occupations show blackened tissues resulting from particulate matter.

Ionic material

This is material containing atoms which may have a positive or negative charge as a result of gaining or losing electrons. Such atoms or groups of atoms are called ions or electrolytes. Ionic material is designated by the relevant charge shown against the atom, thus Na^+, K^+, H^+, Cl^-, $NH2^+$, $COOH^-$, etc.

(In order, these are positively charged sodium and potassium ions, hydrogen ion, chloride ion negatively charged, amine group positive and carboxyl group negatively charged.) Ions like these are continuously moving into and out of the cell as they are often required or eliminated products from the thousands of chemical reactions occurring in cells.

In solution

Substances which are capable of dissolving in a liquid are called solutes – the liquid is the solvent and the solvent dissolved in the solute is a solution. Water is the most common molecule in the human body (nine out of every 10 molecules are water). Water is the most important solvent in the human body and most chemical reactions involve molecules dissolved in water.

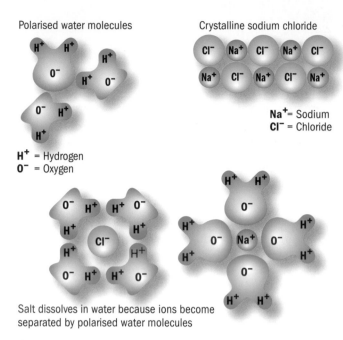

Figure 13.9 Salt dissolving in water.

Water is composed of two hydrogen atoms linked by chemical bonds to one oxygen atom. The hydrogen atoms have slight positive charges and the oxygen a slight negative charge so that water exists as a polar molecule. When a substance like salt (sodium chloride) is introduced into water, the water molecules are attracted to the positively charged sodium ions and negatively charged chloride ions and these become surrounded by water molecules. Sodium and chloride ions separate from the crystalline salt and thus are said to be dissolved.

Molecules having enough polar bonds or ionized groups will dissolve in water and are therefore hydrophilic. Molecules with electrically neutral groups do not dissolve in water and are hydrophobic. Such molecules will dissolve in non-polar solvents such as carbon tetrachloride (which is used as a dry cleaning solvent for grease stains on clothes).

Colloidal forms

A colloid consists of larger particles (but which are too small to be seen with a light microscope) which are dispersed or scattered throughout a medium (gas, liquid or solid).

Reflect

PVA glue (a whitish sticky material) can flow but more slowly than liquid – this is a colloid. If you have ever seen anyone make original starch (not spray starch) for stiffening collars, this is a colloid too. Uncooked egg white is a clear colloid.

■ Protein sols

Cytoplasm is an example of a colloid caused by the protein molecules which are not readily dissolved in water, so it is a protein sol. Blood plasma is another protein sol because of its plasma protein content. Polysaccharide molecules can also produce colloids when mixed with water. They are not readily soluble as the molecules, like proteins, can be too large to simply dissolve.

■ Emulsions

An emulsion occurs when one liquid is dispersed in droplets in another, such as fat in milk. Emulsifying agents cause one liquid to form very small droplets which increases the surface area. This is what happens when bile salts are added to fats in chyme in the small intestine – the fats break up into thousands of tiny globules producing a milky appearance. This provides an enormous surface area which the pancreatic enzymes, dissolved in the water of the chyme, can act upon, causing fat digestion to break down to fatty acids and glycerol. (See Book 1, Unit 5.)

Movement of materials

You have learned about states of matter and materials and now you will learn about the ways in which materials are moved into and out of cells.

Diffusion

You know that molecules, atoms and ions are in constant random motion and that this is most marked in gases and liquids because they are further apart. When there is a large number of molecules of a substance and a small number in another area, with no effective barrier between them, this random motion will cause the numbers to even up. This is known as **diffusion.**

A definition of diffusion is:

The movement of molecules from a region of high concentration to a region of low concentration.

Notice the emphasis on concentration – these must be different and this is known as a **concentration gradient**. The greater the concentration gradient the faster will be the rate of diffusion. Clearly, this will not happen instantly and so time is also important. As the numbers of molecules become more evenly distributed, the *net* movement of molecules will slow down and eventually stop.

This is said to be a state of **equilibrium**. However, it is important to understand that random motion is still occurring – it is just that as many move in one direction as in the other (in other words there is no net movement in one direction).

In the body, diffusion often takes place through cell membranes, but these are freely passable to the diffusing molecules provided that the barrier is thin. Note that in the lungs there are only two simple squamous epithelial cells separating the dissolved gases in the alveoli from the blood in the pulmonary capillaries.

There is no source of energy required for diffusion of molecules.

Key terms

Diffusion The movement of molecules from a region of high concentration to a region of low concentration.

Concentration gradient The difference between opposing concentrations.

Equilibrium The state of having no net movement of molecules because the concentrations have evened up.

Facilitated diffusion

Some materials diffuse through the cell membrane by a related process known as **facilitated diffusion**.

To facilitate something means to make it easier and the protein channels in the cell membrane assist in transporting molecules such as glucose and urea into and out of cells. Clearly, not only is the concentration gradient important here but also the number of channel proteins capable of allowing the materials through. The channel proteins have a shape containing a special receptor site for the molecule to be transported and then change shape to prevent further molecules binding until it is released on the opposite side of the membrane. One of the most vital systems depending on facilitated diffusion is the transport of glucose across cell membranes into the cell. Without the existence of the carrier proteins, the cell is virtually impermeable to glucose. When the glucose is released into the cytoplasm, it is almost immediately metabolized, thus maintaining the concentration gradient.

Key terms

Facilitated diffusion Diffusion down a concentration gradient that is dependent on energy-using carrier molecules or channel membranes.

Reflect

In the absence of insulin, a hormone produced by the pancreas, target cells are impermeable to glucose penetration.

Is it likely that insulin binds to the carrier proteins to cause them to open on the tissue fluid side?

Osmosis

Osmosis is a special type of diffusion of water molecules. It can be defined as:

The movement of water molecules from a region of high concentration (of water molecules) to a region of low concentration (of water molecules) through a selectively permeable membrane.

Once again there is a concentration gradient *but* it is only concerned with numbers of water molecules. In addition, there is mention of a selectively (sometimes also called partially) permeable membrane. You can think of permeable as meaning 'leaky'; a freely permeable membrane will allow most small molecules to pass through. A **selectively permeable membrane** allows some molecules through but not others. The molecules are usually too large.

Imagine a U-shaped tube in which there is a barrier of selectively permeable membrane in the centre. One limb of the tube contains water and the other a solution containing large molecules, say a protein solution in equal volumes. The presence of the protein molecules takes up a lot of space – consequently there are less water molecules in that limb. There is a high concentration of water molecules on one side and a low concentration on the other. Water molecules will move through the selectively permeable membrane towards the low concentration on the 'protein' side, resulting in unequal volumes. This will continue until equilibrium has been reached.

Theoretically, a pressure could be supplied to the top of the protein solution to prevent water molecules passing through the selectively permeable membrane from the water limb. This is known as the **osmotic pressure** of the protein solution.

Key terms

Osmosis The movement of water molecules from a region of high concentration to a region of low concentration (of water molecules) through a selectively permeable membrane.

Selectively permeable membrane A membrane such as the phospholipid bilayer which allows some molecules to pass through by osmosis but not others.

Osmotic pressure The pressure exerted by large molecules to draw water to them. Plasma proteins in blood plasma have an osmotic pressure necessary to return tissue fluid.

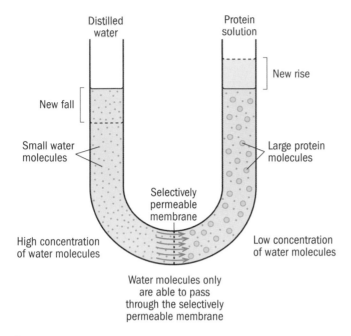

Distilled water

Protein solution

New rise

New fall

Small water molecules

Large protein molecules

Selectively permeable membrane

High concentration of water molecules

Low concentration of water molecules

Water molecules only are able to pass through the selectively permeable membrane

▲ Figure 13.10 Osmosis.

Cell membranes can act as selectively permeable membranes to some substances. Osmosis occurs in the distal convoluted tubules of the kidney nephrons as they pass through a region of high sodium concentration in order to concentrate urine (see page 192).

Active transport

There are many examples of materials passing through living cells against a concentration gradient and neither diffusion nor osmosis can account for this type of movement. This is **active transport**; the word active is used because this is an energy-using process powered by the release of energy from ATP in the cell (from the mitochondria). Carbohydrate digestion in the small intestine produces glucose and this may require active transport across cells of villi against a concentration gradient.

Key terms

Active transport The movement of materials against a concentration gradient using energy from ATP.

Endocytosis

This is the process of taking materials which are outside of the cell into the cell by **phagocytosis** or **pinocytosis**.

Phagocytosis literally means cell eating and pinocytosis means cell drinking. The process demonstrates the fluid nature of the cell membrane rather well. Regions of the cell membrane fold into the cell or invaginate forming a pouch. The neck of the pouch gets narrower and eventually pinches off so that the material and a small volume of tissue fluid are enclosed within the cell in a membrane-bound pocket or vesicle. Larger particles such as bacteria and cell debris (from damaged cells) are taken in this way; as the endocytic vesicle moves through the cell it will merge with lysosomes and the material will be digested and broken down to basic raw materials.

Endocytosis can also be used to transport proteins and other chemicals across a cell to be released on the other side. Pinocytosis encloses only tissue fluid, or tissue fluid plus some specific molecules the cell requires. The specific molecules bind to carrier proteins in the membrane.

Pinocytosis occurs in all cells but phagocytosis occurs only in special cells such as macrophages and granulocytes (white blood cells also called phagocytes). Endocytosis and **exocytosis** require energy from ATP to accomplish the tasks.

Key terms

Phagocytosis The engulfing and destruction of cell debris and foreign bodies by mobile cells which produce arm-like extensions to surround the material.

Pinocytosis A process similar to phagocytosis but involving pinching off a vesicle filled with tiissue fluid to take into the cell.

Endocytosis Transport of materials from the outside of a cell to the inside.

Exocytosis The reverse of endocytosis, i.e. transporting materials from inside the cell to the outside.

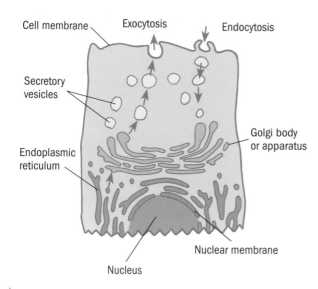

△ Figure 13.11 Endocytosis and exocytosis.

Exocytosis

As you will anticipate from the name, exocytosis means the process of releasing materials from the inside of the cell to the tissue fluid. Membrane-bound vesicles move through the cell to the cell membrane and fuse with it, releasing the contents as they do so. It is a way of introducing secretory molecules into body systems and also a method of replacing the cell membrane used up in endocytosis. This method is used for molecules that cannot pass through the cell membrane by diffusion or osmosis.

Factors affecting movement

The influences on movement will be considered in the next section. However, the availability of energy from ATP, and the fluidity of the cell membrane, are clearly important for all processes except for diffusion and osmosis. The surface area and thickness of any intervening selectively permeable or freely permeable membranes will affect the rates of diffusion and osmosis. There are also complex cellular stimuli that cause endocytosis and exocytosis to occur that are beyond the scope of this unit.

Influences on movement of materials

There many known influences on why materials move in cells, into cells and out of cells and possibly many influences that are not yet known too. You will learn about some known influences.

Size

You have already learned that molecular size is important in osmosis; that a larger molecule cannot move through a selectively permeable membrane such as a protein like albumin, one of the plasma proteins. You have also learned that protein molecules cannot pass simply by diffusion and osmosis and are often transported across a cell by endocytosis.

The size of any surface for transport is vital as it must be large enough to allow sufficient molecules or ions to be transported to accommodate the metabolic processes in a cell. For this reason, the surface-area-to-volume ratio for any cell is critical. Surface area is the area of cell membrane which must support the internal cytoplasmic and nuclear activities. Cells cannot just keep on growing larger as the area of cell membrane will not be adequate for exchanging materials for the volume of the cytoplasm.

Theory into practice

Take a jelly cube (or a cube of plasticine). Measure the length, width and depth of its sides and calculate the surface area and volume. Cut the cube into four even quarters and repeat the calculations.

1 Calculate the surface area/volume relationship of the original cube.

2 Calculate the surface area/volume relationship of the quarter cube.

3 Comment on the results.

4 Explain what this means for cell metabolism.

5 When the optimum size of a cell has been reached, what will happen next?

Size will also be important in terms of width and length of a surface carrying out transport of materials. Here are some examples.

- The surface area of single-celled alveoli in the lungs, if spread out flat on a surface, would total the area of a football pitch.
- The surface area of the villi in the ileum of the small intestine would be similar.
- There are over a million nephrons in a small organ like a kidney.

All these demonstrate the need for an enormous surface area for transport that must be folded and folded to make organs capable of compacting into the human body.

Distance

As with size, so with distance. Any disease that affects the distance to be travelled reduces the efficiency of the transport process. For example, dissolved gases such as oxygen and carbon dioxide pass across the alveolar/capillary interface with ease in health. However, a patient with pneumonia has extra fluid and mucus in the alveoli and may suffer considerably from the lack of oxygen. Such a condition, often known as **cyanosis**, results in a bluish-purple tinge to blood vessels visible in the nail beds, ear lobes, cheeks and lips.

Pneumoconiosis, the dust disease of the lungs, produces fibrosis and scarring. Again, this results in cyanosis and of course respiratory difficulties.

Key terms

Cyanosis Bluish colour of the skin and mucous membranes indicating poor oxygenation of blood.

Pneumoconiosis Industrial disease caused by inhaling dust particles over a period of time.

Diffusion can distribute molecules quickly over a short distance but is very slow over more than a few centimetres. Vander, Sherman and Luciano (1990) state:

It takes glucose 3.5s to reach 90 per cent equilibrium at 10 μm (10 thousandths of a millimetre) away from a source of glucose, such as the blood, but it would take over 11 years to reach the same concentration at a point 10 cm away.

Temperature

Increasing the temperature also increases **kinetic energy** (the energy of motion) and so molecules will move faster in diffusion and osmosis. The average speed of molecules depends on temperature and the mass of the molecule.

Key terms

Kinetic energy The energy of motion.

Vander et al (1990) report on diffusion thus:

At body temperature, an average molecule of water moves at about 2500 km/h whereas a molecule of glucose, which is ten times heavier, moves at about 850 km/h. In solutions, such rapidly moving molecules cannot travel very far before colliding with other molecules. They bounce off each other like rubber balls, undergoing millions of collisions every second. Each collision alters the direction of the molecule's movement, so that the path of any one molecule becomes unpredictable.

Conversely, cooling temperatures means that less kinetic energy is available, resulting in the slowing down of molecular movement.

Active transport, endocytosis and exocytosis systems will increase too, up to a point. However, as they depend on energy systems, carriers and the nature of the fluid cell membrane, a continually increasing temperature will begin to change the shape of protein molecules rendering them inactive.

Concentration gradient

This has been referred to in the section on diffusion.

Osmotic potential

This is the power of a solution to gain or lose water molecules through a membrane. Weaker or more dilute solutions have higher osmotic potentials than concentrated solutions; it follows therefore that pure water has the highest **osmotic potential**. When tissue fluid returns to the blood, it does so by osmosis because the plasma proteins in blood plasma have a lower osmotic potential than the aqueous tissue fluid – the single-celled capillary wall acts as the selectively permeable membrane.

Key terms

Osmotic potential The power of a solution to gain or lose water molecules through a membrane.

In context

Under normal circumstances, some protein molecules inevitably escape from capillaries into interstitial spaces (spaces between cells filled with tissue fluid). In other circumstances associated with diseases of the renal system, excess protein can accumulate in the interstitial spaces.

1   **Explain one circumstance that could cause more protein than normal to accumulate in interstitial spaces.**

2   **Explain the change in osmotic potential of tissue fluid caused by excess protein.**

3   **What effect would this have on the return of fluid from tissue fluid to the blood? What sign would doctors notice? Can you give this a clinical name?**

Cells are capable of accumulating materials in low concentration from the surroundings and also capable of eliminating water found in high concentration outside the cell. In this way, osmotic potential energy is transformed from chemical energy.

Electrochemical gradient

Cells have a difference in electrical charge across the cell membrane, the exterior of the cell membrane carrying positive charges and the interior negative charges. This

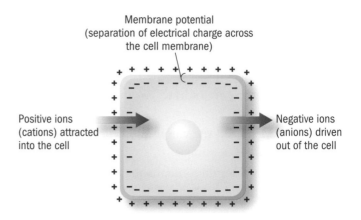

▲ Figure 13.12 The electrochemical gradient operating across a cell membrane.

is often referred to as a **membrane potential** and it will affect the diffusion of ions across the membrane. The result of this is that positively charged ions like sodium and potassium will be attracted into the cell and negatively charged ions such as chloride ions will be repelled. This force operates even when there is no concentration gradient. This is often referred to as the electrochemical gradient.

Key terms

Membrane potential The potential difference across a cell membrane caused by different ions.

Permeability of cell membrane

Most charged or polar molecules and ions diffuse across the phospholipid bilayer very slowly or even not at all, whereas non-polar molecules (those not carrying electrical charges) diffuse quite rapidly. This is possible because they dissolve in the fatty acid chains or the lipid layer of the cell membrane. Materials such as dissolved oxygen, carbon dioxide, fatty acids and steroid molecules diffuse in this way quite easily and rapidly. It appears then that the lipid part of the membrane acts as a selective barrier. Polar ion movement is dealt with in the next section.

Channel proteins

The rates of entry of non-polar molecules through the cell membranes are very similar in different cells. This is not so for polar ions and molecules; different cells 'import' these at different rates and overall they are much faster than one would expect given their relative insolubility in the lipid bilayer. Experiments have shown that an artificial bilayer membrane containing no protein results in virtual impermeability to ions such as sodium, potassium, chloride and calcium. However, real cell membranes are permeable to these ions. This suggests that the protein channels are responsible for the permeability of the cell membrane to polar ions and molecules. Shapes of membrane protein channels are varied and related to the ions they allow through. The channels are extremely small so preventing other molecules from passing. The channels are selective as gate-keepers and permeability to particular ions depends on the number and variety of protein channels in the cell membrane of particular cells.

Carrier molecules

You have already learned about **carrier molecules** in the section on facilitated diffusion. There are many types of carrier molecules in membranes, each specific to a particular substance or group of substances by way of its characteristic binding site. For example, amino acids and sugars have different binding sites and carrier proteins. Once again, the rate of movement will be influenced by the number of carrier proteins in cell membranes and by the number of binding sites occupied with transporting molecules at any one time.

Key terms

Carrier molecules Molecules that bind to others, facilitating their transport.

Assessment activity 13.2

P2 Explain the ways in which materials move into and out of cells.

1   What are the processes which enable materials to enter and leave cells?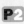

Grading tip for P2

Explain the processes of diffusion, facilitated diffusion, osmosis, active transport, endocytosis and exocytosis, illustrating your answer where this helps understanding. If you intend going further for merit then after each explanation of process, follow with:

M2 Explain the factors that influence the movement of materials into and out cells.

2   What changes the processes enabling materials to enter and leave cells? **M2**

Grading tip for M2

For each process in P2, explain the relevant factors influencing the movement of materials. For example, size, distance, temperature and concentration gradient are all relevant to diffusion. This will give your writing structure and coherence.

D1 Analyse the role of the phospholipid bilayer in terms of the movement of materials into and out of cells.

3   How is the phospholipid bilayer involved in the passage of materials to and from the cells?

Grading tip for D1

You need to read through the whole of this section on movement of materials and attempt some Internet research as well. There is plenty of scope in the text to discuss the movement of polar and non-polar molecules/ions through the bilayer, illustrating your writing with examples and bringing in channel proteins and carrier molecules as well.

In this section, you will learn about the importance of water, its role in the body and its unique properties. The distribution of water into body compartments and the types of material which are found in water are also included. The section will examine the role of electrolytes and the maintenance of pH in the body.

Constituents of body fluids

Water

Remember!

Earlier in this unit, you learned that nine out of every 10 molecules, in the millions of molecules contained in the human body, are water molecules. Clearly, water is crucial in the maintenance of living tissue, living processes and life itself. You have learned about water's chemical composition and the fact that it is a polar molecule (the hydrogen atoms carry a slight positive charge and the two oxygen atoms negative charges).

Water is the main component of all body fluids comprising at least 90 per cent of blood plasma, lymph, urine, saliva, digestive juices, bile, cerebrospinal fluid and tissue fluid. Without water, the fluids could not flow and this is essential for the onward progression of all these fluids. Stagnant fluid (i.e. fluid which does not flow because it has no outlet) is always a focus for infection which becomes potentially life-threatening. Water is essential to life because it provides the medium for all metabolic reactions and the transport of essential substances around the body.

Water molecules are constantly being moved between fluid compartments of the body. You will learn later that although some water is made as a by-product of metabolism, this is not sufficient to maintain life, so water is an essential nutrient of the diet.

Solutes

Remember!

Solutes are substances that dissolve in a solvent to produce a solution.

There are many solutes dissolved in water in body fluids. We are going to explore the major solutes.

■ Glucose

Glucose belongs to the class of organic molecules known as carbohydrates which have the general formula of $Cn(H_2O)n$, where n represents any whole number. As you see, there is a link between the name of the group and its

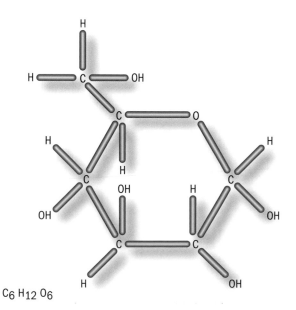

$C_6H_{12}O_6$

▲ **Figure 13.13 The structure of glucose.**

chemical construction because each carbon atom has the elements of water or hydrate attached to it. In glucose, the n is 6 so the accepted formula for glucose is $C_6H_{12}O_6$. A better representation can be seen in Figure 13.13 as this shows the two-dimensional shape of glucose (it is actually three-dimensional but this cannot be easily shown on paper). Five carbon atoms and an oxygen atom form a ring with hydroxyl and hydrogen groups attached to each carbon atom.

Glucose is a monosaccharide (this means single sweet), disaccharides contain two such rings linked together and polysaccharides many rings.

Glucose tastes sweet and is the most common carbohydrate in blood.

Reflect

Sucrose is a disaccharide consisting of two molecules of glucose linked together by a chemical bond. Sucrose is very sweet and is the type of sugar made from plants that we add to tea and coffee.

Starch and glycogen (so-called animal starch) are polysaccharides that are less sweet.

Where in the human body is glycogen found?

The normal range of blood glucose is from 4.5–5.6 mmol per litre or 70–110 mg per 100 mls.

■ Urea

Urea is a metabolic waste product of surplus amino acids.

Dietary proteins are digested to amino acids and absorbed into the blood. Both proteins and amino acids contain nitrogen atoms in their amino group ($-NH_2$) and excess amino acids cannot be stored because of the nitrogen component.

The nitrogen-containing amino group is converted into ammonia (NH_3) inside cells and then is easily transported through the cell membranes into tissue fluid and ultimately blood whence it is transported to the liver. In the liver, ammonia combines with carbon

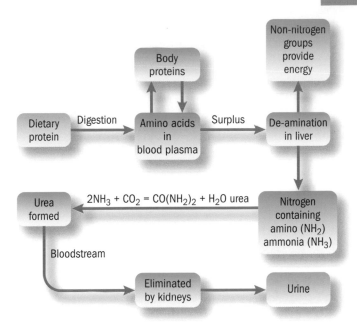

▲ **Figure 13.14 The formation of urea.**

dioxide to form urea. It is important to realise that ammonia is poisonous to cells if allowed to build up and, comparatively, urea is far less toxic. Urea is continuously released back into the bloodstream and removed via the kidneys as a component of urine.

The normal range of urea in the blood is 2.5–6.7 mmol per litre or 8–25 mg per litre.

Electrolytes

These are compounds which, when dissolved in water, **dissociate** (split) into ions. These ions are electrically charged particles capable of conducting electricity – hence their name. For example, salt (sodium chloride) will split into positively charged sodium ions and negatively charged chloride ions (see page 170). It is important to understand that atoms are electrically neutral because the number of electrons (negatively charged) orbiting around the nucleus, and the number of protons (positively charged) in the nucleus, are equal. However, if an atom

Key terms

Dissociate To split into ions.

gains or loses an electron, it gains a charge and becomes an ion. Some atoms can gain or lose more than one electron and gain the relevant number of charges, for example, calcium loses two electrons to become Ca^{2+}. Collectively these ions are referred to as electrolytes. Ions can form from either atoms or molecules by the process of **ionisation**. Ions with a positive charge are called **cations** as they would migrate towards the cathode in electrolysis and negatively charged ions are **anions** as they would migrate to the anode.

Key terms

Ionisation The process of forming ions.

Cations Positively charged ions like sodium and hydrogen.

Anions Negatively charged ions like chloride and hydroxyl.

Some common cations and anions are shown in the table below.

Atom	Symbol	Cation	Anion
Hydrogen	H	H^+	
Sodium	Na	Na^+	
Chlorine	Cl		Cl^-
Potassium	K	K^+	
Calcium	Ca	Ca^{2+}	
Hydroxide	OH		OH^- (hydroyl)
Magnesium	Mg	Mg^{2+}	
Hydrogen carbonate (bicarbonate)	HCO_3		HCO_3^-

Table 13.2 Common cations and anions.

Carbon, oxygen and nitrogen atoms do not dissociate into ions.

■ Acids, bases and salts

Hydrogen has a single proton in the nucleus and a single electron in orbit. When the electron is lost it becomes a positively charged ion as it has one single proton (see Table 13.2).

Substances that give rise to hydrogen ions in solution are known as **acids**.

Key terms

Acid A substance giving rise to hydrogen ions in solution.

An acid is defined as a molecule capable of giving up a hydrogen ion in solution and having a pH (see page 182) less than 7 (pH7 is pure water).

The stomach produces an acid known as hydrochloric acid HCl which ionizes in solution thus:

$$HCl \rightarrow H^+ + Cl^-$$

Another important acid produced by increased respiration is carbonic acid formed when carbon dioxide dissolves in water of plasma. An enzyme called carbonic anhydrase catalyses this reaction and it can go forwards or backwards. This is represented by a double arrow. Carbonic acid then dissociates into hydrogen ions and hydrogen carbonate ions.

$$CO_2 + H_2O \Leftrightarrow H_2CO_3$$
$$H_2CO_3 \Leftrightarrow H^+ + HCO_3^-$$

Strenuous exercise, therefore, increases the acidity of the blood. At this point, you need to understand the difference between strong acids and weak acids as this is important in the maintenance of the acid-base balance. A strong acid, usually an inorganic acid, has most of its molecules in the dissociated state, i.e. there are large numbers of hydrogen ions present. A **weak acid**, usually an organic acid, has only a small number of dissociated molecules. In effect, if a **strong acid** could be converted to a weak acid, many hydrogen ions would be removed into complete molecules so acidity would be less.

Key terms

Weak acid An acid which does not dissociate very much.

Strong acid An acid which greatly dissociates.

Any substance that can accept hydrogen ions or remove them from solution is known as a **base**. Bases have also been called alkalis. Hydrogen carbonate in the above reaction acts as a base because it can accept hydrogen ions removing them from solution.

A **salt** is formed from the reaction between an acid and a base – the hydrogen atoms become replaced by a metal group.

Key terms

Base A substance which accepts hydrogen ions.

Salt A substance produced by the action of an acid and a base.

Sodium chloride is formed from the action of hydrochloric acid on sodium hydroxide (a strong base). Sodium chloride is a salt – note that this is a chemical group of compounds (forget that sodium chloride is also known as salt – this is because it is a salt).

NaOH	+	HCl	=	NaCl	+	H_2O
Sodium hydroxide		Hydrochloric acid		Sodium chloride		Water

Remember!

How does sodium chloride act in water? (See page 170.)

Roles of electrolytes

Essential minerals

To be called essential, a mineral must be essential for health and not be able to be made in the human body. There are seven major minerals that are considered essential to the body.

- Calcium and phosphorus are major components of bone and teeth but calcium is also needed for muscle contraction and blood clotting.

- Potassium is a major constituent of cells.
- Sodium is a major constituent of blood and tissue fluid.
- Sulphur is a component of many amino acids and proteins. It is necessary for collagen formation (in bones and tendons) and keratin in nails and hair.
- Magnesium is also found in bones and teeth. It is used in muscle contraction and is an activator for many important enzymes.
- Chloride tends to follow sodium and is required for hydrochloric acid manufacture in the stomach.

Numerous other minerals are essential but only in very small quantities. These are known as trace elements and comprise: iron, iodine, copper, zinc, manganese, cobalt, chromium, selenium, molybdenum, fluorine, tin, silicon and vanadium.

In control of osmosis/osmotic pressure

Sodium salts are a major constituent of blood and tissue fluid. Every time they enter a cell (through protein channels, for example) they are rapidly expelled by an ATP-energised pump. Chloride ions perform in a similar way. Potassium salts, on the other hand, are major intracellular (inside the cell) ions and when they leak out of the cell membrane, they too are rapidly returned. These salts assist in controlling osmosis through the cell membrane. When the osmotic pressure outside the cell is equal to that inside the cell, they are said to be isotonic to each other. As much water moves into the cell as moves out.

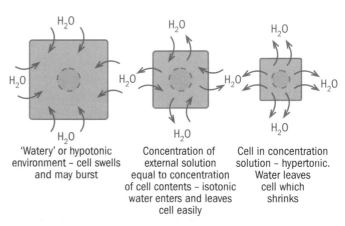

▲ **Figure 13.15 Cells in different osmotic environments.**

However, if cells are in more dilute solutions, the osmotic pressure is higher and water molecules will pass, by osmosis, from outside to inside, causing the cell to swell and possibly rupture. A swollen or damaged cell cannot function efficiently. Conversely, if cells exist in a more concentrated solution with a lower osmotic pressure than the cell contents, water molecules will leave the cell resulting in dehydration and shrinkage. Once again, the cell cannot function effectively and may die. Sodium and potassium salts play a major role in controlling osmosis and osmotic pressure. The brain and the kidneys regulate the quantities of sodium and potassium salts in body fluids.

Remember!

Pure water has the highest osmotic potential. Solutes in water alter osmotic potential.

Maintenance of acid-base balance

This will be considered in detail in the next section. However, electrolytes have important roles in the maintenance of the balance between acids and bases in the body. This is accomplished by buffers in body fluids. A buffer is a chemical system that acts to prevent change in the concentration of another chemical substance.

Buffer systems consist of a weak acid and their soluble salt. You will recall that weak acids mainly remain as molecules and only a few dissociate. The salt, however, readily dissociates producing large numbers of negatively charged ions. These ions readily accept hydrogen ions if more are produced as a result of metabolism, thus removing them from solution and keeping pH more or less constant. Hydrogen carbonate and hydrogen phosphate are particularly important.

Acid-base balance

In this section, you will learn about the pH scale and buffer systems in more detail and why it is so important to keep acidity and alkalinity within a narrow range of variables.

This is a measure of the quantity of hydrogen ions in a solution. It is an artificial logarithmic scale based around the ionisation of water. When water dissociates it produces equal numbers of H^+ and OH^- ions and each has been determined as 1×10^{-7} mol dm^{-3}. (Note that dm^{-3} = 1 litre.)

This is such a small number that the pH scale was derived. It is based around the pH of water at 7 which is neither acidic nor basic. By making the scale logarithmic (denoted by the p) and reciprocal $1/\times$, the scale became easier to understand.

$$pH = -\log[H^+] \text{ or } 1 \div \log[H^+]$$

The greater the quantity of hydrogen ions, the greater the acidity and the lower will be the pH.

The pH scale begins at 1 and ends at 14 with 7 being the neutral point. Any substance between 1 and 7 is acidic in nature and from 7 to 14 a substance is a base.

Strong acids have a pH near to the bottom of the scale such as 1–3 and strong bases have pH's nearer to 14.

Importance of maintaining hydrogen ion concentration in body fluids

The importance of buffer systems in maintaining and stabilising the pH of cellular and body fluids cannot be over-emphasised. You have learned that metabolic activities are controlled by thousands of cellular and digestive enzymes and that enzymes only work efficiently within a narrow range of pH. Enzymes alter the rate of chemical reactions; in the human body, most enzymes speed up the rate of reactions many times. For example, carbon dioxide is carried in blood plasma mainly as the hydrogen carbonate and, without the presence of the enzyme carbonic anhydrase to improve the rate of formation of hydrogen carbonate, (see page 180 for the equation), the elimination of carbon dioxide would be too slow to support life. Failure to keep blood pH between 7 and 8 usually results in death.

Buffer systems

Blood and tissue fluid are buffered at around pH 7.2–7.4 by the system incorporating carbonic acid and sodium hydrogen carbonate as the weak acid and sodium salt of the weak acid.

$H_2CO_3 \Leftrightarrow H^+ + HCO^{3-}$ (small dissociation)

$NaHCO_3 \Leftrightarrow Na^+ + HCO^{3-}$ (large dissociation)

Extra hydrogen ions caused by metabolic reactions, such as vigorous exercise or diet, are accepted by the large numbers of hydrogen carbonate ions to form H_2CO_3 which exists mainly as molecules. In due course this will further push the reaction to the left and CO_2 and H_2O will be formed. The CO_2 will be removed through increased ventilation.

Conversely, if the hydrogen ion concentration becomes too low, the buffer releases hydrogen ions into solution to keep the pH constant.

The main buffer which prevents large fluctuations in cells is the dihydrogen phosphate and monohydrogen phosphate buffer system. (Note that di- means two and mono- means one.) This system operates around pH 7.2.

Reflect

pH of blood is normally kept within the range 7.2 –7.4. Does this mean that blood is slightly acid or slightly alkaline?

The phosphate buffer system operates mainly through kidney function. Tubular cells of the renal nephrons are stimulated to produce ammonia when the blood is becoming too acid. The ammonia replaces the sodium in the dihydrogen phosphate causing increased acid secretion in urine. The pH of urine can vary from 4.0 to 8.0.

Finally, an important buffer operating in cells and plasma is that utilising proteins. At one end of a protein chain there is an amino group and at the other end there is a carboxyl group.

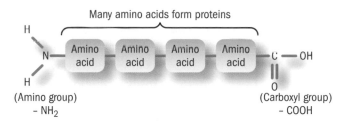

▲ Figure 13.16 Amino and carboxyl groups of proteins.

When there is a fall in pH, and therefore a corresponding rise in hydrogen ion concentration, the amino groups will accept the extra hydrogen ions. Conversely, where there is a rise in pH, the carboxyl groups will dissociate to release hydrogen ions to restore pH.

Role of water

You have learned that water is the main constituent of body fluids (page 178) and this section will examine the important properties of water in relation to this role.

In relation to properties

■ Specific heat capacity

Specific heat capacity is the amount of energy required to raise 1 kg of a substance by 1°K. The Kelvin scale is the SI temperature scale. You do not need to worry about the Kelvin scale if it is new to you. Water has a high specific heat capacity which means that it takes a lot of energy to raise 1 kg of water one degree of temperature.

Reflect

Have you noticed that, even on a very hot day on the beach when the sand burns your feet, the sea still feels cold? Can you explain this now?

This means that even in hot climates warm-blooded animals like humans will not have a massive rise in temperature – nor will they cool down too quickly. Water also has a high heat of vaporisation, meaning that it takes a lot of energy to convert liquid water into water vapour. This property is useful as it means that, when sweat is evaporated from the skin surface, a lot of heat energy from the skin surface is used up, thereby cooling the skin.

■ Solvent

Water is an excellent solvent for many important substances in the body and you learned how this happens on page 170.

■ Surface tension

Water also has a high surface tension, meaning that the quantity of water in contact with air or other material tends to have the smallest possible area. A fine watery film between the two pleural surfaces (one covering the lung and one lining the inside chest wall) creates a tension that literally pulls the lung surface along when the ribs move upwards and outwards during inspiration.

Distribution of water

In physiology, the weight of an average person is calculated at 70 kg and about 60 per cent of this body weight would be water. This produces a figure of about 42 litres of total body water.

Total body water comprises the water inside cells, known as intracellular water (28 litres) and that which lies outside cells called extracellular water (14 litres).

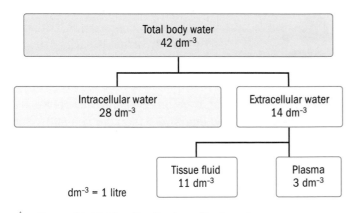

▲ Figure 13.17 The distribution of body water.

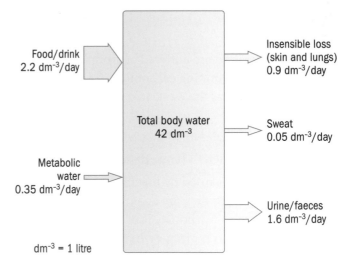

▲ Figure 13.18 Average daily water gain and loss.

These two figures probably surprised you as we tend to think of body water as blood, lymph, tissue fluid and urine and not as water inside cells. In fact only one third of water is in plasma and tissue fluid. Tissue fluid, also known as intercellular and interstitial fluid, is actually the majority component of extracellular fluid, being 11 litres compared to 3 litres of plasma. Tissue fluid is of course derived from plasma and has the same constituents apart from plasma proteins. Tissue fluid is a protein-free plasma filtrate. Lymph comprises about 10 per cent of the tissue fluid from which it forms, the remainder returning to plasma. Tissue fluid is not called lymph until it enters the branching network of the lymphatic vessels.

Role of tissue fluid in homeostasis

Tissue fluid plays an integral part in **homeostasis** (maintaining the constancy of the **internal environment**).

Key terms

Homeostasis Maintaining a constant internal environment around cells.

Internal environment This is the physical and chemical composition of blood and tissue fluid which surrounds body cells.

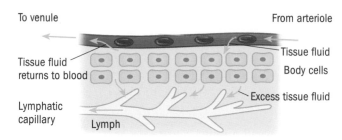

To venule
From arteriole
Tissue fluid
Tissue fluid
returns to blood
Body cells
Lymphatic
capillary
Excess tissue fluid
Lymph

▲ Figure 13.19 The formation and removal of tissue fluid.

Tissue fluid is driven out of the arterial end of a capillary by the remaining blood pressure after the blood has been driven through the medium muscular arteries and arterioles. At this stage it has a high dissolved oxygen concentration and low carbon dioxide. It is also loaded with nutrients such as glucose, amino acids and salts. Tissue fluid circulates around and between cells (hence the name intercellular fluid) distributing raw materials by diffusion, osmosis, facilitated diffusion, etc. Waste metabolic materials pass in the opposite direction from cells into tissue fluid and, if allowed to accumulate, would cause serious disruption and eventually cell and body death.

However, having collected the metabolic waste, most tissue fluid re-enters the venous end of the capillaries because the plasma proteins (still inside the capillaries) exert an osmotic pressure drawing the fluid back into the capillary. This is assisted by the low blood pressure at the venous end because of the volume of fluid forced out at the arterial end. The waste materials are carried away to be excreted via the lungs or the liver and kidneys. Some proteins do escape the capillary (about 2 per cent) and, as they cannot either be allowed to accumulate or re-enter the capillary, they are removed together with any surplus tissue fluid and waste products via the lymphatic system. In this way, the tissue fluid has a role in maintaining the stability or constancy of the internal environment.

Assessment activity 13.3

P3 Describe the distribution of water in the body and the functions of constituents of body fluids.

1   How is water spread throughout the body and what are the functions of its solutes?

Grading tip for P3

You might start with an annotated diagram of a container showing the various 'water' compartments of total body water, providing a short description in the annotations and lists of the solutes found in each compartment. This could be followed by text describing the functions of each solute.

M3 Explain the contributions of water and solutes to the maintenance of a constant internal environment for cells.

2   How do water, glucose, urea and electrolytes help in homeostasis?

Grading tip for M3

This work can be added on to the work for P3 as it will be a logical progression. If you want to, you can add the contribution to homeostasis as a sub-heading after each solute function. You will definitely need to discuss acid-base balance and the functions of buffers in this section. You may need to read on further into the last section on homeostatic processes in relation to water balance.

You have learned about the many features of water and solutes and you will now place this in context with reference to the renal system and how water is regulated to maintain homeostasis.

Water intake

Water is obtained from three sources for the body:

- fluids that are drunk
- water in food
- water produced as a by-product of metabolism.

It will obviously vary from day to day but, generally speaking, an individual takes in approximately 1.2 litres in fluid such as water, soft drinks, beverages and alcoholic drinks like wine and beer. Surprisingly, as much as 1 litre is taken in as food; even the driest cracker has water in it and vegetables and meat have a high proportion of water.

Only about one third of a litre is produced from chemical reactions such as the oxidation of glucose and lipids. The total intake per day is around 2.5 litres.

In the previous section on the control of osmosis/osmotic pressure (see page 181) you learned about the effect of water gain on cells.

Water output

Water is lost from the body in four ways:

- Through the skin – there is a constant loss from the skin that an individual is not conscious of. This is caused by evaporation and is known as insensible water loss – it can add up to 0.5 litre. In addition, there can be a variable amount lost through sweating to cool the skin. Clearly this depends on the climate and the season and ranges from about 50 ml to 2 litres.
- From the lungs – air breathed out is saturated with water vapour and this can range from 0.3 to 0.5 litre.

- From faeces exiting from the gastro-intestinal tract – water loss averages about 0.1 litre.
- Through urine – in a temperate climate such as the UK this totals about 1.5 litres.

These figures take no account of loss by unusual circumstances such as vomiting and diarrhoea when water loss can be considerable and lead to dehydration and life-threatening situations (particularly in babies and older people who have less efficient water-regulating systems). It is also worth noting that the volume of urine generally declines in hot weather as extra water is lost as sweat. Menstrual loss in females varies from female to female with the average loss being 60 ml.

In the previous section on the control of osmosis/osmotic pressure (see page 181) you learned about the effect of water loss on cells.

Theory into practice

Try to maintain your own fluid balance sheet for 24 hours. A weekend day is probably best and one where you are not undertaking vigorous exercise.

You can research the volumes of water in the food that you consume by consulting a nutrition manual and you will need two labelled plastic measuring jugs to measure the volumes of fluid and urine (keep them separate). Take the standards for faeces (0.1 litre) and breath (0.4 litre) and the insensible perspiration as 0.4 litre. Assume that metabolic water intake is 0.35 litre.

1 Calculate the total water intake and total water output.

2 Are you in fluid balance? Ignore any difference under 50 ml.

3 If not, explain what would happen if the same imbalance was repeated daily for a week.

Discuss the influence of environmental temperature on your findings.

Renal system

Gross anatomy

The renal system comprises two kidneys, their tubes known as ureters, the bladder and the urethra.

The kidneys lie on the posterior or back wall of the abdomen, above the waist and partly protected by the lowest ribs. There is one on each side of the vertebral column.

Theory into practice

Most people believe that their kidneys are much lower down than they actually are. Try asking five people to point to their kidneys. Then show them the correct positions. If you are unsure, check the positions out on an anatomical model or in Unit 5 of Book 1.

What proportion of your small survey got the position of the kidneys wrong?

What proportion got the liver correct and the kidneys wrong?

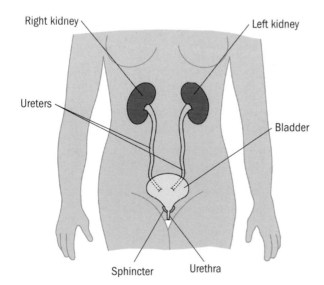

▲ Figure 13.20 The gross anatomy of the renal system.

The bladder is a central pelvic organ connected to the kidneys by two ureters 20–30 cm in length. Both bladder and ureters have a lining of epithelium, surrounded by muscle and fibrous tissue.

The bladder is connected to the exterior by the urethra, which is much longer in males than females. In males, the urethra just below the bladder is completely surrounded by the prostate gland. The urethra in males forms part of the penis.

Associated blood supply

Two short renal arteries enter each kidney directly from the aorta and similarly two short renal veins come from each kidney to join the inferior vena cava. Each renal artery enters the kidney at the indented surface facing the aorta. This is known as the hilum of the kidney and it quickly breaks up into numerous smaller branches which give off tributaries at right angles to supply each nephron with an **afferent arteriole**. Nephrons are the basic functional units of the kidney. The afferent arteriole breaks up into a tuft or knot of capillaries, closely pushed into the first cup-shaped beginning of each nephron, termed the **Bowman's capsule**. The knot of capillaries is called the **glomerulus**. Emerging from the glomerulus is an **efferent arteriole** which is narrower than the afferent arteriole. The efferent arteriole runs close to the tubules of the nephrons breaking up into a separate network of capillaries around the tubules before re-uniting to form branches of the renal vein. As you will learn, this blood supply is of vital importance to kidney function.

Key terms

Afferent arteriole The arteriole preceding the glomerulus.

Bowman's capsule The cup-shaped beginning of a nephron.

Glomerulus The tuft of capillaries located within the Bowman's capsule.

Efferent arteriole The arteriole leaving the glomerulus.

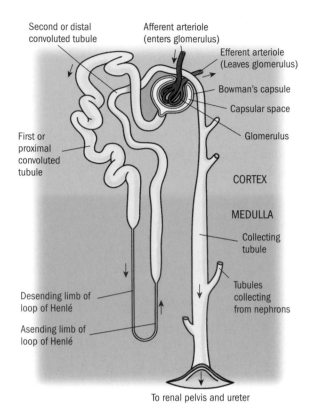

Figure 13.21 A nephron.

Labels on the figure:
- Second or distal convoluted tubule
- Afferent arteriole (enters glomerulus)
- Efferent arteriole (Leaves glomerulus)
- Bowman's capsule
- Capsular space
- Glomerulus
- First or proximal convoluted tubule
- CORTEX
- MEDULLA
- Collecting tubule
- Descending limb of loop of Henlé
- Ascending limb of loop of Henlé
- Tubules collecting from nephrons
- To renal pelvis and ureter

Physiological overview

The kidneys process blood by removing water, urea and excess mineral salts from it to provide a balance to enable the body to function efficiently. In performing these tasks, the kidneys regulate water, electrolytes and acid-base balance and eliminate the waste products of metabolism such as:

- urea from surplus amino acids
- creatinine from creatine in muscle (this acts rather like ATP)
- uric acid from nucleic acids (all plant and animal cells comprising food have nuclei)
- the end products from the breakdown of haemoglobin (from old red blood cells).

Kidneys also remove unwanted chemicals from the blood such as drugs, pesticides, food additives and toxins and secrete hormones such as **erythropoietin**, which controls the production of red blood cells, and **renin**, which influences blood pressure.

■ Urine production

The renal fluid undergoing modification as it passes along the nephron tubules is not called urine until the final changes are made in the last part of the tubule (see the next section). The filtrate enters the Bowman's capsule at a rate of 120 ml/min^{-1} (ml per minute), but urine production averages only 1 ml/min^{-1} dripping into the pelvis of the ureter, demonstrating the enormous changes which have happened in the tubules. Urine then moves down the ureters, partly by gravity and partly by peristalsis, to collect in the bladder.

■ Composition of urine

The composition of urine will vary depending on diet, intake of fluids, climate and degrees of activity.

Theory into practice

Examine Table 13.3 which shows the average percentage composition of plasma and urine.

1 Explain why there are no blood cells or plasma proteins listed in the table.

2 Explain why glucose and amino acids are not listed.

3 Which substances are nitrogen-containing materials excreted from the body?

4 Calculate the concentrations of the following substances in urine:

- urea
- sodium.

Reflect

Sweat produced during vigorous activity is a dilute salt solution.

What changes would you expect in urine content after a 5 km cross-country run in hot weather?

It will perhaps be useful to compare the average composition of urine and plasma in percentages. You can see these in the table below.

Chemical	Plasma %	Urine %
Water	90–93	95
Urea	0.02	2
Uric acid	0.003	0.05
Sodium	0.3	0.6
Chloride	0.35	0.6
Potassium	0.02	0.15
Phosphate	0.003	0.15
Ammonia	0.0001	0.05

Table 13.3 Some principal components of plasma and urine.

■ Storage of urine and micturition

Ureters enter a balloon-shaped muscular organ in the front of the pelvis called the bladder. The lower neck is guarded by a ring of muscle which acts as a sphincter, relaxing to permit urine to be released when the bladder walls are stimulated by the pressure of a volume of urine. Urine is stored in the bladder for a period of time until the volume and pressure stimulate parasympathetic nervous impulses, causing the bladder muscle to contract and urine to be released. The technical term for the release of urine is micturition, although urination is commonly used.

Kidneys

Each kidney is bean-shaped and dark red in colour. The indented area faces the mid-line of the body and is known as the hilum. The ureter and renal vein emerge from the kidney and the renal artery enters the kidney at the hilum. There is a capsule of membrane surrounding the kidney and each is topped by the conical adrenal gland. The kidneys and adrenal glands are surrounded in adipose tissue.

Gross anatomy

When sectioned lengthways or longitudinally, the kidney shows an outer darker cortex and an inner paler medulla. The medulla is composed of a number of cone-shaped pyramids with the tip of the cone projecting into the area where the ureter joins the kidney. This area is known as the pelvis of the kidney (pelvis means a bowl). Urine drips from the medullary pyramids into the pelvis.

The arterioles emerging from the branches of the renal artery tend to follow the border between the cortex and medulla, giving off smaller branches at right angles into

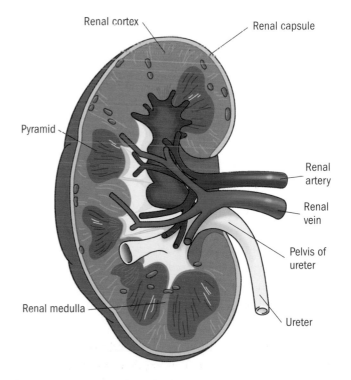

▲ **Figure 13.22 A longitudinal section through a kidney.**

the cortex to supply the million or so nephrons found in the kidney.

Structure and functions of nephrons/kidney tubules

The nephron (see Figure 13.21) consists of a cup-shaped Bowman's capsule linked to a coiled tubule which then runs into a straight hairpin-shaped section called the loop of Henlé, a second coiled tubule and then a straight collecting duct emptying at the conical tip of the pyramid. The coiled tubules and Bowman's capsule are located in the cortex but the loop of Henlé and collecting duct are chiefly located in the medella. The blood vessels associated with the nephrons give the cortex its dark red colour.

The Bowman's capsule is made of two layers of simple squamous epithelium with a small fluid-filled gap between them. The glomerulus is closely associated with the inner layer of the cup.

Reflect

The glomerulus is a tuft or knot of capillaries. Capillaries have walls made of simple squamous epithelium. So there are only two flattened layers of cells separating the blood in the capillaries from the space in the Bowman's capsule.

Where have you found this type of arrangement before?

In fact, the inner layer of epithelial cells have been specially modified and have 'legs' with spaces in between for fluid to escape through. The only barrier to the fluid is the basement membrane of the Bowman's capsule and the capillary wall, which you have learned is selectively permeable. These specially adapted cells are called podocytes and are visible with an electron microscope.

Ultrafiltration

The afferent arteriole (see *Associated blood supply* on pages 187–8) has a larger diameter than the efferent arteriole leaving the glomerulus. This contributes to high pressure in the glomerulus as there is a 'traffic jam' of blood. Due to the shortness of the renal artery coming straight from the aorta, and this 'traffic jam', the blood in the glomerulus has a high pressure that forces out fluid from the plasma. The fluid is a protein-free plasma filtrate – it contains no blood cells and no plasma proteins because they are too large to pass through the capillary/epithelial (podocyte) barrier.

Remember!

In kidney disease, when glomeruli are damaged, protein does manage to pass into the filtrate. This is one of the main signs of kidney damage and is called proteinuria. Protein in urine causes it to froth when passed (just as milk does when it is agitated). An experienced carer can tell that there is protein in urine because of the frothing.

The fluid is now known as glomerular filtrate or renal fluid. The average rate of glomerular filtration (GFR) is

Theory into practice

Cardiac output averages 5 litres or dm^{-3} every minute and of this about 3 litres is plasma. Twenty per cent of plasma in the capillaries is filtered as it passes once through the kidneys.

1 Urine production averages 1 ml/min^{-1}. Calculate the volume passed in 24 hours and compare this with the average volume passed in water output (page 184).

2 Calculate to the nearest whole number how many times the whole of the plasma is filtered every day.

3 Explain how the figure obtained in question 1 is of value in homeostasis.

120 ml/min⁻¹. The process is known as **ultrafiltration** because it takes place under high pressure. The pressure in the glomerular capillaries is 55 mmHg and this has to overcome:

- the filtrate pressure pushing outwards in the Bowman's capsule (15 mmHg) and
- the osmotic pressure of the plasma proteins in the capillaries trying to draw fluid back (30 mmHg)

so the net filtration pressure is 15 mmHg.

Key terms

Ultrafiltration The process driving a protein-free filtrate from plasma from the glomerulus.

Selective reabsorption

You have learned that, on average, glomerular filtration rate (GFR) is 120 ml/min⁻¹ and urine formation is 1 ml/min⁻¹, so it is fairly clear that 119 ml/min⁻¹ must be reabsorbed along the renal tubule. However, reabsorption is different for different substances, so it is called **selective reabsorption**. The first coiled part of the tubule (often referred to as the proximal convoluted tubule or PCT) is where the majority of reabsorption takes place into the capillary network surrounding the tubule. Here seven eighths of the water and sodium ions are reabsorbed. You will also recall that chloride ions tend to follow sodium so that returns as well. In addition, all the filtered glucose and amino acids are reabsorbed, so that there should be none of these molecules leaving in urine. It would be rather pointless to ingest food, digest and absorb the end products, only to have them leave in urine.

The glomerular filtrate is then significantly reduced by the time it reaches the entrance to the loop of Henlé.

Key terms

Selective reabsorption The process whereby some materials are reabsorbed back into the capillary network around the tubules but not others.

Theory into practice

You have learned how some substances are reabsorbed in the proximal convoluted tubule (PCT).

1. Assuming that the dissolved products in glomerular filtrate have negligible volume, calculate the new volume of fluid entering the loop of Henlé.

2. Which nitrogen-containing compounds remain in the fluid after passing through the PCT?

3. Make a list of other substances remaining in the fluid.

4. What will happen to the concentration of substances not reabsorbed?

Take it further

You should also be aware that tubular cells can secrete certain substances from the plasma in the capillary network surrounding the tubule into the lumen of the tubule, the mechanism nearly always being by active transport. This second process of materials entering the tubule (the first being glomerular filtration) is very useful in maintaining homeostasis. Common ions secreted are hydrogen and potassium ions, as well as creatinine. Many drugs are excreted in this way, for example, penicillin. This process is called tubular secretion.

Under what circumstances might tubular secretion of hydrogen ions take place?

Loop of Henlé and the counter-current mechanism

The two limbs of the hairpin-shaped loop of Henlé lie very close together in the medulla. The function of the loop was unknown for many years, although animals living in desert regions were known to possess very long loops and aquatic animals very short loops. The conclusion was reached that the loop was concerned with water conservation. Later, it was discovered that the tissue fluid surrounding the loop was hyperosmotic (above normal osmolarity) and this was due to sodium ions. The mechanism works as follows:

- The tube is full of filtrate at normal osmolarity, say, arbitrarily 300.
- As this fluid rounds the bend of the loop and starts to climb up, sodium ions are passed from the ascending limb into the descending limb by active transport.
- The descending limb fluid now becomes 400 and the fluid leaving the loop becomes 200.
- As this fluid at 400 rounds the bend, more sodium ions are actively pumped across, making the descending limb now 500 and the ascending limb 300 and getting less as the end of the hairpin is achieved.
- The hyperosmotic fluid slowly diffuses into the tissue fluid surrounding the hairpin, but more sodium is actively pumped across to maintain the increased osmolarity.
- Eventually, the sodium ions will find their way back into the blood but the sodium ions keep on coming to maintain the high osmolarity.

This is known as the **countercurrent mechanism.**

The purpose of this hyperosmotic region is to attract water molecules from the filtrate in the collecting ducts, but this only happens under the influence of a hormone. When water molecules are drawn across by osmosis into the tissue fluid and finally the blood, the urine will be more concentrated.

Principles of osmoregulation, the role of the hypothalamus and anti-diuretic hormone

Osmoregulation is one process involved in homeostasis and means controlling the osmotic potential of the blood. In simple terms, it is making sure that the blood is at the right concentration. When blood becomes too concentrated, water is conserved until the correct concentration is restored. Less water is passed in urine, so it becomes more concentrated. When blood is too dilute, more water is passed in urine until the blood concentration is restored. This causes more dilute urine to be passed.

The **hypothalamus** in the brain lies just above the **pituitary gland** and contains modified neurones called

Key terms

Countercurrent mechanism A process involving active transport of sodium ions from the descending limb of the loop of Henlé to the ascending limb.

Key terms

Hypothalamus Part of the brain involved in water balance.

Pituitary gland An endocrine gland chiefly controlled by the hypothalamus in the brain.

Remember!

The limbs of the loop of Henlé are not the only structures in the medulla – the last part of the tubules known as the collecting ducts are tightly packed in the medulla as well.

Figure 13.23 The countercurrent mechanism. ▶

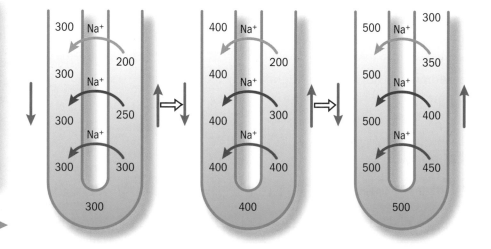

osmoreceptors which monitor the concentration of the adjacent blood. When blood is too concentrated, the osmoreceptors stimulate the posterior part of the pituitary gland to secrete a hormone called **antidiuretic hormone** (ADH). ADH causes the cells of the distal convoluted tubule (DCT) and collecting tubules to become more permeable to water. As the collecting tubule passes through the hyperosmotic area in the medulla, water passes out by osmosis into the tissue fluid and the blood. When the osmoreceptors are not stimulated because blood is too dilute, little ADH is secreted and the tubules behave as if they are waterproofed and water passes onwards into the urine.

Key terms

Osmoreceptors Modified neurones sensitive to the osmotic pressure of blood.

Antidiuretic hormone (ADH) A pituitary hormone causing tubular cells to become more permeable to water.

ADH secretion will be high in a hot climate where water is being lost as sweat to cool the skin. ADH will be low when an individual has been drinking a lot of fluid and not sweating.

Overall, volumes of urine are lower in the summer months than in the winter months.

Reflect

You may have heard about some individuals being on 'water' tablets. These are known as diuretics. A diuresis is a copious flow of urine, so diuretics increase the flow of urine.

Can you suggest one or two conditions in which part of the treatment might be diuretic medication?

Dysfunctions in relation to water balance

Physiological problems arise when the balance between water intake and water output is disturbed and some of these are discussed below.

Oedema

This is when too much fluid accumulates in the body tissues. It may be visible or not. Doctors will look for **oedema** either in the ankles, if a patient can walk about, or at the base of the spine if the patient is in bed. Until there is about 15 per cent extra fluid, the only sign would be an increase in weight. After that, when a doctor presses their thumb into the swollen tissues, an indentation appears which takes some time to disappear. This is known as pitting oedema.

Key terms

Oedema The accumulation of tissue fluid around the body cells.

In context

Ian has severe chronic bronchitis and emphysema brought on by a lifetime of smoking. He has now developed right-sided heart failure. Ian's legs and feet are very swollen. He is being treated with digitalis to strengthen his heart beat and diuretics which increases the output of urine from his kidneys.

1   **Explain what is meant by right-sided heart failure.**

2   **What is the relationship between heart failure and oedema of the legs and feet?**

3   **From your knowledge of osmo-regulation, suggest how and why diuretics might work.**

Heart failure can cause oedema because the heart is unable to drive blood onwards effectively and the pressure builds up in the congested veins. This results in a higher capillary pressure which is now greater than the osmotic pressure of the plasma proteins trying to return tissue fluid to the blood. Consequently, there is an accumulation of tissue fluid.

In renal failure, the kidneys cannot excrete enough sodium chloride from the body and it accumulates in tissue fluids. Sodium chloride attracts water to it and so there is a build-up in tissue fluid and oedema. In kidney disease, where there is damage to glomerular capillaries, protein is lost in the urine. This means that plasma protein content of blood is lower than normal, so the osmotic pressure attracting fluid back to the blood stream is low and oedema results.

Any condition lowering the osmotic pressure of the plasma proteins in the blood can result in oedema – for example, malnutrition in undeveloped countries, alcoholism or cirrhosis of the liver. Similarly, any condition involving salt retention in the tissues will also result in water accumulation, for example, cirrhosis of the liver.

Kidney failure

The kidneys have a reduced ability to excrete water, salts, urea, creatinine and uric acid from the blood in the condition generally known as kidney failure. This can lead to a multiplicity of problems such as disturbed water and acid-base balances, urea accumulation (uraemia), proteinuria, hypertension, anaemia, oedema and chemical disturbances in the blood.

Acute kidney failure can arise as a consequence of physiological shock such as severe injuries, haemorrhage or burns and even a heart attack. Chronic renal failure develops more slowly, arising from long-standing hypertension, diabetes, kidney defects, kidney stones and any condition which obstructs the flow of urine for a long time, such as prostatic enlargement. The number of nephrons also decreases with age. For example, at the age of 20 there are about 700,000 nephrons functioning but by 60 years of age the figure has dropped to around 250,000 in each kidney. At birth, there are a million nephrons in each kidney.

Chronic renal failure is a life-threatening disease and without treatment, coma and death will follow.

No two kidney patients are on exactly the same medication regime, although there will be many similarities. Most will be on diuretics and antihypertensive drugs to increase urinary output and reduce blood pressure. Drugs to correct blood chemistry will depend on the specific disturbance and most will be on a particular diet regime. This will have common features such as:

- high carbohydrate for energy
- low protein to reduce the workload of the kidneys in excreting urea
- no added salt and special cooking methods to remove excess potassium
- limited fluid input to achieve a balance with input.

Inevitably, there is progress towards what is called end-stage renal failure when dialysis or a kidney transplant becomes necessary.

Signs and symptoms might include:

- decreased urine production
- fatigue
- anaemia
- weakness and loss of weight
- nausea, vomiting and loss of appetite.

Renal dialysis

There are two main types of dialysis, **haemodialysis** and **continuous ambulatory peritoneal dialysis (CAPD)**. Haemodialysis involves attaching a client to a kidney

Key terms

Haemodialysis The removal of metabolic waste products from the blood via a kidney machine because the kidneys are seriously damaged.

Continuous ambulatory peritoneal dialysis (CAPD) A different form of dialysis carried out by running dialysing fluid into the peritoneal cavity of the abdomen for several hours and then running the fluid to waste and replacing with 'clean' dialysate.

machine for at least four hours a day, three or four times a week. A client requires a 'fistula' operation several months beforehand – this is usually in the arm. A **fistula** is an artificial connection between an artery and a vein, into which the needle attachment to the kidney machine is made. Multiple layers of special membrane material separate the client's blood from dialysing fluid in the kidney machine.

Key terms

Fistula An artificial connection made between an artery and a vein for attachment to a kidney machine.

Any substance (waste products, toxic materials and excess water) needing to be removed from the blood is in low or zero concentration in dialysate so that the substance passes across by diffusion and osmosis. Any substance not requiring elimination can be kept at a high concentration in the dialysate. The dialysate runs to waste and the 'cleaned' blood is returned to the client.

CAPD uses the inner lining or peritoneum of the abdomen as the dialysing membrane and the dialysate is introduced through a special tap and catheter. The process takes about one hour to complete (twice a day), i.e. to empty the old dialysate and introduce the fresh. The client may walk about with the dialysate inside (hence use of the word 'ambulatory') and carry on with work. Although peritoneal dialysis can take place in hospital, most patients carry out CAPD at home and work.

Reflect

There are thousands of people waiting for organ donations. Only a small percentage of the population carries donor cards. Fatalities occur and in the UK organs are wasted because large numbers of individuals have not thought about this.

Have you considered being an organ donor?

Conversely a few clients have home kidney machines but most haemodialyse in hospital.

Patients can be dialysing successfully for many years. However, the procedure is very expensive and kidney machines are in short supply. The semi-permanent answer is transplantation. Although the surgery and after care are expensive, this is nowhere near the cost of many years of dialysis. Unfortunately there is also a problem with kidney donations as these are in short supply.

Transplantation

In the UK, most transplant organs are only available from recently deceased persons or close relatives.

The composition of the recipient individual's antigenic make-up is determined from blood tests and matched to a donor's make-up so that they are as closely matched as possible. This process is called **'tissue-typing'**.

Failing kidneys are usually left in place and the new kidney placed in the pelvis (groin area) and connected to the bladder by the donor's ureter. The donor blood vessels are connected to branches of the lower aorta and vena cava.

The client begins **immuno-suppressant** medication to prevent rejection and monitoring is carried out by urinalysis, blood tests and ultrasound scanning. The chief danger of rejection is in the first few months after the transplant.

Key terms

Tissue-typing Identifying the protein markers on cell membranes to determine compatibility for transplantation.

Immuno-suppressant Specific types of medication to suppress or reduce the immune response. Given to prevent rejection.

More than 80 per cent of transplants are successful, enabling the client to live a normal life for many years while continuing on immuno-suppression.

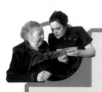

In context

Sarah was a school teacher who contracted influenza. She was off work for two months, still feeling weak and nauseous. Her husband called the GP again, expressing dissatisfaction at Sarah's recovery. After numerous examinations, Sarah was admitted to hospital for diagnostic tests and eventually was told that she had poor renal function due to an undiagnosed long-term hypertension and would need dialysis. The dialysis procedures were explained and Sarah opted for CAPD as this offered the best opportunity for returning to work. After two years of dialysis at home and one episode of peritonitis, Sarah was offered a transplant. This was carried out successfully, although Sarah's

health had never been good enough for a return to work. Her transplant worked efficiently for 12 years but then began to fail. The hypertension during these years had been difficult to control.

Sarah has now returned to haemodialysis and is hoping for another transplant.

1 **Explain the process called CAPD.**

2 **Why is this considered the most appropriate for individuals who wish to continue working?**

3 **Identify and explain the factors which may have led to Sarah's transplant failing after 12 years.**

Transplant organs age faster than normal body organs and, while some transplants may last for over 30 years, many also fail within the lifetime of the recipient. This means that the individual would have to return to dialysis and the long wait for a repeat transplant. Individuals are tissue-typed and placed on a transplant

waiting list. The potential recipient must be in reasonably good health to withstand surgery and not have any other untreatable life-threatening conditions.

Frequently, two kidneys become available for donations and this benefits two people as only one kidney is transplanted at a time in an individual.

Assessment activity 13.4

P4 Describe the gross anatomy and physiology of the renal system.

1 How is the renal system organised, and what are its major functions in the body?

Grading tip for P4

What does gross mean in this context?

You only need to describe the macrostructure of the renal system, not the microscopic system, and give a broad overview of the physiological functions, as you will be discussing these in more detail in the later assessments.

P5 Describe the role of the kidney tubules in the homeostatic control of water balance.

M4 Explain the role of the kidney tubules in the homeostatic control of water balance.

2   What is the precise role of the kidney tubules in regulating the volume of water in the body?

Grading tips for P5 and M4

What is the difference between P5 and M4?

P5 is asking for a description. This means that you are painting a picture using words – stating simply what happens. M4 is asking you to provide details, facts and reasons. If you are attempting a higher grade, you will in this case first describe and then provide details and reasons why, so you will be subsuming P5 into M4. It is important to realise that after the details on ultrafiltration, the PCT absorption of water is not dependant on whether the body is short of water or not. The control happens in the DCT as a result of ADH secretion or lack of it. You will also need to discuss the countercurrent mechanism as this relates to the action of ADH on the DCT.

P6 Describe dysfunctions in relation to water balance and their possible treatments.

M5 Explain dysfunctions in relation to water balance and their possible treatments.

3   What problems can arise in managing the water content of the body and how might these be overcome?

Grading tips for P6 and M5

Which dysfunctions will you describe and explain?

Once again, the difference between the grades is the difference between explaining and merely describing. To achieve high grades, you will need to discuss oedema and kidney failure and explain why water balance is disturbed. Possible treatments will include maintenance medication, different forms of dialysis and transplantation. If you are able to use short case studies to illustrate your work, that will be impressive. Try to visit a dialysis unit or ask a renal dialysis nurse to visit your class as a speaker.

D2 Analyse the impact on the human body of dysfunctions in relation to water balance.

4   What problems do people have when they cannot regulate their water input and output?

Grading tip for D2

How will you interpret the impact on the human body and what is meant by analysis?

Case studies will really help you here or a speaker who has renal problems or experience on a renal unit. You could discuss the implications of dietary restrictions including fluids, the social and emotional problems arising from dialysing, anaemia in kidney disease, the effects of being immuno-suppressed, the problems with iron build-up from treatment to combat anaemia, etc. Analysing these problems will mean providing reasons why these problems arise.

Websites will also provide information on kidney diseases.

Knowledge check

1. Explain the structural and functional differences between rough and smooth endoplasmic reticula.

2. What is meant by the term transcription?

3. How does transcription differ from translation?

4. Explain the terms active transport and facilitated diffusion.

5. Distinguish between intracellular fluid and intercellular fluid.

6. What are the components of a buffer system? Give one example of a buffer system.

7. Explain the pH scale.

8. What is a polar molecule and how is this relevant to the phospholipid bilayer?

9. Explain how anti-diuretic hormone may be important in an endurance race such as a marathon.

10. Explain why fluid and dietary restrictions are important in a patient undergoing dialysis.

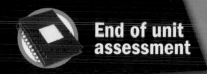
Preparation for assessment

This unit will be internally assessed by your tutors and will probably consist of four assignments.

You need to demonstrate that you meet all the learning outcomes for the unit. The criteria for a pass grade set the level of achievement to pass the unit. To achieve a merit, you must also meet the merit learning outcomes and, to achieve at distinction, every pass, merit and distinction learning outcome must be demonstrated in your unit evidence.

1 The first assignment is based on the microstructure of the cell and its physiology.

Describe the microstructure of a typical animal cell and the functions of the main cell components. `P1`

Use four examples to explain how the functions of the main cell components relate to overall function. `M1`

A well-annotated diagram, supported by some written work, should be sufficient for this purpose. Care should be taken to ensure that you can truly claim authenticity by modifying and labelling any images downloaded from the Internet. You should write any text in your own words. For M1, you should give specific examples of cell types to support your examples of how the functions of the main cell components relate to overall cell function.

For example, you could use a striated muscle fibre with its very large numbers of mitochondria to explain the release of energy for muscle contraction.

2 Your second assignment could be used for P2, M2 and D1 in relation to the movement of materials into and out of cells.

Explain the ways in which materials move into and out of cells. `P2`

Explain the factors that influence the movement of materials into and out of cells. `M2`

Analyse the role of the phospholipid bilayer in terms of the movement of materials into and out of cells. `D1`

You will describe the ways in which materials move into and out of cells (P1) and extend this by including a description of the factors that influence this (M2).

For D1, you need to analyse the role of the phospholipid bilayer in terms of the movement of materials across cell membranes. This will be particularly important in osmosis (as a selectively permeable membrane), endocytosis and exocytosis. You will discuss the protein receptor sites and protein channels and how hormone molecules alter the permeability of the membrane by interfering with the active sites and thus altering the uptake of selected materials.

3 P3 and M3 could be the basis for your third assignment.

Describe the distribution of water in the body and the functions of the constituents of body fluids. `P3`

Explain the contributions of water and solutes to the maintenance of a constant internal environment for cells. `M3`

You could use annotated diagrams supported by a report to describe the distribution of water in the body and the functions of water and solutes (P3). This can be extended and applied to the maintenance of a constant internal environment for cells (M3).

4 Your final assignment is based on the anatomy and functioning of the renal system. It covers P4, P5, P6, M4, M5 and D2.

Describe the gross anatomy and physiology of the renal system. `P4`

Describe the role of the kidney tubules in the homeostatic control of water balance. `P5`

Explain the role of the kidney tubules in the homeostatic control of water balance. **M4**

Describe dysfunctions in relation to water balance and their possible treatments. **P6**

Explain dysfunctions in relation to water balance and their possible treatments. **M5**

Analyse the impact on the human body of dysfunctions in relation to water balance. **D2**

A combination of annotated diagrams and explanatory text will form the basis of your evidence with case studies providing appropriate opportunities to demonstrate evidence of dysfunctions.

Resources and further reading

Baker, M. et al (2001) *Further Studies in Human Biology* (AQA) London: Hodder Murray

Boyle, M. et al (2002) *Human Biology* London: Collins Educational

Givens, P., Reiss, M. (2002) *Human Biology and Health Studies* Cheltenham: Nelson Thornes

Indge, B. et al (2000) *A New Introduction to Human Biology* (AQA) London: Hodder Murray

Jones, M., Jones, G. (2004) *Human Biology for AS Level* Cambridge: Cambridge University Press

Moonie, N. et al (2000) *Advanced Health and Social Care* Oxford: Heinemann

Myers, B. (2004) *The Natural Sciences* Cheltenham: Nelson Thornes

Pickering, W.R. (2001) *Advanced Human Biology through Diagrams* Oxford: Oxford University Press

Saffrey, J. et al (1972) *Maintaining the Whole* Milton Keynes: Open University

Stretch, B., Whitehouse, M. (2007) *BTEC National Health and Social Care Book 1* Oxford: Heinemann

Vander, A.J. et al (2003) *Human Physiology: The Mechanisms of Body Function* London: McGraw Hill

Ward, J. et al (2005) *Physiology at a Glance* Oxford: Blackwell

Wright, D. (2000) *Human Physiology and Health for GCSE*, Oxford: Heinemann

Nursing Times and similar for case studies

Useful websites

BBC
www.bbc.co.uk/science/humanbody

British Heart Foundation
www.bhf.co.uk

NetDoctor
www.netdoctor.co.uk

NHS Direct
www.nhsdirect

Surgery Door
www.surgerydoor.co.uk

GRADING CRITERIA

To achieve a pass grade the evidence must show that the learner is able to:	To achieve a merit grade the evidence must show that, in addition to the pass criteria, the learner is able to:	To achieve a distinction grade the evidence must show that, in addition to the pass and merit criteria, the learner is able to:
P1 describe the microstructure of a typical animal cell and the functions of the main parts **Assessment activity 13.1 page 168**	**M1** use four examples to explain how the functions of the main cell components relate to overall cell function **Assessment activity 13.1 page 168**	
P2 explain the ways in which materials move into and out of cells **Assessment activity 13.2 page 177**	**M2** explain the factors that influence the movement of materials into and out of cells **Assessment activity 13.2 page 177**	**D1** analyse the role of the phospholipid bilayer in terms of the movement of materials into and out of cells **Assessment activity 13.2 page 177**
P3 describe the distribution of water in the body and the functions of constituents of body fluids **Assessment activity 13.3 page 185**	**M3** explain the contributions of water and solutes to the maintenance of a constant internal environment for cells **Assessment activity 13.3 page 185**	
P4 describe the gross anatomy and physiology of the renal system **Assessment activity 13.4 page 196**		
P5 describe the role of the kidney tubules in the homeostatic control of water balance **Assessment activity 13.4 page 197**	**M4** explain the role of the kidney tubules in the homeostatic control of water balance **Assessment activity 13.4 page 197**	
P6 describe dysfunctions in relation to water balance and their possible treatments. **Assessment activity 13.4 page 197**	**M5** explain dysfunctions in relation to water balance and their possible treatments. **Assessment activity 13.4 page 197**	**D2** analyse the impact on the human body of dysfunctions in relation to water balance. **Assessment activity 13.4 page 197**

Physiological disorders

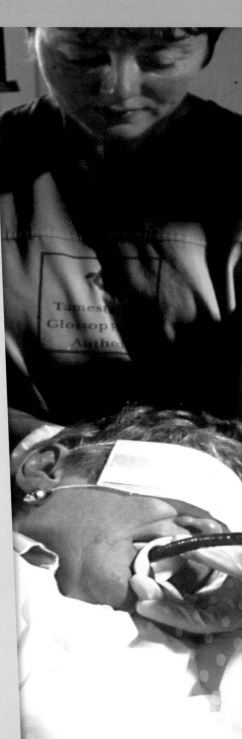

Introduction

This unit provides you with an opportunity to apply your understanding of physiological principles to the authentic experience of individuals affected by physiological disorders.

You will be required to produce two in-depth case studies, describing the course of two individuals' disorders and the signs and symptoms they present. You will research and explain their physiology and the processes involved in reaching a diagnosis.

You will also investigate the roles of professional and support personnel and of informal carers involved in all aspects of diagnosis, treatment and care of the individuals. Finally, you will conduct some secondary research to explore the possible future progression of the disease.

This unit will be valuable for anyone aiming to progress to professional training in the health and social care professions.

There are strong links with several other units in the programme, including Unit 5: *Fundamentals of anatomy and physiology* and Unit 13: *Physiology of fluid balance*.

How you will be assessed

This unit is assessed internally by your tutor.

After completing this unit you should be able to achieve the following outcomes:

- Understand the nature of two physiological disorders
- Understand the processes involved in diagnosis of disorders
- Understand the care strategies used to support individuals through the course of a disorder
- Understand how individuals adapt to the presence of a disorder.

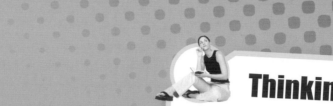

Thinking points

Which subject will you choose for your first case study? You will need to think about both the type of disorder and the individual.

You will need to spend significant time with your chosen subjects and for this reason family members or friends are the most appropriate. Formal consent (usually in writing) must be obtained and verified by an eye witness. If you investigate a disorder of someone in a care setting, then you must obtain the consent both of the individual and of the care setting.

Discuss your ideas with your tutor to ensure that:

- you can meet the requirements of the unit (as someone in the early stages of a disorder may have received only limited medical care)
- you have sufficient physiological understanding of the disorder.

You will need to consider confidentiality at all times, so think twice before including photographs, copies of clinical reports and images such as X-ray films and scans.

Be sensitive to the feelings of the subject of your research. Remember that they are living with the disorder and it doesn't go away once you have finished. To pay regular visits to someone solely to produce a piece of work for a qualification, and never to visit again when it is finished, would be deemed quite uncaring.

Appropriate disorders for your case study

You can study disorders other than those in the following list but you must check out your choice with your tutor.

- diabetes (insulin dependent or non-insulin dependent)
- coronary heart disease
- stroke (cerebral haemorrhage, cerebral thrombosis or cerebral infarction)
- Parkinson's disease
- Alzheimer's disease
- asthma
- emphysema
- motor neurone disease
- multiple sclerosis (MS)
- rheumatoid arthritis
- osteoporosis
- Crohn's disease
- ulcerative colitis
- inflammatory bowel syndrome (IBS)
- cancer – lung, bowel, skin, breast, prostate gland.

Start by making a pattern diagram of all contacts with physiological disorders, including the current stage of each illness and its physiological nature. Check the diagram against the unit requirements and delete any entries that will prevent you from achieving your goals (for example, if the individual's illness is only recently diagnosed or if you will not be able to spend much time with that person). Discuss your diagram with your tutor to select the individual and disorder for your first case study.

Draft a consent form for signature by the chosen individual and an eye witness. Check it with your tutor and save and print out two copies. If you are going to involve a care setting, prepare a form for consent.

Individuals

Two case studies are required so you will need two individuals with different diagnosed physiological

disorders who have been referred to professionals for investigation, have subsequently been diagnosed and are, or have been, receiving treatment and care.

A **diagnosis** is usually made by a doctor. When it is based on the signs and symptoms, it is sometimes called a **clinical diagnosis** and, if these might fit more than one disorder, a **differential diagnosis** is made. A family doctor might need another health care professional's opinion and make a **referral** to the appropriate professional or professional service.

Key terms

Diagnosis The process by which the nature of the disease or disorder is determined or made known.

Clinical diagnosis A diagnosis made on the basis of signs and symptoms.

Differential diagnosis The recognition of one disease from among a number presenting similar signs and symptoms.

Referral Handing over to another professional (usually a specialist) or type of service such as physiotherapy.

As you progress with the requirements of the unit in this chapter, you will follow a case study of Steve, who has chronic renal failure. This should help you determine how to set out and research your own case studies. A disorder which is not in your list has been chosen as an example to leave you free to choose one from the recommended list. Note that details of clinical investigations and measurements for Steve have been largely omitted as being irrelevant to your learning. However, you will need to include these details when you carry out your own investigations.

Investigate

Although a case study is not the same as a research proposal, it has many related issues, such as deciding what methods to use to collect information and data. Ethical issues are just as central and so is the importance of respecting confidentiality of the data obtained.

When you know an individual very well, he or she might tell you that they really do not mind if you write about their details fairly openly. However, it is one thing to say that in advance and another to see your details in print and they may feel differently at a later stage. It is also your duty in health and social care to respect confidentiality and you could give reassurance by saying that you have to plan your case study confidentially as part of your task.

This of course means not using their names, addresses, true age or any details that might be used to identify the individuals. A fictitious name is better than Mr A or Mrs B as these do tend to interrupt the flow of the work.

Primary research

This is first-hand information collected by you. It is likely to involve notes made during your observation of your chosen subject. Best practice would be to make these notes immediately after a meeting as it is intrusive to make notes at the time.

You might note:

- the psychological state of your subject in comparison with other meetings, for example, nervous, tense, happy, anxious, depressed, etc., backed up with evidence from demeanour, body language and verbal communication.
- visible signs and symptoms such as complaints of pain or signs of discomfort backed up with evidence, such as massaging or holding a wrist or knee, etc.
- changes in activities of daily living such as now having Meals on Wheels or a mobility aid
- difficulties in maintaining employment or relationships (these will usually be elicited verbally)

Key terms

Primary research This is information collected by you – not someone else – during the course of your investigation. It might consist of observations or interviews.

- evidence of coping strategies or changes in lifestyle.

Noting your observations immediately after a meeting is easier if you have a memory aid to guide you, so construct a dated diary sheet to fill out after each visit. Use the generic bullet points listed earlier to guide you, leaving a few blank rows to add any particular observations specific to your case study.

Remember!

Be sensitive. Keep any meeting short if you feel the individual is in pain or discomfort.

Another form of primary research useful in compiling your case study is the interview. A semi-structured interview will give you confidence. Plan how many times you will see your subject and what you will ask on each occasion to meet the unit requirements.

Try to keep the interview to an acceptable time scale, perhaps half-hour or hour-long sessions, and be prepared to finish early if there are signs of fatigue or discomfort. You may record your interview if the individual has no objection.

Theory into practice

You have chosen the physiological disorder asthma and your 16-year-old sister for your case study. You plan to carry out six half-hour sessions over a period of three weeks.

Using the unit requirements for a case study, write a rough plan for six interviews stating how you would use the time to collect the information you need.

Secondary research

This is information collected by other people which you will use to help you in compiling your case studies. You may be accessing Department of Health, support group or charity websites for information and statistics. On the other hand, you may be researching your chosen physiological disorder in books such as health encyclopaedias, health and social care textbooks, magazines, professional journals or even media articles. Whatever your source, you must give credit to people who have done the research by acknowledging author and date of publication. At the end of your case studies, you can compile a list of references including any people you have sought information from (seek their permission first). **Secondary research** will back up your evidence, show connections between sections and possibly supply information that you have not been able to find at source.

Key terms

Secondary research This is information collected by other people and used by you in your investigation. It might include published data and statistics, information about the same or related topics or different case studies. Secondary data should always be referenced and acknowledged.

Ethical issues

Ethics refers to a code of moral principles so that any issues which raise questions about morality can be termed ethical issues.

By gaining the consent of your subject at the start of your case study, you have avoided one issue; to be talked and written about without giving consent would be a gross infringement of privacy and decency. You may have been in a situation where someone has said something about you that has made you angry or unhappy and of course you would not wish your subject to be placed in such a position.

Although it will make life more difficult for you, the individual must be aware that he or she can back out of the study at any time. You must also agree to portray any information provided in a fair and honest manner and never deceive your subject. The individual chosen for the

study may request a copy of the study or wish to read it through when you have finished. This should be agreed to. You should also be able to say how many people will be reading the case study and who they are. This is pertinent to keeping your information limited to those who need to know. Never divulge it to your best friend or anyone else. It is also binding for you not to enquire about someone else's case study. However, you obviously will need to discuss your work with your tutor and your subject must be aware of this.

Lastly, you must ensure that the individual is protected from harm. This may sound silly at first, because you are not intending to carry out any physical investigations. However, you have already learned about the need for sensitivity, and careless questions may cause psychological harm or stress – the individual might even become anxious about some of the questions you have asked once you have left. You may become over-enthusiastic and let an interview go on for too long, causing fatigue and exhaustion. Being asked lots of questions may seem like an interrogation and you must guard against this. This is another reason why you should plan your interviews so that you don't become a nuisance, calling back again and again, because you forgot something you need to write about.

Respect for confidentiality of data obtained

The confidential information relating to the disorder of your case study subject, and the confidential information

Theory into practice

You need to be aware of ethical issues and respect the confidentiality of all information supplied to you for the purpose of writing your two case studies.

Compile a short leaflet demonstrating how you will manage ethical issues and confidentiality. Discuss the leaflet with your subjects and note any concerns they may have. Note that even if a subject expresses a lack of concern about confidentiality, you still have an ethical duty to observe the principles discussed earlier.

divulged by your subject, have been supplied to you to assist in your work. Such information must not be divulged to peers, friends or relatives and it is your ethical duty to keep the information private. Remember that the subject should be aware that you may need, from time to time, to discuss the nature of your work with your tutor.

Physiology

You will remember that physiology is the science that deals with the functions and activities of life or living tissue and the physical and chemical phenomena that are involved.

Body systems affected

You will need to write about the body systems affected by the disorder. There may be more than one – in fact there may be several systems involved with a complex disorder. However, you will only be required to identify and explain the major systems affected.

In diabetes, for example, this would include the endocrine and digestive systems (role of pancreas, liver and carbohydrate digestion). At some stage, you might need to discuss how diabetes affects the cardiovascular and nervous systems but it would be adequate to only describe the organs and tissues that are involved.

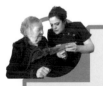

In context

Steve suffers from chronic renal failure. The major body system involved is the renal system although other systems such as the cardiovascular and musculo-skeletal systems can become involved.

1 **Describe the body system involved in renal failure.**

2 **Using secondary research, investigate the physiological changes caused by renal failure.**

3 **Research probable causes of renal failure.**

Table 14.1 gives a summary of the major systems that are involved in all the physiological disorders listed in the specification and reproduced on page 202.

Disorder	Major body systems involved
Diabetes	Endocrine and digestive systems
Coronary heart disease	Cardiovascular and respiratory systems
Stroke	Cardiovascular and nervous systems
Parkinson's disease	Nervous and musculo-skeletal systems
Alzheimer's disease	Nervous system
Asthma	Respiratory system
Emphysema	Cardiovascular and respiratory systems
Motor neurone disease	Nervous and musculo-skeletal systems
Multiple sclerosis (MS)	Nervous and musculo-skeletal systems
Rheumatoid arthritis	Musculo-skeletal system
Osteoporosis	Musculo-skeletal system
Crohn's disease	Digestive system
Ulcerative colitis	Digestive system
Inflammatory bowel disease (IBS)	Digestive system
Cancer	• Respiratory system – lung • Digestive system – bowel • Skin • Reproductive system – breast • Reproductive system – prostate

Table 14.1 Disorders and the major body systems involved.

You will find it helpful to revise the appropriate body system by returning to Book 1, Unit 5: *Fundamentals of anatomy and physiology*.

Structural and physiological changes caused by the disorder or its treatment

After an overview of the body system, you will need to explain how the disorder has affected the anatomy of the system, either **macroscopically** or **microscopically,** or both if appropriate.

Macroscopic changes that can be seen without the aid of a microscope.

Microscopic changes that cannot be seen without using a microscope.

For example, if you are investigating breast cancer, you will need to identify and explain how the macroscopic structure of the breast might change. The breast might be enlarged, swollen or distorted. The skin overlying the breast might appear dimpled, called *peau d'orange* because it resembles the skin of an orange. The nipple might become inverted (sunken) or there could be a bloody discharge from the nipple ducts. You would then go on to explain the microscopic changes usually arising as a result of a **needle biopsy** or **lumpectomy**. The pathologist looks for evidence of abnormal cells.

Another example, motor neurone disease, might show muscle wasting macroscopically and degeneration of nerve fibres and muscle fibres microscopically.

As well as structural changes, there are likely to be physiological changes resulting from the disorder too. For example, in motor neurone disease, there is muscle weakness, commonly beginning in the hands or the legs. Other physiological disturbances are cramps, unusual stiffness or irregular, spontaneous contractions of areas

Needle biopsy This is when a fine needle is inserted into a lump or organ to remove material for microscopic examination. Needles may have cutting tips to remove small sections of tissue or have a hollow stem for removing fluid (containing cells). The material is prepared for microscopic examination. The search is for abnormal cells which might be enlarged, peculiarly shaped or have actively dividing nuclei.

Lumpectomy An operation to remove a suspect lump which is then sent for microscopic examination.

Muscle wasting Observable diminishing muscle mass.

of muscle. In a stroke, caused by an interrupted flow of blood to part of the brain or bleeding in the brain, there can be weakness or paralysis of one side of the body, slurred speech, visual disturbance, difficulty in swallowing, confusion and headaches. With a stroke, the effects depend on the actual part of the brain that is affected.

Treatment can cause both structural and physiological changes too. Nearly all invasive procedures will inevitably cause some structural damage. Invasive procedures involve cutting or piercing the skin or inserting instruments or material into the body.

In context

Steve had suffered from high blood pressure (hypertension) for many years and his doctor had prescribed medication (anti-hypertensives) to reduce his blood pressure. Several years ago, while on holiday, he began to feel generally unwell and suffered from severe headaches. On his return, he saw his doctor who found that his blood pressure had become dangerously high. Steve was referred to a specialist in renal disorders (nephrologist). Among other tests, Steve had a kidney biopsy to examine the condition of the microscopic

nephrons in his kidneys. The nephrons were severely damaged and his kidney function tests demonstrated that kidney function was rapidly decreasing. There were both structural and physiological changes due to the disorder of chronic renal failure.

1   **Explain the purpose of any biopsy.**

2   **Name three other disorders where the taking of a biopsy is useful.**

3   **Assess the value of biopsies.**

Biopsies, injections and blood transfusions are examples of invasive techniques. Physiotherapy after injuries such as fractures, or in conditions like arthritis or early stages of motor neurone disease, can reduce joint stiffness, retrain muscles after a stroke, reduce muscle spasms and minimise pain and inflammation. Clinical drugs can restore blood chemistry as insulin does in diabetes, hormones do in endocrine disorders and iron supplements in anaemia.

The range of treatment for disorders is vast and you will need to explain how the treatment and the disorder affect the anatomy and physiology of the body for your chosen disorders.

Psychological effects

Many of the disorders you will study are long-term non-communicable (not infectious) disorders with limited treatment and management. Some might be curable in the accepted sense, such as breast cancer or coronary heart disease, but many will progressively get worse, such as Alzheimer's and Parkinson's diseases.

Disorders like these can have psychological effects as well as physiological effects and most of these will be negative effects such as bouts of **depression** and anxiety. Service users will naturally be concerned for themselves but also for their family and especially dependents.

Pain is often associated with worry, depression and fear of the unknown. When a diagnosis has been made, the perception of pain and its effects is often less, especially if the sufferer can be reassured.

Individuals have very different **pain thresholds**, especially if they have been incapacitated or ill for a long time and are 'used' to the pain experience.

Key terms

Depression Extreme sadness or melancholy. Reactive depression occurs as a result of illness. Some types of depression have no known cause.

Pain threshold The level at which the agony becomes unbearable. Individuals have different pain thresholds and the levels can be affected by past experiences of pain.

In a few disorders, such as multiple sclerosis, the service user may have periods of intense or exaggerated well-being (which is not justified) interspersed with periods of depression. This state of exaggerated well-being is known as **euphoria**.

Key terms

Euphoria An inflated sense of well-being when circumstances do not warrant it.

When you are carrying out your primary research for your case studies, you must observe and record the changes in mood by your subject. You can confirm an observation sensitively if need be, with a gentle open question. Do not ask baldly whether they are depressed or have bouts of depression, you are almost certain to get agreement which may or not be expanded upon. Volunteered information is different and you may be able to gently explore this further. Do not persevere if it is clear that the service user does not wish to discuss the subject.

Reflect

Have you ever felt down as a result of an illness? It is common to feel tiredness and weakness, for example, after influenza or food poisoning.

Research the effects of depression and compare them with how you felt. Depression has more signs and symptoms than a temporary feeling of unhappiness.

Influences on development of disorder

After a disorder has been diagnosed, the cause may be apparent or not. In most cases of the types of disorders you may be studying, the causes will not be transparent but there may be underlying factors or influences which have played some part.

Some factors are discussed below:

Inherited traits

As knowledge and understanding of inheritance grows, we are aware that many disorders such as cystic fibrosis, phenylketonuria (PKU) and Down's syndrome are inherited from one or both parents or that a mutation of a gene or chromosome has occurred at or before conception. Other medical conditions are not openly inherited in this way but research has shown that they tend to run in families and there is said to be an inherited trait that predisposes family members to certain conditions.

Breast cancer is a well-known disorder that runs in some families and it is not uncommon nowadays for female family members to have breast removals or mastectomies as a preventative strategy.

Multiple sclerosis also runs in families. Research has shown that relatives of individuals with multiple sclerosis are eight times more likely to develop the condition as those without an affected family member. There are also inherited traits in osteoporosis and relatives are advised to take preventative measures by leading a healthy lifestyle including no smoking and moderate alcohol intake, a calcium-rich diet and significant exercise. Post-menopausal women may be prescribed hormone replacement therapy as the female hormone oestrogen is important in maintaining bone density.

Lifestyle choices

You learned above that lifestyle choices are important in preventing osteoporosis in vulnerable individuals and you will be well aware of the role smoking plays in the possibilities of developing lung cancer. Excessive exposure to ultra-violet light is a major factor in the development of skin cancer and still a summer tan is seen as evidence of 'health' and looking well. Only very slowly are we becoming used to the idea of using a high-factor sun screen and covering up exposed skin, especially around noon, in the summer months. It is

taking a long time to change the summertime culture among young adults in the UK.

People with sedentary lifestyles and jobs who do not regularly take exercise are prone to coronary heart disease, diabetes and strokes.

Diets rich in saturated fats and refined sugars influence the development of non-insulin-dependent diabetes, coronary heart disease and stroke. Diets rich in meat and fat and low in fibre are thought to be significant in the development of bowel cancer. Emphysema is regularly associated with chronic bronchitis as a result of smoking.

You are almost certainly going to find that some lifestyle choices influence at least one of the physiological disorders you will choose.

Employment

The work of an individual can exert an influence on the development of the disorder. We are now very familiar with the effects of exposure to asbestos. In the past, many environments contained asbestos as it was heavily used to reduce the risk of fire. Catering establishments, schools, many manufacturing plants and even homes were built using asbestos. An aggressive form of cancer called mesothelioma became linked to asbestos exposure and this caused cancer of the pleura lining the lungs.

Pharmacists, because of the fine dust from the dispensing of drugs, frequently develop allergies and asthma. Teachers previously exposed to chalk dust can develop similar problems. Military personnel have developed serious illness from harmful chemicals used in warfare. Miners exposed to coal and rock dust are prone to bronchitis and emphysema as well as pneumoconiosis, a disease which results in severe scarring of the lungs.

You have already learned about skin cancer from sun exposure but of course many employees work outside – gardeners are particularly prone to skin cancer.

Many workers had contact with chemicals that we now realise predispose them to cancer, such as benzene and benzene products. These are known as carcinogens. Neither must we forget about professional sportspeople, ballet dancers and acrobats, all of whom experience excessive wear of joints and muscles and injuries which may progress to arthritis. Mohammed Ali, who has Parkinson's disease, is not alone in the boxing world in suffering from a cerebral disorder.

You will need to find out whether employment has been a factor in the development of the disorders in your case studies.

In context

Steve had spent his early adult life as an officer in the army and he served in Africa, Malaya and Korea. Steve had several bouts of malaria during this period and also suffered from yellow fever. He has had problems with kidney stones in the past.

He also smokes cigars regularly and in the army was a cigarette smoker. Steve has been overweight for many years now, although he was a fit, sports-loving, athletic man in his early adulthood. He doesn't worry much about healthy eating.

Since leaving the army, Steve has had a career in engineering sales. He now drives for long distances and is away from home for considerable periods.

1 **Discuss the effects of lifestyle factors on Steve's health and well-being.**

2 **Explain how Steve's employment may have had an effect on his health.**

3 **Evaluate the possible influences on Steve's physiological disorder.**

Diet

You have learned about the influences of some dietary choices on the development of diabetes, coronary heart disease and strokes in the previous section of lifestyle choices. People who do not eat healthy, balanced diets are prone to obesity, bowel disorders and bowel cancer. Fibre is thought to be particularly important in preventing gastro-intestinal disorders and the current 5 A Day health promotion campaign, which encourages people to eat more fruit and vegetables, is attempting to introduce more fibre into the diets of UK people (as well as preventing obesity).

Convenience foods have come under attack in recent years due to their high saturated fat and sugar content. So-called healthy meals, advertised as being low in fat, are often high in refined sugar and can result in dental disease and diabetes.

Alcohol, as well as being a major cause of road accidents and a significant factor in unwanted pregnancies and criminal activities, may lead to cirrhosis of the liver, a serious life-threatening disorder. Alcohol is contraindicated (should not be mixed) with many types of medication.

Environmental influences

Under this heading, you might consider the quality of air and water, noise and light pollution, housing, crime levels, climate, altitude, natural and man-induced radioactivity levels, etc.

Fortunately in the UK, most environmental influences are strictly regulated and their influences on disease are minimised. However, poor quality housing, particularly

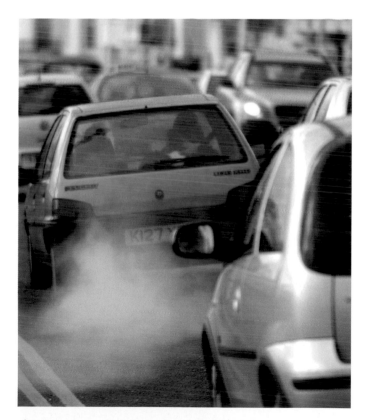

▲ Polluted air can make the symptoms of asthma worse.

rented accommodation, still exists in many large inner cities and can lead to the spread of tuberculosis, respiratory illnesses and infestations. Air pollution, including fumes from traffic, while not believed to cause asthma, certainly makes attacks more frequent and severe.

Research has shown that more cases of cancer occur in inhabited areas close to some nuclear plants. Mobile phone masts and wind farms are coming under increasing scrutiny for effects on the health of nearby inhabitants, but as yet no definitive proof has been acknowledged.

The possible environmental effects on the development of disorders are vast and so you will need to investigate this carefully for your chosen disorders.

Signs and symptoms

Physiological disorders will be characterised by the **signs** and **symptoms** experienced by the individuals suffering from the disorders.

Key terms

Sign An objective indication of a disorder noticed by a doctor (or nurse).

Symptom A feature complained of by the service user or patient.

It is not possible to explain every sign and symptom for all the disorders you might investigate but some common manifestations could include those shown in Table 14.2.

Common signs	Common symptoms
Pallor/red flush/jaundice	Pain/discomfort/ general malaise
Sweating/dehydration	Thirst
Trembling/tremors	Palpitations
Smell (breath, body)	'Pins and needles'
Changes in appearance of urine/ faeces	Paralysis
Changes in heart rate	Headache
Changes in breathing rate/wheezing	Visual disturbances
Rash/spots	Unsteadiness/muscle weakness
Changed blood pressure	Changes in urination
Changes in sensation	Changes in bowel habit
Loss/gain in weight	Loss/gain in weight
Changes in consciousness	Cough
Changes in mobility	Seizure
Changes in skin/mucous membranes, for example, colour, texture, etc.	Presence of lump/blood
Changes in temperature	Nausea/vomiting

Table 14.2 Common signs and symptoms.

In context

Steve had no signs of a disorder and only noticed that his headaches happened more frequently and were more severe. He generally felt unwell but could not describe why, except to say that he always felt tired.

Steve showed some signs and symptoms of an enlarged prostate gland – a common problem in older men.

1   Many people complain of 'just not feeling right'. Find out the correct medical term to describe this.

2   Do people with high blood pressure always suffer from headaches?

3   Where is the prostate gland and what are its functions?

In each case study of a physiological disorder, you will describe and explain the signs and symptoms characteristic of the illness.

Take it further

Find out the symptoms associated with an enlarged prostate gland. How can this be differentiated from prostate cancer?

Assessment activity 14.1

For each of your chosen disorders, carry out the following tasks:

P1 Describe the course of two different physiological disorders as experienced by two different individuals.

1 Describe the events which relate to the illness from the start of symptoms to the present day. How did your chosen subject suspect that something was wrong and how did his or her health change from that day to now? **P1**

Grading tip for P1

Do you feel that you have an understanding of the progression of the disorder? Try to collect the information together in time order, such as:

What made the person go to the GP in the first place? What were the actions carried out by the GP at the first and subsequent visits? How long before referral? What happened after referral?

P2 Describe the physiology of each disorder and factors that may have influenced its development.

2 Explain the structure and physiology of the main body systems which are involved.

3 Explain the signs and symptoms of the disorder.

4 Identify and explain the factors which have influenced the development of the disorder. **P2**

Grading tip for P2

Are the possible causes and signs and symptoms making sense now you understand more of the physiology of the systems involved? This will be the opportunity to carry out some secondary research to extend your knowledge and understanding. You can access websites on the Internet for increased depth and breadth.

M1 Explain how the course of the disorder in each individual relates to the physiology of the disorder.

5 How will you relate the developing illness to the way in which the normal functions of the body are disturbed? **M1**

Grading tip for M1

What is the physiology of the disorder? This means describing what is being disturbed in the body, either macroscopically or, more likely, microscopically. Then you will need to relate this to the original and ongoing signs and symptoms.

There can be several stages between the first time an individual visits their GP with a complaint and the diagnosis being reached.

Referral

Occasionally, a doctor will examine a patient and be extremely anxious about the diagnosis and telephone or provide a letter for immediate attention by hospital doctors, usually consultants.

When the patient has private health insurance or is financially well off, he or she can be seen within a day or two at a private health hospital.

More usually, however, the family doctor will see the patient a few times before deciding on referral to a consultant or specialist in that field of medicine or continuing to treat the patient at the surgery. There may be several weeks before the patient can actually be seen by a specialist consultant or his team. In either case, the family doctor may also arrange for the patient to have X-rays, blood tests, physiotherapy or other services. A GP will refer a patient whose diagnosis is in doubt, needs specialist treatment or whose condition is urgent and/or serious.

Investigations

Any investigations carried out will be specific to each disorder but will always include a medical history and standard blood tests, such as a blood count and haemoglobin level (see *Blood tests* below).

Medical history

This is the process where the doctor listens to what the patient has to say and asks appropriate questions about the patient's symptoms and any previous disorders that might have an influence on the development of the disorder.

This account from the patient can be extremely vital in providing the clues to the nature of the illness and, in an ideal world, should not be rushed. The doctor is searching for significant clues that will form the pattern for establishing the exact nature of the complaint or diagnosis. In many instances, the doctor can elicit information that will point to two or more conditions and he or she will then try to establish which one is the most likely (this is known as a differential diagnosis).

It is important to establish the likelihood of the illness. If the patient is in pain or distress some form of treatment may be necessary. The treatment itself might then mask the original symptoms and make the diagnosis more difficult.

After recording the medical history, the doctor will carry out a physical examination. This may be short or extended, depending on the nature of the disorder. For example, the doctor is extremely unlikely to examine anything other than the chest area if a patient is complaining of difficulty in breathing. A patient who has symptoms related to the digestive tract will have the abdominal area examined. During a physical examination, the doctor is likely to listen to the patient's heart and lungs and measure blood pressure, especially if the patient has not been seen before or for a long time.

Palpation

This is a technique for feeling organ shapes, sizes and surfaces with the hands. It is particularly useful on the abdomen because doctors are taught to examine for larger than normal organs such as the liver, spleen, bladder, etc. Areas of unusual tenderness or rigidity are noted, together with any abnormal masses or lumps.

Blood tests

Samples of blood can be obtained in two ways, by venepuncture (inserting a syringe needle into a vein) or by a finger prick using a small, sterile lancet. Venepuncture is used when several millilitres of blood are required for clinical analysis. An examination of blood provides a good indication of the health and well-being of a patient. Many substances normally present in blood can be reported on including:

- haemoglobin level (for anaemia)
- levels of blood salts, technically known as electrolytes (for renal disorders, diabetes, metabolic bone disorders)
- hormone levels (for pregnancy, endocrine disorders)
- blood gases, such as oxygen and carbon dioxide (for respiratory disease)
- specific enzyme tests (for heart attacks)
- plasma proteins (for bleeding disorders)
- pH (for renal disorders, diabetes – see page 182).

A special test known as a blood cell count will reveal whether the different types of blood cells are present in normal quantities and appearance.

The finger prick test is used when only small quantities of blood are required for measuring the presence of a particular substance. For example, diabetics use small quantities like this soaked into paper in a special device for monitoring their blood glucose. Health visitors will use a heel prick on newborn babies to collect tiny amounts of blood to test for phenylketonuria (PKU test).

There are also other special blood tests for various different purposes, for example, blood culture to determine whether septicaemia or blood poisoning is present.

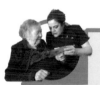

In context

At the first consultation after referral, a detailed medical history and physical examination was followed up by blood and urine tests.

Blood tests showed that some chemical constituents were higher than normal and there was a small degree of anaemia. Urine tests showed that Steve's urine was loaded with protein (normally absent).

Steve's blood pressure was 195/120.

1 **From your knowledge of physiology, explain the source of protein in this disorder.**

2 **Outline the connection between blood chemistry and urine constituents.**

3 **Explain the physiological significance of finding protein in urine.**

Urine tests

The physical characteristics (such as colour, smell, clarity, pH, concentration) and chemical composition of urine (glucose, **urea**, protein, drugs, hormones blood, etc.) can reveal underlying conditions such as kidney diseases, pregnancy and diabetes. More specific tests can estimate kidney function and inherited metabolic disorders. Urine, like blood, can be cultured to detect microbial infections.

Key terms

Urea A nitrogenous substance resulting from the liver breaking down excess **amino acids** from the digestion of proteins. Nitrogenous material not required for metabolism cannot be stored in the body. If allowed to accumulate, urea is toxic to body tissues and can result in death.

Amino acids The nitrogenous end products of protein digestion normally used to build up new structural and physiological body proteins such as enzymes and hormones. However, many Western diets contain too much dietary protein, and after digestion the unwanted amino acids will be broken down by the liver and eliminated by the kidneys.

Radiological investigations

You will most likely have seen plain black and white X-rays which are ideal for viewing the skeleton in a non-invasive way. Modern equipment produces high quality images without exposure to much radiation.

Despite this, all radiation is harmful and every effort is made to minimise exposure. Radio-opaque materials can be used to fill hollow organs, such as the alimentary canal, and if the part is viewed from more than one angle, filling defects (black areas not filled by the radio-opaque material) caused by tumours and polyps, or bumps caused by ulcers or erosion, will be displayed. The most common radio-opaque material is a barium compound and a service user will drink this (a barium meal) or have it poured into the rectum as an enema (barium enema) depending on whether the upper or lower part of the alimentary canal needs to be examined.

Different radio-opaque substances can be introduced into the cardiovascular system to display particular blood vessels – this is known as angiography. Radio-opaque iodine compounds are used to display the urinary tract as these can be excreted by the kidneys and show the pelvis of the ureters (where the ureter enters the kidney), the ureters, bladder and urethra. This is useful to determine whether there are any blockages to the passage of urine.

Scans

The most common form of scan is an ultrasound scan and the technology is now so advanced that it is used for many things. Most people associate ultrasound scans with pregnancy monitoring, but they are also used for visualising the liver, gall bladder, pancreas, breast and kidneys. Ultrasound works by bouncing high frequency sound waves off internal organs but has difficulty where there is a lot of gas, such as in the lungs, or a casing of bone like the adult brain (new-born babies' brains can be scanned through the so-called 'soft spot'). It is used to

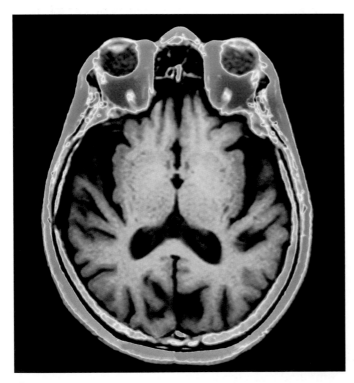

▲ Brain and skull scan taken at eye level.

detect tumours, foreign bodies, cysts and abnormalities of structure. Ultrasound scanning is considered very safe.

MRI (magnetic resonance imaging) scans are also safe because they do not use radiation either. Powerful magnetic fields and radio waves are used to provide high quality three-dimensional images of organs and structures within the body. Equipment is still not available everywhere as it is very expensive.

CT or CAT (computerised (axial) tomography) scans use X-rays passed at different angles through the body, transformed using a computer to produce cross-sectional images (slices). This is particularly useful in producing serial slices of brain tissue but is also used for other organs.

Function tests

These are tests that have been specially designed to determine the degree of function of particular parts of the body, to assist with diagnosis and assess the value of treatment. Function tests for an organ may include imaging techniques as well (see *Radiological investigations* and *Scans*).

Liver function tests are commonly ordered by GPs and specialists to assess liver function in service users who are suspected of having liver damage, liver disease or a partial loss of function. These tests look for chemical compounds that the liver manufactures or breaks down and are helpful in distinguishing between a disease of the liver and a blockage of the bile duct. Bilirubin is made by the liver from the breakdown of old, unwanted red blood cells and passed into bile. When bile flow is blocked, bilirubin levels will be higher than normal. Albumin is a plasma protein made by the liver and passed into blood. When liver cells are damaged or diseased, albumin levels will be lower than normal.

Kidney function tests clearly will include an examination of the urine (see urine tests). More precise results can be obtained from clearance tests.

Urea and creatinine are two substances excreted into urine by healthy kidneys. In a clearance test, the service user collects all urine over a 24-hour period in a plastic container and the amount of creatinine excreted can be compared with the blood levels to determine how well the kidneys are removing creatinine (or urea).

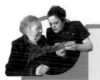

In context

The clinical specialist determined from the initial consultation and clinical investigations that Steve had a renal disorder and ordered further kidney function tests, including a creatinine clearance test.

The result showed that Steve had only 40 per cent of normal kidney function.

1 **How had the specialist reached his diagnosis?**

2 **Outline the process involved in a creatinine clearance test.**

3 **Investigate how far a person's liver can deteriorate before symptoms arise.**

Key terms

Reflexes These are automatic responses to stimuli. The patellar or knee-jerk reflex is a common reflex that doctors use as a test. It enables doctors to determine whether there is damage to the nervous pathway and also whether the speed of nervous impulses is increased or decreased.

EEG or electroencephalogram This is a tracing of the electrical activity of the brain. An abnormal rhythm may be found in epilepsy, dementia (Parkinson's disease) and brain tumours.

Brain function tests assess mental state and abilities, sensation and **reflexes**. Electrical activity can be measured by **EEG** and movement and muscle tone estimated.

Pancreatic function tests can include enzyme measurements in blood or the duodenum.

Reproductive and endocrine function tests can measure hormone levels in the blood.

Measurements

Certain measurements are taken routinely, such as pulse rate, breathing rate, blood pressure, body temperature and body weight and height (see Book 1, Unit 5).

Blood pressure should only be measured by a competent operator.

The force blood exerts on the walls of the blood vessels it is passing through is known as the blood pressure. It can be measured using a special piece of equipment called

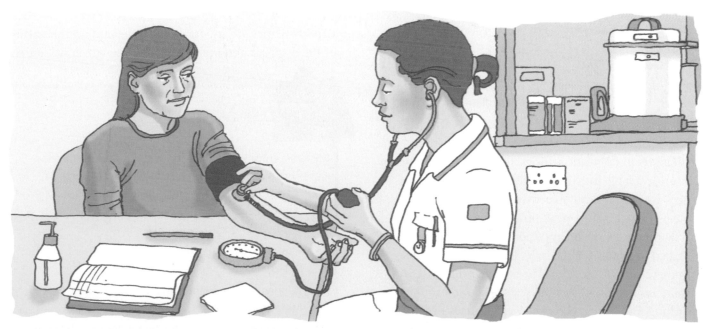

▲ Figure 14.1 Taking blood pressure using a sphygmomanometer.

a sphygmomanometer, often abbreviated to 'sphygmo' (pronounced sfigmo).

Other measurements are taken that are specific to particular disorders. For example, service users with asthma are encouraged to monitor their own disorder by peak flow measurements.

Peak flow measurement is now important in lung function testing and is quite easy to do. It measures the maximum speed of expiration and is associated with the calibre of the subject's main airways. A baseline is

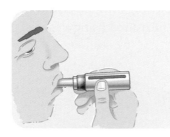

▲ **Figure 14.2 Measuring peak flow.**

often obtained using a medical spirometer with a skilled operator and then a simple peak flow meter is used, particularly in domestic settings, for monitoring. Special sizes are available for children. Electronic peak flow meters are available but expensive. Many children and adults with asthma use peak flow meters twice daily to monitor their condition and modify their therapy. They are asked to record the readings and take the records with them on visits to clinics or hospitals. Patients with chronic bronchitis and emphysema will also monitor their lung function in the same way. Athletes in training and patients requiring physiotherapy of the chest may also find peak flow readings useful.

Monitoring

Individuals with physiological disorders will all be subject to monitoring of some description. This will depend on the state of health of the service user, the particular disorder and the current stage of the diseases.

Regularity of checks by professionals

Some checks might only take place annually whereas others might happen weekly (fairly unusual) or even daily if there is an acute phase. The setting will clearly be a factor in monitoring; when the service user is in hospital, monitoring will occur daily with a specialist team visiting perhaps every other day. A patient in a quiet phase of MS (known as a remission) might only visit the GP once every two months and the specialist once a year. When a relapse (reoccurrence of the disease) occurs, monitoring intervals will be greatly shortened. Most commonplace infections that are treated by a GP with prescribed antibiotics are checked on again one week later and often a GP will only ask a patient to come back if the infection is not responding to treatment (a reflection of the pressure on the NHS).

Repeat measurements

Repeating measurements will also depend on the nature of the disorder and the treatment being given. When

In context

Steve continued to visit the renal outpatients once every two months. At every visit, he was weighed, had blood pressure measured and supplied a 24-hour collection of urine. He then attended the phlebotomy department for venepuncture.

1 **Explain the purpose of a phlebotomy department.**

2 **Why would renal patients be weighed at every out-patient visit?**

3 **What is the purpose of a 24-hour urine collection?**

service users are dispensing their own treatment, as instructed by the medical professionals, they are likely to repeat measurements very frequently. For example, asthmatic and diabetic patients will measure peak flow and blood glucose levels probably more than once a day. A person with hypertension in the early stages of treatment may attend the surgery or health centre blood pressure clinic once a week and keep a diary of their own BP measurements in the meantime.

Modern measuring devices, such as a blood glucose meter, can store many measurements in their memory so that professionals can get information on the fluctuation or stability of the levels over a period of time.

Repeat investigations

Generally, investigations are more costly and time-consuming to repeat than measurements. This means that they are less likely to be so frequent.

Investigations are likely to be repeated if the result of an earlier investigation was inconclusive and professionals feel that information can still be obtained to either make a diagnosis (if this is still in doubt) or to check on the results of a particular treatment. Inconclusive biopsies can be a common reason for repeat investigations, such as in some forms of cancer. Repeat X-rays are common to check on skeletal healing of abnormalities, fractures, etc.

Repeat investigations will also shed light on the progress of some diseases, with or without treatment being involved. Lung investigations through X-rays are quick and easy to do in the following up of a disease such as tuberculosis.

Monitoring, then, is a vital way of checking on the disease processes, treatment being given and the health and well-being of the service user. In your case studies, you will need to investigate the type, regularity and purpose of monitoring the service user's health.

Assessment activity 14.2

For each of your chosen disorders, carry out the following tasks:

P3 Describe the clinical investigations carried out and measurements made to diagnose and monitor the disorder in each individual.

1   What measurements and investigations are appropriate to your chosen disorder?

Grading tip for P3

Your chosen individuals will be able to help you with the monitoring by describing the procedures carried out during an out-patients appointment (and at home – diabetes, asthma). However, if the disease is long-standing, the memory of diagnostic investigations and measurements may be distant. Some of the equipment may not have been invented at that time! You can make a list from your sources of secondary information or use the information above to prompt memory recall. It would be useful to identify the potential of modern methods of diagnosis, such as CT and MRI scans, even though the equipment was not available or called upon in your case study.

M2 Explain possible difficulties involved in making a diagnosis from the signs and symptoms displayed by the individuals and the results of their investigations.

2   What problems arose in making a final diagnosis from the presentation of the signs and symptoms and the results of all the tests?   **M2**

Grading tip for M2

How long did it take doctors to confirm a diagnosis?

Some disorders are notoriously difficult to diagnose, especially in the early stages. Disorders such as MS and Alzheimer's disease fall into this category and initially diagnosis may be made by eliminating other disorders with similar signs and symptoms. Forgetfulness is a common symptom of later adulthood and could be seen as a normal part of the ageing process. On the other hand, asthma, coronary heart disease and diabetes can be diagnosed more easily, although there are always some patients in which it can be difficult. If you have chosen coronary heart disease for your investigative study, you will learn that some patients in later adulthood do not display the characteristic signs of a heart attack. ECG traces take time to display the changes shown, making diagnosis more difficult.

Small strokes can have confusing effects and in elderly people can prove challenging to diagnose. People with MS may display symptoms for only a short while and then have a remission lasting for many years or never have another occurrence.

Take time to research this properly.

14.3 The care strategies used to support individuals through the course of a disorder

In this section, you will learn about:

- the different care settings that the service user will experience
- the individuals responsible for the care
- the type of care that will be given.

The information here can only be generic as there are many types of physiological disorder that you may be investigating. You can use this information as a 'pick and mix' selection to apply to your case studies.

Care settings

A care setting is the name given to any location where care is dispensed. Care settings will change as an individual with a disorder is diagnosed, treated and care-managed.

GP surgery

This is likely to be the first or primary setting in which the patient initially seeks help for symptoms they are experiencing. There might already be a long-term relationship between the patient and the doctor, which is advantageous to both. A medical history will be taken, if not already known, and the doctor will ask relevant questions about the new symptoms.

The doctor will quickly have a possible list of disorders that the patient may be suffering from as a result of their questioning and will then carry out a physical examination to support or decrease their differential diagnosis. The physical examination will be enhanced by routine measurements such as BP, body temperature, pulse and breathing rates.

The doctor may decide quickly that the patient needs to be referred to hospital specialists, write a letter explaining the findings at the initial consultation and make an out-patients appointment with an appropriate specialist or consultant at the earliest opportunity. More usually, however, the doctor will arrange to use services allied to the hospital for X-rays, blood tests or other early investigations and request that the patient returns at a date when these results are likely to be available.

After further consultations, the doctor might still refer the patient to hospital or treat the condition for a time.

In context

Steve continued to visit his GP but less frequently as the GP was informed by the hospital after each out-patient appointment. The GP continued to dispense Steve's considerable list of medicines and held medication review appointments with him about twice a year.

1 **Explain the importance of keeping a GP informed about hospital visits.**

2 **Why is it important to review medication regularly?**

3 **Explain the psychological importance of maintaining contact with the GP.**

Health centre

More and more GP surgeries are grouping together in purpose-built health centres where extra services and facilities can be offered. Such facilities might include maternity services, counselling, alternative therapy sessions, various specialised clinics, phlebotomists, mobility aids specialists, family planning, health

promotion, etc. Such services relieve the pressure on hospitals, serve the local community well and may save patients having to travel long distances to hospitals. They are often located close to pharmacies so that medication is more easily obtained.

Hospital care

Service users may access hospital care as out-patients or in-patients.

People with serious disorders such as cancer will be admitted as soon as possible for investigations and treatment. Where the condition is less acute, they may make out-patient visits for a long time, for example, in cases of Parkinson's disease or Alzheimer's disease. Diabetic patients may be admitted for a short period to stabilise the condition with appropriate medication.

Hospitals have varied facilities and it may be necessary to be taken from one hospital to another for specialist facilities such as scans. This is usually for a short period only. Smaller hospitals have limited facilities and specialist consultants may visit, for example, for one day every month.

Service users are likely to be admitted as in-patients for any surgery except for minor complaints.

Own home

Most people who are ill would prefer to stay in their own homes while being cared for, especially if they have a loving family around. Older people often have a fear of hospitals or going into residential care and would prefer to stay at home, with familiar things around them. They often feel that if they leave home, they will not return.

Many of the disorders listed on page 204 will allow people to be cared for at home until the later stages of the illness. Where special aids are required, such as stair lifts, bath hoists and disabled access, these can be provided after a professional assessment. It is also more cost-effective for the NHS for people to continue independent living for as long as possible. Services such as home carers, Meals on Wheels and chiropody can be arranged to support people in their own homes as part of a care package of assistance.

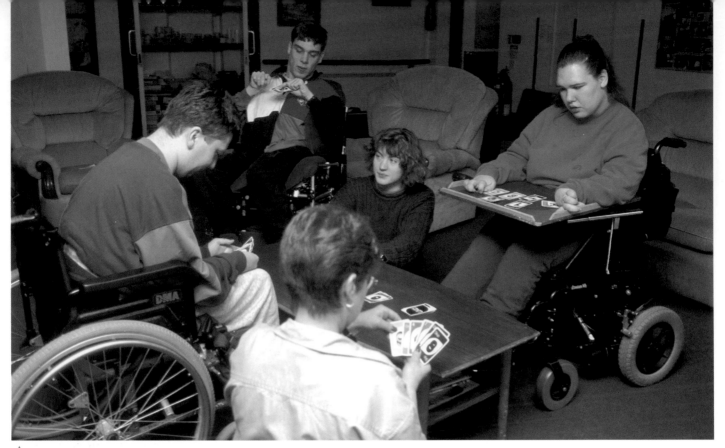

▲ Care strategies may include social care settings.

Social care settings

People suffering from late stages of disorders like Parkinson's and Alzheimer's diseases, rheumatoid arthritis, stroke and coronary heart disease may have to be cared for in a social care setting such as residential care because of increasing disability and the need to keep them safe. Other people may be able to stay at home and go to a day care setting several times a week for specific care, company and relaxation. This can be particularly important if the family is working during the day or the individual lives alone.

People

You have looked at a general range of care settings above but mainly it is the people who work there that are fundamental to the caring process and we can look at only a few.

General practitioner

You have learned about the role of the GP under GP surgeries in the previous section.

Clinical specialist

Clinical specialists have taken further qualifications in their particular field of medicine and become an 'expert'; you may be more familiar with the term consultant.

They are often called by their specialist field with '-ist' on the end, so a cardiologist specialises in heart disorders, a nephrologist in kidney disorders and a rheumatologist in bone diseases. These types of clinical specialists are usually physicians – people who practice medicine as opposed to surgery.

A doctor who has specialised in heart surgery will be a cardiac surgeon, a kidney surgeon is a renal surgeon and a bone surgeon is an orthopaedic surgeon.

Then you will get specialists for some particular life stages; a paediatrician is an expert professional in diseases of children and a geriatrician is concerned with diseases of elderly patients.

An oncologist is a specialist in tumours and a radiologist studies both the diagnosis and treatment of disease using radiological techniques.

There are clinical specialists in biochemistry, haematology, pathology and cytology, who service users rarely see but who work behind the scenes in departments that assist other clinical specialists.

The list of clinical specialists is very long and, if you meet an '-ist' name you do not recognise, either ask a professional (or the service user) or consult a dictionary.

Clinical specialists cannot see every service user and usually head a team of people consisting of registrars, senior house officers and house officers in descending order of rank. The specialist will often see the service user on a first visit to make a diagnosis and order investigations.

Nurses

Many years ago, nurses used to be seen as the 'handmaidens' (servants) to doctors. Now they are rightly recognised as expert professionals in individualised client/patient care, emanating from sound research and knowledge-based practice.

Like doctors, there are several tiers of nurses, all working to a value-based system. The system of nurse education underwent significant reforms several years ago and is now a recognised degree programme. Nurses also specialise in different programmes such as mental health, children, health visiting and midwifery, to mention only the major branches.

Nurses are taking on more and more of the traditional roles of doctors, such as prescribing medicines. Nearly every individual receiving care will have contact with nurses at most levels. Service users rely on nurses to meet their everyday caring needs as they tend to see doctors infrequently.

Professions allied to medicine

These include:
- occupational therapists
- physiotherapists
- radiographers
- radiotherapists
- chiropodists

to name only the major branches. The education programmes of all these professions are specialist degree programmes.

Occupational therapists are rehabilitation experts, and although this may involve rehabilitation looking towards employment or getting back to work, their work is also vital to ensure that service users have the abilities and competencies to manage at home. For example, an occupational therapist will be involved in the care of any service user who has musculo-skeletal problems before they can transfer from hospital to home. They will assess the service user and, if necessary, visit the home to see which mobility aids will assist in everyday living.

Physiotherapists are concerned with the treatment and rehabilitation of movement, mainly muscles, by the use of heat, light, electricity, massage, remedial exercises and manipulation.

Radiographers, not to be confused with radiologists (see *Clinical specialists*), are professional health care workers in either a diagnostic X-ray department or a radiotherapy department. They position the service user for the correct angle of the radiation and manage the process of radiography or radiotherapy. Radiotherapists will be important to cancer patients in particular.

Chiropodists, also sometimes known as podiatrists, care for the feet and treat diseases of the feet. The care of feet is particularly important for older diabetic service users as they are prone to gangrene from open cuts (inflicted by scissors when cutting toenails).

Pharmacists

Pharmacists work in hospital settings dispensing medication for in-patients and some out-patients, and also in pharmacies or chemist shops serving communities. Pharmacists are allowed to give advice and some forms of treatment to the community. Many offer extra services such as BP or blood glucose monitoring.

People use pharmacists for more or less instant advice because it is less frightening and more informal than going to the surgery. It's also more convenient to pop in while shopping and people 'don't like to bother the doctor with unimportant things'! Hospital pharmacists will advise hospital doctors on inappropriate combinations of drugs and side-effects and often confer with others at a 'case conference' where multi-disciplinary health professionals discuss the best form of care for a particular service user.

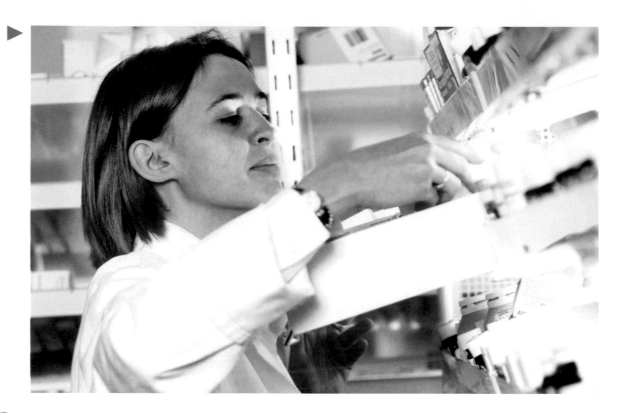

Pharmacist at work. ▶

Phlebotomists

A phlebotomist is a person skilled in taking one or more blood samples by puncturing a vein, usually close to the inner side of the elbow, and withdrawing blood through a syringe. Many blood samples have to be placed in special bottles for specific tests and taking blood from some individuals is notoriously difficult! Most phlebotomists work in hospital settings and although nurses are also competent in taking blood samples, the sheer volume of blood that needs to be taken from all the service users would occupy the time of many nurses so specialist care workers are employed.

Laboratory personnel

Blood samples, urine samples, stool samples, biopsies, etc., all have to be analysed and hospital laboratories employ many people. Service users rarely see laboratory personnel.

Care assistants

Care assistants undertake most of the care associated with daily living and will, in a hospital setting, be the carers most involved in meeting the needs of service users. They undertake more practical National Vocational Qualifications. Many progress after achieving these qualifications to degree programmes in nursing. Care assistants are also employed to carry out similar tasks in social care and domestic settings.

Counsellors

Counsellors provide guidance and psychological support, usually for a specific problem, but also where feelings and attitudes are important. Counsellors work in cancer care, abortion and HIV support as well as many other areas. Such areas might include mental health, family therapy, marriage guidance, sexual difficulties, substance abuse, terminal illness, disability and bereavement.

Although sessions are usually with one individual, there can also be group therapy sessions.

Counselling can be of great benefit for people with MS, motor neurone disease, cancer and stroke conditions. It helps people to take a realistic view and to remain positive in difficult circumstances.

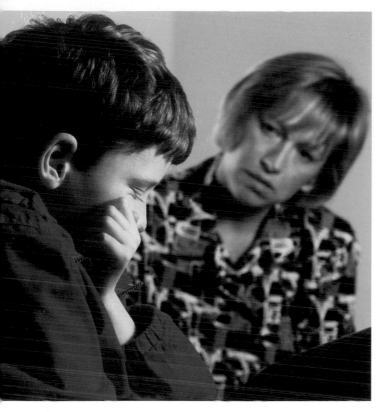

▲ **Counselling can be part of the care strategy.**

Informal carers

So far in this section we have looked at formal carers, those individuals who work in the health and social care field as professionals. Informal carers are individuals who have not taken any care qualifications but nevertheless carry the main burden of looking after a family member, relative or friend who is not fully independent. Informal carers are family members (sometimes children), friends, neighbours, faith-based

Reflect

Have you ever cared for somebody or observed a close friend or relative caring for an individual?

Think about the qualities an informal carer needs and the personal sacrifices they make.

organisation members, etc. There are massive numbers of informal carers doing a fantastic job, often 24 hours a day, seven days a week, with very little support either financially or practically. Many informal carers are tied, unable to work or enjoy free time but do so selflessly.

Clearly, this is a very important source of care for individuals with physiological disorders.

Take it further

What feelings might an individual with a chronic illness have when they can no longer carry out their own daily activities and need informal care from someone else?

Lay carers

Lay carers are individuals who are outside the health professions and not necessarily known to the service user. They include informal carers and voluntary workers from organisations which may be faith-based such as the St Vincent de Paul society (SVP) or those specialising in disorders such as Mencap for learning disabilities. They are not paid for attending to an individual with a disorder but may be part of a care plan.

Care

The different care strategies for physiological disorders are numerous and will depend on the particular disorders that you choose. However, certain strategies are useful in many disorders. We will look at some below.

Medication

There are many types of medication – too many to include all of them – but some include:

- analgesics (painkillers)
- antibiotics (to combat infection)
- anti-inflammatory drugs
- antihypertensives (to lower BP)

- metabolic dysfunction drugs (to correct or limit impaired chemical functions)
- immunosuppressive drugs (to suppress the immune response)
- carcino-chemotherapeutic drugs (to combat cancer, may be used in conjunction with radiation therapy)
- anti-allergic drugs (to suppress symptoms of allergic reactions)
- diuretics (to increase urine flow, thus removing surplus fluid from the body)
- bronchospasm relaxants (asthma and emphysema)
- hormone replacements
- muscle relaxants (stroke, MS)
- anti-depressants
- drugs for cardiac failure, angina, arrhythmias (changes in the heart's rhythm).

You will need to explore the types of medication used in your chosen disorders.

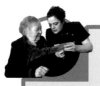

In context

The pharmacy personnel are very important to Steve as he frequently finds that he is short on particular medications – he is not well-organised. He takes antihypertensives to lower his BP, iron to counteract anaemia, diuretics to eliminate fluid and chemicals to adjust his blood chemistry (metabolic dysfunctional medication). The hospital nutritionist has offered advice on a 'renal' diet. This involves limiting protein intake, avoiding potassium-rich foods and a restricted fluid intake.

1 **Outline the dietary advice that nutritionists might give to patients with osteoporosis and coronary heart disease.**

2 **Some of Steve's medication is similar to that given to patients with coronary heart disease. Suggest reasons for this.**

3 **Pharmacists often offer services other than dispensing prescriptions from doctors. Investigate the increased services offered by pharmacists.**

Aids

Mobility aids may be required in arthritis, stroke, motor neurone disease, MS and in other conditions when the individual with the disorder is becoming frail and requires support. Such aids may be walking sticks, Zimmer frames or wheelchairs. People may need a variety of other aids such as stair lifts, bath hoists, support splints (to support weak muscles), special chairs, special cutlery and untippable dishes. Aids should be supplied to enable people to manage their daily living activities for as long as possible to retain their independence, self-respect and dignity.

Some people, especially those with lung cancer, bronchitis and emphysema and coronary heart disease, may require oxygen cylinders at home to ease breathing difficulties.

Surgery

Surgical operations may play a significant part in the ongoing progress of the disorders. A service user may have a heart bypass operation (see Figure 14.3) if they have coronary heart disease. This is where a short length of leg vein or artificial tubing may be joined to a section of healthy coronary artery to avoid a blockage and rejoined beyond the obstruction, so forming a bypass. This is often done two or three times if the coronary arteries are seriously diseased – so-called double or triple bypass operations.

Tumours will often be removed, especially in the early stages of cancer. Removing a lump from the breast (a 'lumpectomy') or the whole breast (mastectomy) may be needed to try to halt the spread of the disease. Removal of the prostate gland in males (prostatectomy) may be required in some cases of cancer.

Skin cancers are usually surgically removed and parts of the lung in the early stages of cancer only.

Surgery may play a part in the management of bowel cancer, Crohn's disease, ulcerative colitis and inflammatory bowel disease if symptoms are severe and not responding to other treatment. When parts of the bowel are removed, the service user may be left with a temporary or permanent **ileostomy** or **colostomy** after which faeces are passed into a bag attached to the abdominal wall and removed periodically.

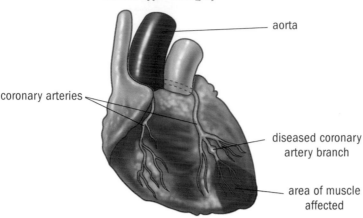

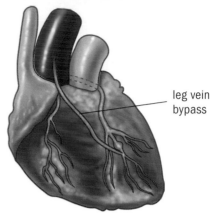

Figure 14.3 ▶
Heart bypass
surgery.

Before bypass surgery

aorta

coronary arteries

diseased coronary
artery branch

area of muscle
affected

After bypass surgery

leg vein
bypass

Key terms

Ileostomy An artificial opening from the ileum to the abdominal wall to evacuate faeces and bypass the large intestine.

Colostomy This is the same as an ileostomy except that the artificial opening is from the colon. The artificial opening is known as a stoma and faeces are evacuated into a bag attached to a belt or by adhesive.

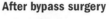

Transfusion

Anaemia can be a feature of several physiological disorders, such as MS, ulcerative colitis and also if surgery has been used to treat the main disorder. Whole blood transfusions may be necessary to correct the impaired oxygen carriage and give a better quality of life. Saline (a physiological salt solution) transfusions may be given to carry some forms of medication, correct dehydration (which can occur in diabetes) or shock after surgery.

In context

About one year after the initial consultation, Steve's kidney function was deemed to be very borderline for health, even with drugs. The nephrologist referred Steve to a renal surgeon to have a fistula (see page 195) made in his arm, ready for haemodialysis. This was carried out under a local anaesthetic. Steve started haemodialysis about nine months later as the fistula had to mature and get larger. Haemodialysis means being attached to a kidney machine to have the blood 'cleansed' of toxins for a minimum of four hours, three times each week. At this point, Steve was still working in sales so he needed to haemodialyse in the evenings, starting at 6 p.m.

Steve was tissue-typed and placed on a transplant list.

Two years later, a suitable donor kidney became available and Steve successfully underwent transplant surgery followed one week later by a prostatectomy. He had several units of blood transfused to correct his anaemia and to make up for blood loss during the surgery. Steve recovered quickly and was able to go home about ten days later.

1 **Explain the possible psychological effects of having to dialyse.**

2 **Investigate what is meant by tissue-typing before transplant surgery.**

3 **What types of drugs do all transplant patients have to take for the rest of their lives?**

Professional advice

You will understand that this can be extremely varied and may extend from reviewing lifestyle factors (such as smoking in respiratory and cardiovascular disease) to dietary advice (such as a recommendation to increase or lower the amount of fibre in the diet). Advice may be given on the degree of activity to be undertaken and the correct use of aids. Advice will be given by doctors, nurses, people in professions allied to medicine, pharmacists and dietitians, to name but a few.

Advice may be verbal (given at consultations) or written in the form of instruction leaflets, information leaflets or simply how to take medication correctly, such as before food, after food and the dosage. Particular advice is given before many clinical investigations, such as bowel cleansing before **endoscopy**.

Key term

Endoscopy This is a clinical investigation to make a direct observation of a hollow organ or tube. The endoscope is a flexible or rigid tube fitted with light transmitting fibres. It can incorporate a camera, scissors and biopsy forceps.

Support for managing the disorder

You have already learned about professional advice and aids but support may come in the form of visits to or from specialist organisations, or volunteers concerned with the disorder itself, such as the Alzheimer's Society, Age Concern, Mencap, Multiple Sclerosis Society, British Diabetic Society, British Colostomy Association and Arthritis Care. All these voluntary organisations have websites where information can be obtained to support service users and their families.

There are also specialist nurses who are designated to help service users in their own homes, such as health visitors, stoma nurses (dealing with the management of ileostomies and colostomies), diabetic nurses and of course school nurses who help a lot of children with asthma. Macmillan nurses help cancer patients (especially in the later stages) and you will learn about other support in counselling, complementary therapy programmes and rehabilitation programmes.

Counselling

See counsellors on page 224.

Many chronic disorders such as MS and motor neurone disease may lead to bouts of depression. Counselling is often used to alleviate the symptoms and help the service user to overcome these periods and develop a more positive approach.

In context

Apart from taking several types of medication, Steve managed to live quite normally, taking holidays abroad, visiting friends and relatives and attending monitoring appointments. Ten years later, the transplant clinic nurse practitioner started to request more frequent blood tests because the levels of some chemicals, such as potassium, calcium and urea, were higher or lower than normal and the urine began to contain protein. The transplant was beginning to fail. Medication was adjusted and, with support, Steve struggled along for another year before he agreed to return to haemodialysis once more. Steve gave up his employment several years ago.

1   **Explain why Steve would be reluctant to return to haemodialysis.**

2   **Explain the psychological effect of returning to haemodialysis.**

3   **Evaluate the contribution of the transplant clinic nurse practitioner in supporting Steve during this year.**

Rehabilitation programmes

These are particularly important after a heart attack or coronary thrombosis and stroke and aim to return the service user to independent living as much as possible. Programmes may include professional advice on maintaining a healthy lifestyle, relaxation techniques, physiotherapy, occupational therapy and psychotherapy as necessary. Complementary therapies may prove useful in improving health and well-being in cancer service users. It is clearly wise to attempt to re-educate or improve the quality of life of a service user to prevent further incidents of ill health where this is possible. For example, another heart attack might be prevented by dietary changes and an exercise regime.

Complementary therapies

Complementary therapies include practices such as aromatherapy, reflexology and naturotherapy. You will be able to find more details of these on the Internet. A brief outline will be given here.

Aromatherapists choose special oils impregnated with plant extracts for external massage. The practice is used particularly in psychosomatic and stress-related disorders.

Reflexologists massage the feet in the belief that parts of the body are reflected on the soles. Many will use herb-impregnated oils as they work.

Naturopaths believe that symptoms are related to the body attempting to eliminate the build up of waste toxins in the body. Consequently, to be healthy, you must only consume natural foods and avoid environmental pollutants.

Acupuncture is a form of Chinese medicine where needles are inserted into the skin to treat disorders. Traditional doctors may suspect that the needles act as a counter-irritant (in the same way as heat pads and pain-relieving creams) causing temporary relief by distraction.

Many people suffering from chronic disorders may use complementary therapies to relieve symptoms even if these are temporary.

Assessment activity 14.3

For each of your chosen physiological disorders, you will need to:

P4 Describe the care processes experienced by each individual case and the roles of different people in supporting the care strategy.

1   What types of care strategies have been given to your chosen individual and how did the actions of the different carers promote care of the individual?

Grading tip for P4

Over a long period of time, there may have been several care strategies and a large number of professional people involved. How will you decide who to include?

Assuming that the service user has visited the GP initially, been referred to a clinical specialist, had surgery and investigations and is now living at home making out-patient visits, then these are the areas on which to base your response. Don't forget to include the people the service user never sees, such as laboratory technicians analysing blood and urine. A laboratory technician may only require one or two lines explaining the role, but you will give a more detailed account of the clinical specialists and GP roles. Before you start, check out the D1 requirement below as it is easier to do this at the same time.

D1 Evaluate the contributions made by different people in supporting the individuals with the disorders.

2 What are the strengths and weaknesses of the assistance given to the individual by the different carers?

Grading tip for D1

What is meant by *evaluation* here?

In P4, you were only asked to describe the roles of support people but here you are required to tease out the strengths and weaknesses of their contributions to support. You can use primary research from your service user here because they will be the only person who can state, for example, how valuable the physiotherapy was to them. Some surprising results may be learned. For example, it may be that the care assistant provided more help in the form of social and emotional support than the clinical specialist and that this was of greater importance to the patient than physical support.

14.4 How individuals adapt to the presence of a disorder

Over a period of time, usually years rather than months, an individual will adapt to the presence of a particular disorder. Changes will be made depending on the stage that the disorder has reached and individuals will develop coping strategies to help themselves manage the changes.

Difficulties

Adaptations may be in several forms, such as changes in the way individuals go about their daily living activities, changes in their mobility, work and relationships. There will be social and emotional adaptations too; many people with serious disorders can no longer enjoy sexual relationships or go on holidays.

Changes in activities of daily living

These will vary tremendously depending on where the difficulty lies. You have already learned that changes may be necessary in the content of the diet – this can be difficult when the individual lives in a family group and special consideration must be made for one person, leading to feelings of guilt. Sleep patterns at night may be disturbed and insomnia becomes a problem; lights and reading material may have to be provided as well as separate sleeping accommodation. When people are unable to dress or bathe themselves, clothing may need to be adapted to Velcro-type fastenings, hoists and stair lifts to be installed and rooms re-assigned for different use. Many families lose their sitting room by converting it into a bedroom on the ground floor. Taps are hard to turn on for people with severe rheumatoid arthritis, so special lever taps become necessary and screw tops can be a nightmare without special can-opening devices. Telephones and alarms may need to be installed in different rooms.

Individuals may need to depend on others for shopping and must be very well organised when they are making lists of what they need. Spontaneity can be taken out of life as forethought becomes important.

Individuals suffering from Alzheimer's disease are prone to wandering, often in the night, and have no idea where they are or where they live. This means that they must be accompanied on trips out, or not go at all. Diabetic patients have to be careful not to miss meals or they may have hypoglycaemic attacks. Nor must they get too engrossed in activities and forget to take their insulin.

All manner of adaptations become necessary and you will have to be both observant and curious to investigate adaptations to daily living.

Mobility

Mobility will change for many disorders from being fully mobile to various degrees of disability over time. MS often shows initially as a dragging of one leg and this may go away for a time (a remission), returning at various intervals (relapses). The symptoms vary in severity from person to person.

In motor neurone disease, the gradual wasting of muscles leads to increasing degrees of disability and in later stages, the individual is unable to move, swallow or speak. It is important to realise that, although an individual is severely incapacitated at this stage, intelligence and awareness are still present.

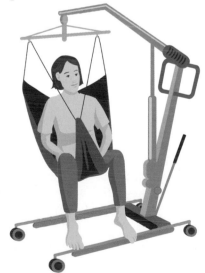

▲ **Figure 14.4 Using a hoist**

Current treatment for rheumatoid arthritis reduces the deformities which used to occur in joints. Mobility aids also enable people to live reasonably independent lives, although some people may use wheelchairs. A person who has experienced a stroke, leading to paralysis of muscles in their limbs, may regain some movement with physiotherapy but may also need mobility aids and/or a wheelchair.

Osteoporosis, which leads to multiple fractures as bone becomes more brittle, can similarly lead to problems with mobility.

Employment

Employment difficulties may arise due to periods of illness and pain leading to time off work. Some employers will be sympathetic and provide resources and aids such as wheelchair access or special chairs where this is possible. Large firms are more likely to have a human resources department which will assist with resources. With smaller firms there are often more problems as they generally cannot afford to have employees absent for long periods.

Many individuals with chronic disorders may need a rest in the afternoons or find the trauma of working just too much and turn to part-time working or no work at all. This may lead to financial difficulties as they have to survive on benefits.

The Disability Discrimination Act (1995) requires employers with 15 or more employees to treat disabled people equally with non-disabled people in all employment matters. This means making any reasonable changes to the premises, job design, etc., that may be necessary to accommodate the needs of disabled employees. It is likely that disabled people do not have the same promotion prospects as non-disabled people.

Relationships

Some partnerships are so strong that they can survive any number of difficulties and the chronic illness of one partner. Yet others fall at the first fence as some people seem not to be able to bear being close to ill health. Other relationships survive for several years and then falter as the long-term strain becomes too much. Much may depend on the ages of the couple if sexual relationships are not possible and the relationship changes from being intimate and sexual to a caring relationship. Older people are often more able to cope. However, many couples enjoy a sexual relationship without a penetrative experience and feel fulfilled. Sexual therapists may be able to help.

The relationship is likely to become lop-sided as one partner is forced into making the majority of decisions and tending to the needs of the other, day after day, month after month, year after year. This can be very demanding for the 'well' partner and the relationship can regularly go through bad patches.

Relationships with children can be very rewarding but also have tense periods as the parent is not able to do what other parents do and the child may resent this. Money may be short because of the illness and there could be a lack of material wealth, not fully understood by children. Relationships with older parents can be difficult as they might have been brought up in an era when disabled people were not encouraged to manage their own lives – this makes them want to do everything for the service user. Cloying sympathy with someone always ready to do the task for you does not help in the end.

Coping strategies

People are famously inventive and, consciously or unconsciously, they develop ways to help themselves manage. These are known as coping strategies. One of the main ways to help individuals cope with their situation is to provide them with accurate information about their condition so they know what to expect.

Family and friends

Being able to meet and talk about concerns and anxieties with family and friends often lessens the fear of the unknown. An old proverb states 'a problem shared is a problem halved' and this is very true. Just simply vocalising the problem helps but the person also has the added advantage that loved ones will frequently think of ways to help so that the problem ceases to exist. Family and friends will also accompany the individual to monitoring and other medical appointments so that the time passes more quickly and someone is at hand to offer reassurance.

When an individual is almost or permanently house-bound, having contact with the activities in the outside world helps to prevent an inward-looking mentality. Family and friends will offer practical support, as well as emotional and social support, by doing household chores and shopping.

Counselling

You have already learned about counselling by professionals but it can also come from health professionals such as nurses and doctors with experience of the disorder and also from friends and family. Problems should be aired as they are frequently founded on false beliefs. For example, a severe pain may be kept quiet for fear that an individual has cancer; this is a common belief. Pain in most cancers is a very late occurrence and, for this reason, pain is less likely to be caused by cancer than other diseases.

Assessment activity 14.4

For each of your chosen physiological disorders carry out the following tasks:

P5 Explain difficulties experienced by each individual in adjusting to the presence of the disorder and the care strategy.

1 What are the problems caused to the service-user by the disorder and the different types of care? **P5**

Grading tip for P5

How will you investigate the difficulties arising from the care strategies without undermining confidence?

The difficulties arising from the disorder can be managed by asking open questions such as:

How do you cope from day to day?

How do you get around?

Asking about relationships can be intrusive but if you know the individual well, you may know the answer. It can be very awkward if you are considerably younger than your chosen person. A simple closed question might elicit further information, but if it doesn't, the individual is showing that they are unwilling to pursue relationships.

Have your relationships changed? If you can say … *with your partner, children* (name them), *etc.,* you may get a better response. Individuals may not wish to discuss this because of the fear that anything said might get back to the relative. You could reassure them of confidentiality but you must abide by their decision.

Difficulties arising from the care strategy can be simply:

How do you find going to the … hospital, GP, physiotherapy, etc., whichever is appropriate.

M3 Explain how the care strategies experienced by each individual have influenced the course of the disorder.

2   How have the different types of care made a difference to the development of the disorder?

Grading tip for M3

How many care strategies will you cover?

Try to choose about three care strategies so that you are asking, for example, about the effect of the physiotherapy on the individual's mobility or perhaps how having a colostomy has improved their quality of life. You will tailor the question appropriately to the disorder and the care the patient has received.

D2 Evaluate alternative care strategies that might have been adopted for each individual.

3   What other care strategies might have been used and what benefits or disadvantages might they have provided?

Grading tip for D2

How will you investigate what else could have been tried?

You need to know this before you can judge the strengths and weaknesses of the alternative strategy.

For example, in Steve's case study, he could have had **CAPD** instead of haemodialysis. However, CAPD would have been difficult for him as he has arthritic fingers and is not happy to manage personal care other than normal personal hygiene. CAPD can be done at home (strength) and individuals can still go away on holiday. However, it carries an increased risk of peritonitis infection (weakness) and the bulky dialysis fluid has to be taken with you (weakness). You can go about your daily activities while dialysing (strength) and even continue work. With haemodialysis, there is instant feedback from the kidney machine about important chemistry statistics and injections can be given through the machine (strength).

The patient (or carer) might be aware of alternative courses of action and, of course, your secondary research will highlight methods of treatment and care strategies.

Key terms

CAPD (continuous ambulatory peritoneal dialysis) This type of dialysis depends on running dialysing fluid into the abdomen through a special valve and allowing the composition of the fluid to change over several hours. The waste fluid is then run out and fresh put in. This usually happens twice a day.

4   What are the similarities and differences in the ways you think that your two case study disorders will develop?   **P6**

Grading tip for P6

Do you think that one of the patients might be in denial or, worse, ignorance?

Your secondary research must equate with the responses from the individual so do this first.

You can ask an open question such as:

What do you think will happen in the future?

You then need to compare the future of both your patients. This will be the first time your two case studies have been interlinked. One individual may have a progressive, terminal illness (such as Alzheimer's disease) whereas the other may believe that the disorder may disappear as they grow older (asthma). In your points of comparison, use words like 'whereas', 'however' and 'but' to illustrate the comparison.

Lifestyle changes

A person who becomes increasingly disabled through a chronic illness will inevitably make changes to his or her lifestyle. These may be dietary changes to minimise discomfort, as in inflammatory bowel disease or Crohn's disease. They may move from a house to a bungalow or ground floor apartment close to shops or public transport if mobility is a problem. Activities may change from, for example, fell walking to using exercise equipment in the home. Surfing the Internet may become an absorbing pastime, as 'talking' in chat rooms can replace leisure time in a club. Going to support meetings of a voluntary organisation or day centre can become the hub of social activities, and so on.

Mobile hairdressers and chiropodists can be accessed for well-being and most shopping can be done on the Internet and delivered to the door.

Complementary therapies

You have learned about the importance of complementary therapies in the reduction of stress and these may be important for reducing stress incurred by the symptoms of the disorder and frustration at not being able to do as much as before. They are also important in imparting a feeling of well-being.

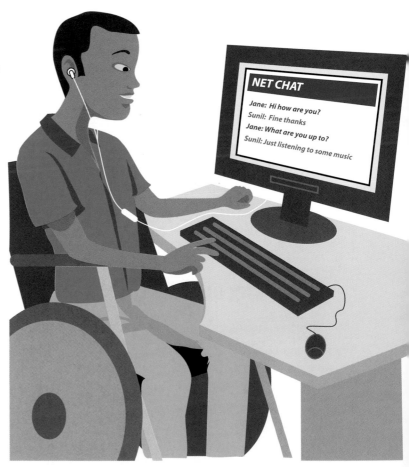

▲ Figure 14.5 Visiting chat rooms can be a good way to meet other people when mobility is limited.

Prognosis

A prognosis is a forecast of the probable course and outcome of the disease and the prospects of recovery as indicated by the symptoms and nature of the disorder. In other words, what is likely to happen in the future. To complete this section, you will need to be extremely sensitive when you are interviewing your client and/or their carers. Alternatively, you could just use secondary research to arrive at your own prognosis.

Likely progression of the disorder

The likely progression of the disorder will depend on the specific disorder, the individual and the stage when diagnosis and treatment began. For example, asthma in a child frequently clears up in adolescence and adulthood whereas diabetes doesn't improve but can be managed so well that side-effects such as cardiovascular disease and infection are kept to a minimum. Cancer prognosis often depends on the stage reached before a diagnosis was made and also on the type of cancer. Some forms of cancer are particularly aggressive and have spread widely through the lymphatic system before being detected. Parkinson's and Alzheimer's diseases, emphysema, motor neurone disorder, MS and rheumatoid arthritis are likely to get progressively worse, although modern treatment can now slow down the deterioration significantly.

Bowel disorders may be resolved if surgery has removed the diseased section or may go on to get worse. Heart bypass individuals may, particularly with lifestyle changes, not have any reoccurrence of heart problems. However, there is no guarantee that another section of artery will not become damaged so that the process must be repeated. When a section of cardiac muscle dies from a lack of oxygen and nutrients, this can never recover and may lead to disorders of rhythm which need to be controlled by drugs. Strokes are caused by cerebral bleeds or thromboses. These may leave lasting damage if brain cells die from 'starvation' or some recovery may be possible if blood is reabsorbed over time or other nerve pathways can be brought into use through training.

Possible impact on chosen individual

You will either know or get to know your chosen individual quite well and be able to form a judgement about the possible impact on them. Some people who have had chronic illness for many years take each day as it comes. They have had to bear increasing pain and disability problems and do so without complaint, making us feel ashamed when we complain of toothache or a headache.

Other people become frustrated, bitter and angry at being incapacitated, especially if there is a lack of support. Fear of the unknown is stressful and people worry about who will look after them, especially if they live alone. Many worry about having to go into residential care when they can no longer manage. This can mean losing their possessions, including their home.

In context

Steve is dialysing regularly and his health has improved. He is currently waiting for a dialysis slot to be available nearer to his home as he travels by ambulance to a large city hospital 30 miles away. He has expressed a desire to go on the waiting list for another transplant. This is unlikely to happen due to his age. Steve will spend the rest of his life on dialysis. Heart disease and infections are possible complications which may end his life. He is still taking immunosuppressive medication.

Although a good proportion of his life is spent in a hospital environment, Steve remains cheerful and hopeful. Dialysis is not as effective as it could be and his fistula may need to be renewed by another operation.

1　**Why might infection be life-threatening to Steve?**

2　**What precautions could Steve take to avoid infections?**

3　**What psychological effect might Steve experience if he was told that a transplant was out of the question?**

Possible changes to care strategy

During the progress of a disorder, different care strategies will be required. This may entail care planning by a social worker who will involve all interested parties, including the service user. The social worker will monitor the care plan in order to see if the needs of the individual are being met and if new needs are arising. The care plan will be reviewed in the light of any changed requirements and strategies will change to meet the new needs.

Knowledge check

1 Name the main body systems affected by the following disorders:

- MS
- Alzheimer's disease
- coronary heart disease.

2 Explain the term *palpation*.

3 Name two factors which may influence the development of a disorder.

4 Which types of scans do not expose the service user to radiation?

5 Explain the role of a phlebotomist.

6 Name three purposes of a blood test.

7 Describe one form of complementary therapy.

8 Name the types of medication used for the following purposes:

- to remove excess fluid from the body
- to lower blood pressure
- to suppress the immune response.

9 Explain the terms *diagnosis* and *prognosis*.

10 Explain the purpose of two measurements.

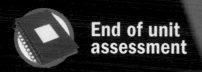

Preparation for assessment

This unit will be internally assessed by your tutors and should consist of two case studies of individuals with dissimilar physiological disorders. The case studies will be quite separate until the final learning outcome (P6) when you are required to compare the future development of the two disorders.

You need to demonstrate that you meet all the learning outcomes for the unit. The criteria for a pass grade set the level of achievement to pass the unit. To achieve a merit, you must also meet the merit learning outcomes and to achieve at distinction, every pass, merit and distinction learning outcome must be demonstrated in your unit evidence.

Describe the course of two different physiological disorders as experienced by two different individuals. **P1**

Try to find two dissimilar disorders to investigate. You must maintain strict confidentiality throughout. You will need access to the service users, so friends, neighbours or relatives you know well will be easier than people in care settings. You must get their permission and use sensitivity at all times. A list of suitable disorders is provided and you are advised to choose two of these. Other disorders can be used but ensure that you have sufficient depth and breadth in your knowledge and understanding of the relevant physiology to achieve the grade you desire. Photographs, clinical reports and images are not required as they may breach confidentiality.

A possible format you could use to tackle this is outlined below.

Start by providing a brief profile of your chosen person and describe the signs and symptoms that prompted the first appointment with the GP. Explain any clinical investigations and measurements made at this visit. If a diagnosis was reached, this is the opportunity to describe normal and abnormal physiology associated with the disorder. Discuss the possible influences on the development of the disorder. **P2**

Continue with the criteria in the order below.

Describe the physiology of each disorder and factors that may have influenced its development. **P2**

You will need to explain the 'normal' physiology of the main body systems affected and the abnormal physiology or pathology of the disorder. You will research the possible causes and influences on how the disorder developed.

Explain how the course of the disorder in each individual relates to the physiology of the disorder. **M1**

In this merit criterion, you will connect the abnormal physiology of the disorder to the events that have occurred to the service user during the illness.

Describe the clinical investigations carried out and measurements made to diagnose and monitor the disorder in each individual. **P3**

After a discussion with your service users, you will use secondary research to provide further details on the clinical investigations and measurements used originally to make a diagnosis and then during the monitoring of the disorder. Give examples of measurements for the disorder. It does not matter if they are not the actual measurements for the individual; you are unlikely to have access to clinical records and the service user is unlikely to remember actual readings over a period of time.

Explain possible difficulties involved in making a diagnosis from the signs and symptoms displayed by the individuals and the results of their investigations. **M2**

Even though the diagnosis may have been clear in one or both of your service users, those of others with the same disorder might have been less clear-cut. Secondary research will usually describe circumstances when the diagnosis is more difficult and cannot just be related to signs and symptoms and clinical investigations. MS and Alzheimer's disease can be very difficult to diagnose and often this is done by default, i.e. eliminating other disorders.

Describe the care processes experienced by each individual case and the roles of different people in supporting the care strategy. `P4`

Time is an important factor here as well as the stage of the disorder. In a very long-standing disorder, you might look at current care strategies and the people who support the individual. If the disorder is of shorter duration, you could incorporate care strategies employed along the way.

Evaluate the contributions made by different people in supporting the individuals with the disorders. `D1`

You can cover this as you are working on P4, by describing the strengths or benefits of the supporters and also the disadvantages or weaknesses of the support. You must base these judgements on evidence.

Explain difficulties experienced by each individual in adjusting to the presence of the disorder and the care strategy. `P5`

You will often find that people adjust to having a disorder quite well but that they dislike going for monitoring appointments, blood tests, etc., and just feel they want to be left alone. You will investigate such adjustments mainly through your primary research.

Explain how the care strategies experienced by each individual have influenced the course of the disorder. `M3`

In this criterion you are finding out (using primary and secondary research) whether the care strategies have helped the individual to improve their health, quality of life or the progress of the disorder.

Evaluate alternative care strategies that might have been adopted for each individual. `D2`

In most disorders, there are other care strategies that could have been tried. For example, you will know that

major or minor surgery, chemotherapy and radiation therapy can play a part in the treatment of breast cancer. Not all are used for every individual. You can investigate this for your disorders using primary and secondary research. The service user might have chosen not to accept certain care strategies.

Compare the possible future development of the disorders in the individuals concerned. `P6`

You must show that you can compare your two disorders by relating points of similarity or difference in this section that deals with the progression of the disorders.

Resources and further reading

Baker, M. et al (2001) *Further Studies in Human Biology* (AQA) London: Hodder Murray

Boyle, M. et al (2002) *Human Biology* London: Collins Educational

Givens, P., Reiss, M. (2002) *Human Biology and Health Studies* Cheltenham: Nelson Thornes

Indge, B. et al (2000) *A New Introduction to Human Biology* (AQA) London: Hodder Murray

Jones, M., Jones, G. (2004) *Human Biology for AS Level* Cambridge: Cambridge University Press

Moonie, N. et al (2000) *Advanced Health and Social Care* Oxford: Heinemann

Myers, B. (2004) *The Natural Sciences* Cheltenham: Nelson Thornes

Pickering, W.R. (2001) *Advanced Human Biology through Diagrams* Oxford: Oxford University Press

Saffrey, J. et al (1972) *Maintaining the Whole* Milton Keynes: The Open University

Stretch, B., Whitehouse, M. (2007) *BTEC National Health and Social Care Book 1* Oxford: Heinemann

Vander, A.J. (2003) *Human Physiology: The Mechanisms of Body Function* London: McGraw Hill

Ward, J. et al (2005) *Physiology at a Glance* Oxford: Blackwell

Wright, D. (2000) *Human Physiology and Health for GCSE*, Oxford: Heinemann

Nursing Times and similar for case studies

Useful websites

BBC
www.bbc.co.uk/science/humanbody

British Heart Foundation
www.bhf.co.uk

British Lung Foundation
www.lunguk.org

NetDoctor
www.netdoctor.co.uk

NHS Direct
www.nhsdirect

Surgery Door
www.surgerydoor.co.uk

Voluntary organisations exist for almost all the diseases on the list for this unit. You can find the addresses and websites in a library or by surfing the Internet. They provide helpful information and recommend literature as part of their services. For example:

British Heart Foundation

British Lung Foundation

Motor Neurone Disease Assocation

The Alzheimer's Society

GRADING CRITERIA

To achieve a pass grade the evidence must show that the learner is able to:	To achieve a merit grade the evidence must show that, in addition to the pass criteria, the learner is able to:	To achieve a distinction grade the evidence must show that, in addition to the pass and merit criteria, the learner is able to:
P1 describe the course of two different physiological disorders as experienced by two different individuals **Assessment activity 14.1 page 213**		
P2 describe the physiology of each disorder and factors that may have influenced its development **Assessment activity 14.1 page 213**	**M1** explain how the course of the disorder in each individual relates to the physiology of the disorder **Assessment activity 14.1 page 213**	
P3 describe the clinical investigations carried out and measurements made to diagnose and monitor the disorder in each individual **Assessment activity 14.2 page 219**	**M2** explain possible difficulties involved in making a diagnosis from the signs and symptoms displayed by the individuals and the results of their investigations **Assessment activity 14.2 page 220**	
P4 describe the care processes experienced by each individual case and the roles of different people in supporting the care strategy **Assessment activity 14.3 page 229**		**D1** evaluate the contributions made by different people in supporting the individuals with the disorders **Assessment activity 14.3 page 230**
P5 explain difficulties experienced by each individual in adjusting to the presence of the disorder and the care strategy **Assessment activity 14.4 page 232**	**M3** explain how the care strategies experienced by each individual have influenced the course of the disorder. **Assessment activity 14.4 page 233**	**D2** evaluate alternative care strategies that might have been adopted for each individual. **Assessment activity 14.4 page 233**

GRADING CRITERIA (*Cont.*)

To achieve a pass grade the evidence must show that the learner is able to:	To achieve a merit grade the evidence must show that, in addition to the pass criteria, the learner is able to:	To achieve a distinction grade the evidence must show that, in addition to the pass and merit criteria, the learner is able to:
P6 compare the possible future development of the disorders in the individuals concerned. **Assessment activity 14.4 page 234**		

Applied sociological perspectives

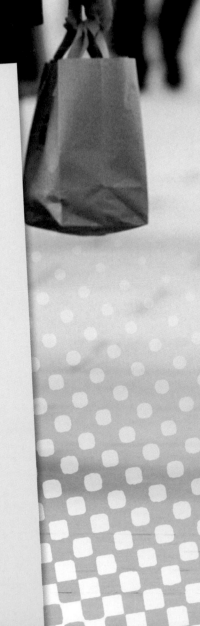

Introduction

This unit builds on and extends your understanding of the topics introduced in Book 1, Unit 7: *Sociological perspectives*. In particular, it explores the impact of poverty and other social inequalities on the health and well-being of individuals and groups in modern Britain.

The unit opens with a discussion of the terms used to describe and analyse inequalities in societies. This is followed by a discussion of the nature and extent of recent changes in the size and make-up of the population and their impact on health and care provision. Finally, you will study the links between social inequalities and health and well-being.

Those of you who have completed Unit 7: *Sociological perspectives* will be familiar with some of these ideas and this approach to analysing the health of the nation; here you will have the opportunity to apply this and additional knowledge to a wider range of social groups. This will include the evidence for the higher incidence of truancy, teenage pregnancies, mental illness and suicide, among the disadvantaged in our society.

How you will be assessed

This unit will be internally assessed by your tutor. A variety of exercises and activities are included here to help you to prepare for assessment. There will be opportunities to apply your sociological knowledge, and especially your knowledge of the effects of inequality and disadvantage, on social groups that are supported by the health and care services. This will include older people,

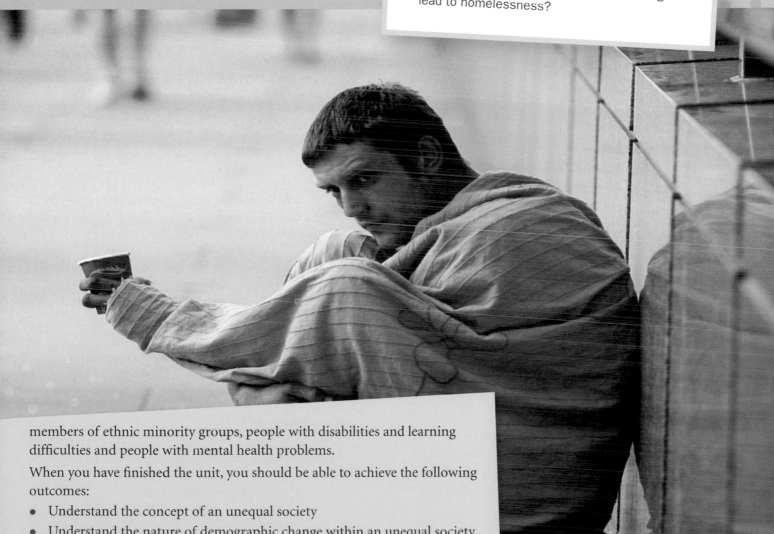

Thinking points

People suffer from a range of social problems, such as substance misuse, discrimination and homelessness.

- How might these problems affect a person's physical, intellectual, social and emotional well being?
- How might social attitudes towards them affect them?
- Are there any services in your school or college to support students with problems that might lead to homelessness?

members of ethnic minority groups, people with disabilities and learning difficulties and people with mental health problems.

When you have finished the unit, you should be able to achieve the following outcomes:

- Understand the concept of an unequal society
- Understand the nature of demographic change within an unequal society
- Understand potential links between social inequalities and the health and well-being of the population.

Social inequalities

Social inequalities are a characteristic of almost all societies and of many social groups within societies. That is, some people or groups of people are seen as having a higher status or as having more prestige than others. **Social stratification** is the term used by sociologists to describe these hierarchies. In geology, the earth's strata refer to different layers of rock which are laid on top of each other. In sociology, the term is used to describe hierarchies and inequalities in societies, where some groups have higher status than others. Those who are identified as being of higher status are more wealthy with easier access to the possessions and the way of life most valued in society.

Key terms

Social stratification A term borrowed from geology (i.e. the earth's strata) which describes the hierarchies in society and how some groups have more status and prestige than other groups.

Reflect

Which social groups in our society do you think have the highest status? Compare your list with others in your group.

In African countries following colonisation, and in America prior to the civil war, groupings were crucially based on race, with black communities having lower social status than the white ones. Some might say that such hierarchies remain, despite legislation.

Theory into practice

Find out which groups are protected from discrimination by legislation in our society.

Reflect

How effective do you think legislation is in combating discrimination against those groups?

In India the Hindu caste system identifies five clearly defined social strata ascribed at birth. There is no inter-marriage and very little social contact between the castes. There is no possibility of **social mobility**, i.e. improving or indeed changing your position in society at all. It is a closed system of stratification. Indian governments in recent years have attempted to remove the inequalities of the caste system but with limited success. The five social strata are:

- Brahmins – the highest caste, the priestly caste
- Kshatriyas – the military, rulers and administrators
- Vaisya – merchants and farmers
- Sudras – manual workers
- The untouchables or social outcasts – the people who have almost no status and who have no caste at all.

Key terms

Social mobility The process of moving from one social stratum to another. Social mobility can be either upward mobility or downward mobility.

In feudal England the different strata were called estates and were based on the ownership of land. The monarchy, knights, barons and earls were in the highest estate, the church and clergy were in the second and the merchants, peasants and serfs were in the lowest estate.

Social class is the form of stratification that describes the social hierarchies in most modern industrialised societies. It is based largely on economic factors linked with income, the ownership of property and other forms of wealth. Sociologists have been particularly interested in the link between our social class position and other aspects of our lives. In this unit we will consider the link between social class and the incidence of substance abuse, crime, abuse, mental illness, teenage pregnancies, bullying and eating disorders.

The official classification of social class used by British governments to measure and analyse changes in the population began in1851. Death rates were analysed using the broad classification of occupations into social 'grades' (later called social classes).

The five social classes identified by the Registrar General in 1921, based largely on perceived occupational skill, remained in place until 2001. These categories were used by government statisticians and others to analyse population trends until very recently and to compare levels of health and ill health, life expectancy, lifestyle choices and life events by social status or class. The five social classes were:

Class 1	Professional class
Class 2	Managerial and technical occupations
Class 3	Skilled occupations Non-manual (3N) Manual (3M)
Class 4	Semi-skilled occupations
Class 5	Unskilled occupations

Table 19.1 The Registrar General's scale of social class, 1921–2001.

Since 2001, the National Statistics Socio-Economic Classification (NS-SEC) has been used for government official statistics and surveys. It is still based on occupation but has been altered in line with employment changes and has categories to include the vast majority of the adult population including:

Class 1	Higher managerial and professional occupations
Class 2	Lower managerial and professional occupations
Class 3	Intermediate occupations
Class 4	Small employers and own account workers (mainly the self-employed)
Class 5	Lower supervisory and technical occupations
Class 6	Semi-routine occupations
Class 7	Routine occupations
Class 8	Never worked and long-term unemployed

Table 19.2 National Statistics Socio-economic Classification (NS-SEC), 2001 to present day.

Social class differs from the more closed systems of the caste or feudal systems, or those based on race or gender, in that the class differences are more difficult to define. They are not backed by law or regulation and social class barriers are arguably far less rigid. There is the possibility of social mobility. People can rise, or indeed fall, in the class system. For this reason, social class is called an open system of stratification compared to the more rigid systems of the feudal system of social caste where social mobility is very rare and usually prohibited.

Reflect

Identify two likely differences in the lifestyles of people in the highest social classes (social classes 1 and 2 in the NS-SEC scale) compared to the lowest two groups (social classes 7 and 8). Consider the reasons for these differences. You might like to discuss this in groups.

Despite the careful and recent reclassification of social class in modern Britain, there is a view that social class differences have disappeared. There is a feeling that class is of little significance anymore – a view backed by the general improvements in the standard of living, the increase in house ownership and the changes and similarities in leisure activities across our society. However, the British Social Attitudes Survey published in January 2007, *Perspectives on a Changing Society,* found that, when asked, 49 per cent of people still allocated themselves to a particular class, the same figure as in 1964, and only 6 per cent said that class was of no significance at all. This classification (the class to which people think they belong and with which they identify) is called their **self-assigned class**. This is in contrast to the class to which they might be allocated by a researcher or government statistician.

Key terms

Social class The form of stratification that describes the social hierarchies in most modern industrialised societies.

Self-assigned class The social class to which people think they belong or with which they identify.

Take it further

Carry out a 'mini survey' among your family and friends and ask them:

- Do you think there are still different social classes in modern Britain?
- To which social class do you think you belong?

Compare your results with those of the British Social Attitudes Survey 2007.

Compare your sample's self-assigned class with their occupation position in the National Statistics Socio-Economic Classification (NS-SEC).

Remember!

Social class differs from the more rigid stratification systems of the feudal system or the caste system in that social mobility is possible, people can change their social class position.

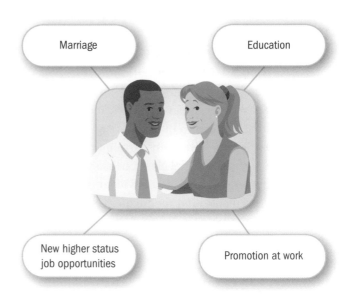

▲ Figure 19.1 Methods of social mobility.

Social inequalities and patterns of health and illness

Despite the difficulties of definition and different views on the continuing significance of class in our society, there is overwhelming evidence that:

- standards of health
- the incidence of ill health or morbidity
- life expectancy

all vary by social group and especially by social class. Members of the higher social classes live longer and enjoy better health than members of the lower social groups. The most influential modern studies that consider the reasons for this difference are the Black Report (1980), and the Acheson Report (1998). Both reports provide detailed and comprehensive explanations of the relationships between social and environmental factors and health, illness and life expectancy. There is also evidence that patterns of health and illness vary with:

- gender
- culture and ethnicity
- disability
- sexuality.

Evidence also shows that:

- men have a shorter life expectancy than women, although women have longer periods of ill health. Life expectancy in the UK has reached its highest level ever for both men and women. Women at the age of 65 can expect to live a further 19.4 years but men aged 65 can expect to live a further 16.6 years only. However, the 2001 census showed that across all social groups, women are more likely than men to report themselves as 'not in good health'

- people from most minority ethnic groups in the UK have greater periods of illness and shorter life expectancy than the host population. In the 2001 census, Pakistani and Bangladeshi men and women in England and Wales reported the highest rates of 'not good' health

- in 2003, MIND published the results of the UK's largest ever survey of the mental health of lesbian, gay and bisexual people. Gay men and lesbians reported more psychological distress than heterosexual people. Recent studies of inequalities in health have revealed gaps in understanding about the health needs of lesbians and gay men and a corresponding lack of services to meet their needs in some parts of the UK

- in the 2001 census, one in six people in the UK (10.3 million) living in a private household reported having a condition that limited their daily activities, a limiting long-term illness. Only about half of disabled people of working age were in work (50 per cent), compared with 80 per cent of non-disabled people of working age.

However, if people from any of these groups are also poor, the differences are even greater.

In 1980, the government suppressed the publication of the Black Report because its findings were so significant and serious in exposing the vast differences in the levels of health and illness between different social classes. Only a small number of duplicated copies were circulated and made available just before an August bank holiday weekend (when they would expect to get very little press coverage). However, this study has been extremely influential and the explanations offered in it are still used by sociologists today when examining and considering these issues.

This approach to considering levels of ill health in the population (i.e. by considering people's social and environmental circumstances) is known as the socio-medical model of health. The shorter **life expectancy** and the relatively higher rates of ill health among the poor are

Key terms

Life expectancy A statistical calculation which predicts the average number of years a person is likely to live. This is usually based on the year of birth but can be calculated from any age.

In context

Paula, John and their three young children live in a detached four-bedroom house in a beautiful and much sought after commuter village. John has a heart condition. He has been made redundant and is not in a position to take further work. They are now in considerable debt. Paula has a low-paid, unskilled job. They are selling their house and will be renting a flat in a poor area of the nearby city. The area is quite run down. There will be no garden, a lot of traffic, a high crime rate and they don't think that they will be able to afford a car.

Discuss the possible impact of this move on the family's health and well-being.

1 **Briefly describe four possible consequences of unemployment for John's social and emotional health.**

2 **Explain how the planned move may impact on the family's health and well-being.**

3 **Discuss how the impact of John's poor health would have been different for the family, if there were no financial worries and they didn't need to move.**

seen as a consequence of the inequalities in society and the life circumstances of the disadvantaged. The poor are more likely to have inadequate diets and live in damp housing, often in inner city areas where the impact of unemployment and environmental pollution is arguably the highest. This is contrasted with the biomedical model of health where disease is seen as mainly caused by biological factors and more recently by our individual lifestyle choices, for example, our diet, lack of exercise, smoking or excessive drinking. In the biomedical model, cures are found by the application of medical science.

The socio-medical and biomedical models of health do not necessarily have to be seen as competing models but as complementary approaches to addressing issues of health and illness.

Theory into practice

Draw a mind map or write a list which summarises the possible range of social and environmental factors that might lead to ill health.

Prejudice and discrimination

Disadvantaged groups in society often become the subject of **prejudice**. Prejudice is a term not easy to define but it refers to a set of attitudes or beliefs about particular social or ethnic groups. People are normally unwilling, unable and often uninterested in changing these attitudes. For example, a prejudiced view would be that men never take their share of domestic responsibilities, they never notice if jobs need to be done and they think that housework is not really their job. If people were really prejudiced, they would not easily change their mind, even if you presented clear examples of men who take a full part in childcare and other responsibilities in the home. Normally, prejudicial attitudes are negative and based on oversimplified views of a group. It is a concept closely linked to the term **stereotyping** which defines a group, in this case

men, as if they all share the same characteristics and ignores their individual differences. When a stereotype is widely held, it is sometimes said that the group is the subject of **labelling**. That is, the stereotypical qualities and characteristics are applied to them, their individual differences are ignored and they are treated accordingly.

Key terms

Prejudice A fixed set of attitudes or beliefs about particular groups in society which people are normally unwilling, unable and often uninterested in changing.

Stereotyping Defining a group of people (for example, women) as if they all share the same characteristics and ignoring their individual differences.

Labelling A term closely linked with stereotyping where the stereotypical characteristics are applied to a person and their individuality is ignored.

Reflect

Can you think of groups who suffer from prejudice? Identify the characteristics that are often linked with those groups. Are they positive characteristics or negative?

In context

Jack is a practice nurse at his local GP's surgery. He holds the view that the non-English speaking patients are all lazy. They use the services but they don't bother to learn English.

1 **Define the terms stereotyping and labelling.**

2 **Explain how these terms could be used to describe Jack's attitude towards non-English speaking patients.**

3 **Discuss how his attitudes might influence the quality of care they receive.**

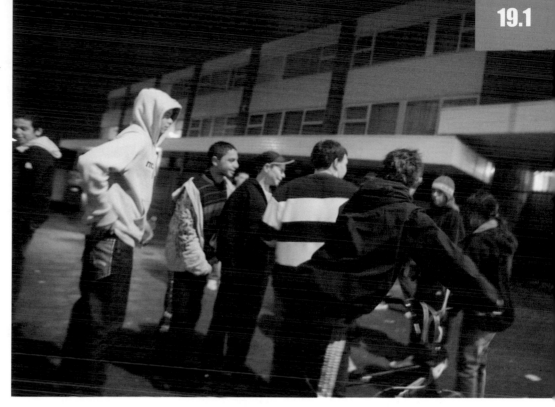

Groups who are discriminated ▶ against can feel marginalised.

Prejudicial attitudes, which in themselves are a state of mind, can easily lead to **discrimination**. This means treating a person differently (usually less favourably) because of particular personal characteristics, for example, their age, race, colour or gender. Groups who are discriminated against can quickly feel **marginalised** by the society or more dominant group. They feel on the edge and excluded from the life and the status enjoyed by the rest of the group or society.

Key terms

Discrimination Treating a person differently (usually less favourably) because of particular personal characteristics, for example, their age, race, colour or gender.

Marginalisation The state of individuals or groups of people who feel on the edge of a society and excluded from the way of life and the status enjoyed by others.

Social exclusion The situation for people who suffer from a combination of linked problems such as unemployment, poor housing, high crime rates and poor health.

Reflect

Can you think of an occasion or a time when you felt discriminated against? What did this feel like? How did you react?

Social exclusion is a term closely linked with issues of inequality, discrimination, stereotyping and marginalisation. However, it refers to wider issues of participation in society. The Social Exclusion Unit (set up by the Labour government in 1997) defined exclusion as:

> *Social exclusion is a shorthand term for what can happen when people or areas suffer from a combination of linked problems such as unemployment, poor housing, high unemployment, poor skills, low incomes, high crime environments, bad health, poverty and family break down.*

The Social Exclusion Unit was set up to address the problems that arose from inequality and its consequences for individuals and groups in society. The problems were seen as having interlinked causes and the Social Exclusion Unit was seen as a way of addressing them. When launching the unit, Tony Blair was quoted as saying that social exclusion is:

> *… about more than financial deprivation. It is about the damage done by poor housing, ill health, poor education, lack of decent transport, but above all lack of work.*

> *Independent*, 8 December 1997

The Centre for Economic and Social Inclusion is an independent organisation which is concerned with promoting social justice, social inclusion and tackling disadvantage. They conduct research, develop ideas and help to design the delivery of services for people and communities that face disadvantage.

Remember!

Prejudice refers to a set of normally negative attitudes about particular groups of people. These negative attitudes may lead to stereotyping, labelling and discriminatory behaviour.

Assessment activity 19.1

P1 Describe the concept of an unequal society.

M1 Explain the concept of an unequal society.

1   Describe and explain the concept of an unequal society. Use examples from news stories and your placements to illustrate the points you make. Examples may include groups perceived as unequal due to their:

- social class
- culture or ethnicity
- age
- disability
- sexuality.

 P1, **M**1

Grading tip for M1

To achieve the merit grade you will need to provide clear examples to illustrate the sociological concept of inequality and explain how it might impact on the life of individuals and their families. Make sure that, where appropriate, you use the formal sociological terminology introduced in this section in your answer (for example, stereotyping, prejudice, labelling, discrimination, marginalisation and social exclusion).

19.2 The nature of demographic change within an unequal society

Demographic change

Demography is the technical term used to describe the study of changes in the size and structure of the population. Social scientists, commercial institutions, governments and other policy makers all study changes in the size and make up of the population. At first they were concerned with measuring:

- natural changes in the population – changes in the birth rates and death rates
- changes in migration (emigration and immigration).

Now demographers examine wider changes in, for example, educational achievements, employment, spending patterns and the use of leisure time.

Changes in the birth rate

Natural changes in the population include changes in the **birth** and **death rates**. The birth rate, measured as a proportion of live births per thousand of the population, fell during the twentieth century from an average of some six children per family in 1870 to 1.7 children in 2007. The 2001 census (for more information on the

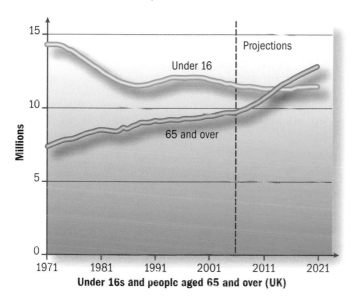

Figure 19.2 The recorded number of people under the age of 16 and over the age of 65 in the UK in 2004 (source: website of Office for National Statistics).

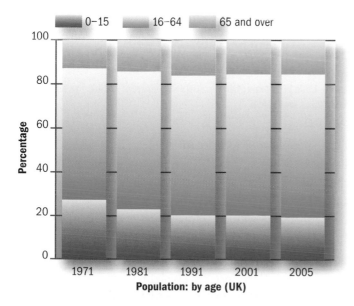

Figure 19.3 16 per cent of the UK population are aged 65 or over (source: National Statistics Online).

Key terms

Birth rate The number of live births per thousand of the population over a given period, normally a year.

Death rate The number of deaths per thousand of the population over a given period, normally a year.

census, see page 254) showed that by 2015 for the first time there are likely to be fewer children under the age of 16 than people over the age of 65. In 2004 there were 11.6 million young people under the age of 16 in the UK (a decline of 2.6 million since 1971) and 9.6 million over the age of 65, an increase of 2.2 million. (The source for this information can be found at the website of the Office for National Statistics.)

It is not possible to explain this trend with full certainty but it is reasonable to account for it by considering the changing social circumstances of the twentieth century.

- In the late 1960s, women were able to take much greater control of their fertility with the wider availability of reliable contraception, particularly the contraceptive pill. Not only was contraception more available, the discussion of sexual issues became more acceptable. In addition, the weakening influence of the church contributed to the use of contraception becoming acceptable and much more commonly used.

- The increased availability and use of efficient contraception took place at a time when women were becoming more independent. More and more women were taking paid work outside the home, thus having more control over their lives and arguably their bodies. If women were to have a career and some personal independence, they did not necessarily want large families.

- Children were becoming increasingly expensive. The school leaving age was raised to 16 in 1973 and a higher proportion of young people were choosing to continue their education and training into their twenties. So, for economic reasons, people were deciding to have smaller families.

- With the introduction of the NHS, and improvements in care services, large families were no longer seen as necessary in caring for parents in their old age. The NHS and social care provision were expected to be in place for the elderly.

The **infant mortality rate** is defined as the number of deaths of babies under the age of one year, per thousand live births over a given period, normally a year. **Perinatal mortality** refers to babies who die during the first week of life. The number of babies who die in infancy declined in the UK during the twentieth century but the numbers are still higher than those of other developed countries. Infant mortality rates are often used as an indicator of the general health and well-being of the population as a whole. If they are high or rising in a particular country or location, or among a particular social group, this would be seen as a possible indicator that levels of general health and well-being may be declining within those groups. A high infant mortality rate will often point to inadequacies in a range of social and economic services and to higher levels of poverty and economic hardship.

Key terms

Infant mortality rate The number of deaths of babies under the age of one year, per thousand live births over a given period, normally a year.

Perinatal mortality rate The number of deaths of babies who die during their first week of life per thousand live births over a given period, normally a year.

Theory into practice

Using a flip chart, create two spidergrams which identify:

- the likely reasons for the differences in infant mortality rates in countries with the highest and lowest figures
- the likely reasons for the fall in the infant mortality rate in the UK in the past 100 years.

Since the mid-nineteenth century there has been a steady fall in the death rate or, to look at this another way, an increase in life expectancy.

The fall in the death rate in the mid-nineteenth century is certainly linked to the public health measures of the time including improved sanitation and cleaner water (in place from the 1840s onwards). In the twentieth century, further public health measures included:

- improved housing
- child immunisation programmes
- improved diets
- the introduction of the NHS and other welfare services
- a general increase in the standard of living.

	Years			
	At birth		At age 65	
	Males	Females	Males	Females
England	76.9	81.2	16.8	19.6
Wales	76.3	80.7	16.4	19.2
Scotland	74.2	79.3	15.5	18.4
Northern Ireland	76.0	80.8	16.4	19.3
UK	76.6	81.0	16.6	19.4

Table 19.3 Life expectancy, 2003–5 (source: Office for National Statistics website).

Many people over retirement age lead busy and active lives. Many remain in paid employment and contribute to a wide range of voluntary and community activities. Lots of retired people give very practical support to their children and grandchildren and often say that they don't know how they found the time to work!

Growing older is a natural process and, while it may lead to slower reactions, poorer eyesight, loss of hearing and restricted mobility, this need not itself be an issue or a problem. However, it does become a problem if there is insufficient support and if day-to-day activities become more of a challenge. The fall in the death rate, or the fact that people are living longer, presents new and pressing issues for health and care workers.

Theory into practice

Search through newspapers, magazines, websites and any other forms of mass media for positive images of older people. In the first 20 minutes of your next lesson, create a poster display using the images or articles collected.

The implications of an ageing population

For those people over retirement age who do need practical care and support, it is very likely to come from family, friends or neighbours. The 2001 census showed a big increase in the number of people over the age of 85 to over 1.1 million, or 1.9 per cent of the population, and it is this age group who typically need more intensive support in order to live independently. When this support comes from the family, despite changes in attitudes and equality legislation, it is still more likely to be provided by adult daughters than adult sons. Changes in family networks have, however, meant that support from the family is increasingly difficult. Adult children will not necessarily live near to their ageing parents. They might have moved for reasons of

Reflect

Think of an elderly person that you know who needs support because of increased frailty.

- What type of support does this person need?
- Who, if anyone, is providing the help?
- Is the support adequate?

Compare your notes with other members of your group.

employment, education, or in search of suitable and affordable housing. To compound this, modern housing often cannot easily accommodate three generations. In addition, increasing numbers of women are in paid work and unable to provide daily care for elderly parents. The increase in divorce, and the high proportion of lone parent families, place further financial and emotional pressures on adult children and the fall in family size often means that the support needs of ageing parents cannot easily be shared.

Services for older people are of course costly and the increasing numbers bring significant financial responsibilities for the working population. Retirement pensions and the costs of providing appropriate care services have to be met at least partly from the taxes of those in work. This is currently impacting on government policy. High taxes are unpopular but government-funded care has to be paid for.

Through much of the twentieth century, older people who needed more support than that provided by family and friends were cared for in large institutions and often the geriatric wards of hospitals. Many of the hospitals carried the stigma and shame of the workhouse. In the mid-twentieth century, publicity was given to a number of scandals concerning neglect and abuse of people in these large institutions. In addition, academics provided further evidence of the unsuitability of this type of provision for older people. Peter Townsend (1962) carried out a survey of institutional care for old people. He found that people:

- were isolated
- lacked power over their lives
- had little opportunity for personal choices about their day-to-day activities
- often did not need to be there but were there for reasons of poverty, homelessness or because they had no friends or relatives who could provide support for more independent living.

From this followed a number of government reports, notably the Wagner Report (1988). It recommended that care should normally be provided in people's homes and that moving to residential accommodation should be seen as a positive choice, and not as a last resort. This was supported by the Griffiths report *Community Care: Agenda for Action* which provided the thinking behind

The NHS and Community Care Act 1990. This act provided the legislative framework and financial support for planned care in the community. It led to the closure of many large institutions and to the provision of care in people's homes or in smaller establishments more closely linked with their community. The community care services include:

- adaptations to homes
- regular home care services
- meals on wheels
- attendance at day centres or lunch clubs
- full-time care in a residential home (long-term care in large institutions rarely happens now).

Theory into practice

In class, share your experiences of work placement in residential settings. Is it the view that the disadvantages of residential care identified by Peter Townsend still remain?

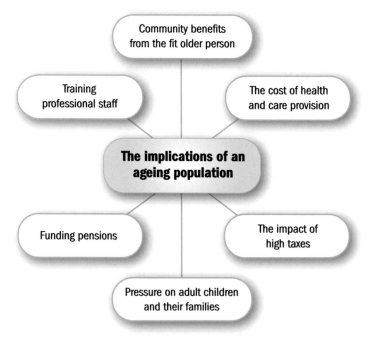

▲ **Figure 19.4 The implications of an ageing population.**

Theory into practice

Find out about the range of community care services for older people in your area.

Migration: immigration and emigration

The first time a question on ethnic origin was asked in a census was in 1991. In the 2001 census, the number of people in the UK from minority ethnic groups was given as nearly 8 per cent of the population. However, Britain has for many years been a nation of many races. There are many factors that lead to emigration. Some people emigrate to escape from war, religious or political persecution, or political instability. Some emigrate to marry, or in search of work, and some for a better standard of living and better educational opportunities. For example, in the seventeenth century, French Huguenot protestants came to Britain to escape religious persecution. Jewish people sought refuge as early as the time of Oliver Cromwell, and then in large numbers at the end of the nineteenth century, and at the time of the Second World War. In that war, men and women served in the British armed forces from Commonwealth countries – notably India, Pakistan and the Caribbean – and from eastern Europe – particularly Poland and Czechoslovakia – and settled down in the country they had fought to defend. In the mid-twentieth century, people from former Commonwealth nations were offered inducements to emigrate to the UK to help solve

Key terms

Immigration The arrival in a country of people who have left their home country and who wish to make the new country their permanent place of residence.

Emigration The movement of people from their home country to make a permanent residence in a different country.

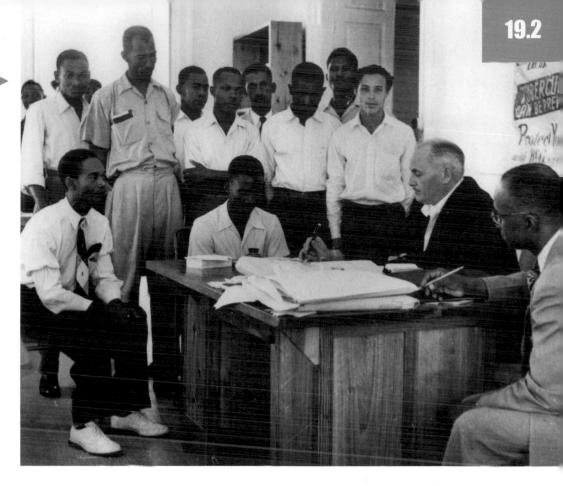

Recruiting manpower in Barbados, 1953.

labour shortages in the health services, textile industries and public transport.

In the late nineteenth century, and until the 1930s, there were more emigrants from the UK starting new lives in other countries than immigrants making their new home in Britain. However, in most years since the early 1930s, the reverse has been the case. There have been more people entering the country than leaving. *Net migration* is a term which refers to the difference between the number of immigrants and the number of emigrants over a given period.

Since the expansion of the European Union in 2004 to include the Czech Republic, Cyprus, Latvia, Lithuania, Malta, Estonia, Hungary, Poland, Slovakia and Slovenia there has been increasing migration from eastern Europe. In 2005, an estimated 185,000 more people entered than left the UK.

In context

You are working in a day nursery in a multiracial community. There is considerable racial tension in the community, with many instances of racially motivated violence and, most recently, race riots.

1 **Identify ways that the nursery could promote racial reconciliation in the community.**

2 **Present your main points as a poster for display.**

3 **Use this work as a basis for a presentation and discussion in your lesson.**

Reflect

Why are governments concerned with studying changes in the size and structure of the population?

Demographic data

Birth and death rates

The impact of birth and death rates on the planning and provision of health and care services was discussed earlier in the unit (see pages 251 to 254).

The census

Every ten years, since 1801 (apart from 1941), the government has carried out a census of the population; this is an attempt to count the total number of people living in the UK. The most recent census took place on Sunday, 29 April 2001. The census is managed by:

- the Office for National Statistics – England and Wales
- the General Register Office – Scotland
- the Northern Ireland Statistics and Research Agency, Northern Ireland.

On the night of the census every household is required, by law, to provide information about the people staying in their house. Those people living in institutions (for example, prisons, hospitals boarding schools or convents) are recorded by the head of the institution and every effort is made to record the number of people who are homeless.

In its earliest forms, the census provided a simple record of the size of the population, the age structure, sex and marital status and the levels of employment. In more recent times, questions have been asked about levels of education, types of housing and housing conditions, car ownership and religion. A record of the size and structure of the population at the time of the last census can be found on the government website www.statistics. gov.uk/census2001. The information gathered on census night included:

- the total population of England, Wales, Scotland and Northern Ireland was 58,789,194

Key terms

The census A compulsory and detailed count of the population in the UK held every 10 years.

- 11.7 million of the population was made up of dependent children
- nearly one in four dependent children lived in lone parent families
- 20 per cent of the population were under 16 years of age
- 21 per cent of the population were over 60 years of age.
- The 2001 census also revealed that there had been a big increase in the number of people over the age of 85 in the population. There were 1.1 million people in this age group, a five-fold increase over the 1951 census.

Electoral registers

Electoral registers, which are compiled by the local council, list the name and address of everyone who is eligible to vote in national and local government elections. People can only vote if their name appears on the register.

Remember!

Changes in the size and structure of the population will be affected by natural changes, i.e. changes in the birth rate and the death rate and also changes in migration, i.e. immigration and emigration.

Using demographic data

Government departments are already making plans for the 2011 census and, for the first time, are discussing the possibility of supplying information via the Internet. Governments need to measure and monitor changes in the size and structure of the population in order to plan provision and anticipate changes in social need. For example:

- an increase in car ownership has implications for transport policies
- an increase in life expectancy has implications for care provision for the elderly

- a fall in the birth rate has implications for child care provision.

Demographic information of this type will be used to set specific targets for planners, for example:

- the number of child care places needed in nurseries and schools over the next decade
- the range and size of provision for older people (and from this information calculate the extent of training needed)
- the size of the building programme needed to meet these demands.

Theory into practice

In groups, draw spidergrams to summarise the implications for governments of the following trends that have been identified in recent censuses of the population:

- a rise in life expectancy
- a rise in the number of one-parent families
- an increase in homelessness
- a wider range of religious practices in our society.

Assessment activity 19.2

P2 Describe recent demographic changes in your home country.

M2 Explain recent demographic changes in your home country.

1 Describe and explain the recent changes in the size and structure of the population. You must refer to:

- natural changes in the population (changes in birth rates and death rates) and
- changes in patterns of immigration and emigration. **P2**, **M2**

> Gain an accurate picture of the size and structure of the population

> Plan and target services to meet population needs

> Monitor changes in the size and structure of the population

> **Demographic data can be used to:**

> Develop future policy directives

> Identify changes in social behaviour

> Set accurate targets for service provision

 Figure 19.5 The uses of demographic data.

Grading tips for P2 and M2

Remember, for the pass grade you are required to describe the recent changes in the size and structure of the population and to achieve the merit you need to *explain* these changes.

To achieve the merit grade you will need to give clear reasons for the changes. For example, an explanation for the fall in the birth rate could be the availability of free and effective contraceptives, and an explanation for the increase in life expectancy could be the development of the welfare state, especially the NHS. You will also need to explain changes in patterns of immigration and emigration, for example, the recent inclusion of eastern European countries in the European Union.

You should provide statistical evidence from your home country. If you live within the UK, you could use statistics for the whole of the UK (England, Wales, Scotland and Northern Ireland) or for Great Britain (England, Wales and Scotland). You may sometimes use data for individual countries within the union.

P3 Use examples to describe the application of demography to health and social care service provision.

2   Describe how demographic data can be used in the planning of health and care services. **P3**

Grading tip for P3

When answering this question, refer to your data on the fall in the birth and death rates, changing patterns of migration and other relevant information on population change. Show how this data should inform the pattern of care provision. For example, increased provision for older people arises from an increase in life expectancy, increased child care provision is due to the increase in the proportion of working parents and responding to the needs of a non-English speaking community arises from an increase in immigration.

M3 Explain the value of the application of demography to health and social care service provision.

3   Explain, with examples, the benefits of using demographic data in the provision of health and social care services. **M3**

Grading tip for M3

Remember that the benefits of using accurate and up-to-date demographic data will be felt by the planners and the care providers (paid and unpaid) and also by the clients and users of health and care services.

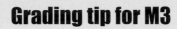

19.3 Potential links between inequalities and the health and well-being of the population

Social inequalities

Regional patterns in health and illness

There are regional variations in patterns of health and illness. Mortality and morbidity rates vary in different parts of the country and also within towns and cities within the UK. It should come as no surprise that it is in the poorer regions and the poorer parts of cities that there are the higher recorded levels of illness.

For example, research has shown that there are regional trends in the incidence of lung cancer across the UK.

Within England, the rates for lung cancer are higher than average in the north west and northern and Yorkshire regions and below average in the south west, south and eastern regions.

Poverty and health and well-being

Poverty is difficult to define. What might seem like poverty to one person could be regarded as riches by another. In our society, if someone cannot afford electrical goods for their home and can never afford a holiday or the occasional meal out in a café or restaurant, it is seen by many as significant deprivation, if not actual poverty. Most people living in Africa would not regard this as a sign of either.

Theory into practice

Write a list of the things that you regard as necessary (i.e. if someone did not have them you would regard them as being in poverty). Compare your list with others in your group. Can you come to an agreement?

The earliest large-scale studies of poverty were conducted at the turn of the twentieth-century. Seebohm Rowntree (1871–1951), a Quaker (and more famously the chocolate manufacturer), studied poverty in his home city of York and Charles Booth (1840–1916) conducted a similar study of poverty in London. Their work has been very influential, not only because they provided the first systematic study of poverty in large cities, but because their rigorous approach to the research, the definitions of poverty they used and their discussions of the impact of poverty on health and social well-being have influenced researchers, governments and policy makers ever since. In his study of poverty in Victorian London, *Inquiry into the Life and Labour of the People in London* (1889–1903), Charles Booth discussed a range of linked issues including the level of wages, unemployment, the quality and type of housing and the health of the poor. Booth and Rowntree were probably the first researchers to make clear the links between low wages, unemployment, disability, poor housing, family poverty and poor health.

Rowntree's measure of poverty was based on information provided by the British Medical Association. Doctors identified the content of the diet necessary to maintain 'physical efficiency'. Rowntree used this as the basis for calculating the minimum income necessary for individuals and their families to remain well. People with an income below this level were considered to be in **absolute poverty**. This level of income was very low, there was no possibility of buying newspapers, presents or even sending letters to family members and certainly no allowance for sweets, toys, alcohol or tobacco.

Key terms

Absolute poverty A term introduced by Seebohm Rowntree, referring to people on a level of income below that which will maintain 'physical efficiency'.

Secondary poverty was defined in this study as a situation where people had an income above the minimum level but who chose to spend their money on other 'unallowable' items. There was a sense in which they were regarded as feckless and irresponsible, and it is possible to see the emergence of the idea of the 'deserving' poor and the 'undeserving' poor – those who chose to spend their money on the non essentials and those who didn't. This approach to defining poverty introduced the concept of the **poverty line,** a level of income below which people were regarded as being in poverty.

Key terms

Secondary poverty A term also used by Rowntree, referring to a situation where people had sufficient money but were in poverty because they spent it on non essentials.

Poverty line A term introduced by Rowntree and still used by policy makers to refer to the level of income necessary to keep people out of poverty.

The idea of the poverty line is still used to inform the benefit system in modern Britain. The level of income support is calculated and set at a level that should allow claimants to sustain good health – a poverty line. On the basis of this very austere definition of poverty, Rowntree found that almost one third of the population of York were in either absolute or secondary poverty. He identified the main causes of poverty to include unemployment, inadequate wages, old age and sickness, large families and the death of the main wage earner.

Rowntree conducted further studies in 1936 and 1950 when more generous definitions of poverty were used – this acknowledged the fact that a healthy life included more than just physical fitness and that social and emotional health were important too. In the later studies he allowed for the purchase of newspapers and books, and for people to have a radio and buy modest presents. Even when he used the more generous criteria, Rowntree found that levels of poverty fell over this period in York to:

- 18 per cent in 1936 and
- 1.5 per cent in 1950.

This led politicians and policy makers to take the view that poverty had almost disappeared. The post-war Prime Minister, Harold Macmillan, famously said, 'We've never had it so good'. However, subsequent studies challenged this view.

Reflect

Which groups of people in our society do you think are most vulnerable to poverty?

Studies of poverty in the second half of the twentieth century approached the issue slightly differently, introducing the concept of **relative poverty**. This defined poverty as a level of income which prevents people participating in the life of the society in which they live. Peter Townsend was key in the development and use of relative poverty in studies of inequality and deprivation. In 1979, Townsend's view was that:

Individuals, families and groups in the population can be said to be in poverty when they lack the resources to obtain the type of diet, participate in the activities and have the living conditions and amenities that are customary or at least widely encouraged or approved, in the societies to which they belong. Their resources are so seriously below those commanded by the average individual or family that they are, in effect, excluded from the ordinary living patterns, customs and activities.

Key terms

Relative poverty A level of income that deprives a person of the standard of living or way of life considered normal in a particular society.

Reflect

Would you feel that a child who attended a nursery was living in poverty if, although generally clean and well fed, they:

- always had clothes and toys that had been passed on
- could not have parties
- didn't have any 'best clothes'
- never went on holiday
- could not afford any of the nursery extras (for example, photographs, outings or events that cost extra money)?

Theory into practice

Using Townsend's definition of relative poverty, write another list of the things that you regard as necessary (without which you would regard a person as being in relative poverty).

Compare your list with your previous list. Discuss your new list with others in your group. Are there significant differences? Can you come to an agreement?

In 1983, London Weekend Television supported a study of poverty known as *Breadline Britain*. The programme was broadcast in 1983. It used the concept of relative poverty, or relative deprivation, developed by Peter Townsend; it was conducted by Joanna Mack and Stewart Lansley. This was updated in and 1991 and again in1999 in David Gordon et al.'s *Poverty and Social Exclusion Survey of Britain* which was produced by the Office for National Statistics and supported by the Joseph Rowntree Foundation.

These large-scale studies attempted to identify both the extent of poverty and those groups most vulnerable to poverty in our society. Briefly, Mack and Lansley measured relative poverty by asking a large sample of the population to identify items that they felt were

Figure 19.6 Groups that are ▶
vulnerable to poverty.

- Older people
- People on long-term benefits
- Lone parents
- **Groups that are vulnerable to poverty**
- People with disabilities
- Long-term unemployed
- People on low incomes
- Unskilled workers

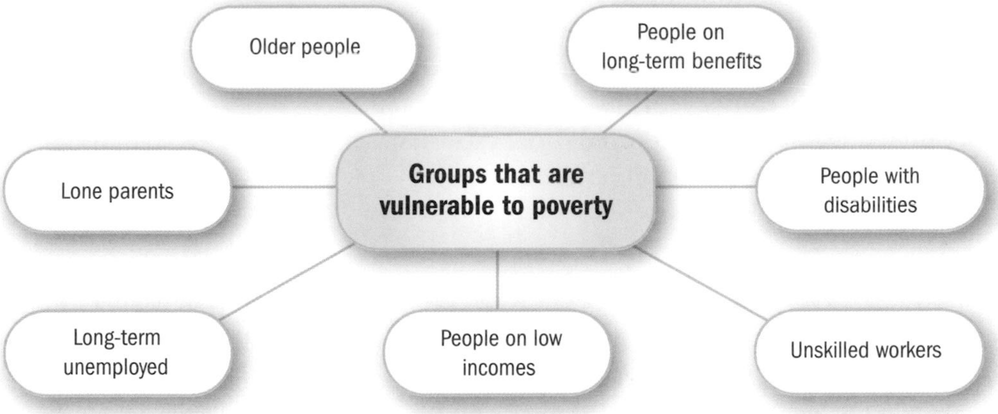

necessities in our society. An item was regarded as necessary if more than half of the respondents claimed it to be so. On the basis of the list, the researchers calculated levels of poverty. Those people who lacked three of the 'socially perceived necessities' were defined as in poverty. By this definition, the numbers in poverty included:

- 7.5 million people (approximately14 per cent of the population) in 1985
- 11 million people (approximately 20 per cent of the population, two thirds of whom relied on state benefits for their main source of income) in 1990.

The 1999 study (2000 Gordon et al) which largely followed the research method of Mack and Lansley found that poverty had increased again. Comparing the 1983 findings to those of 1999, the researchers found that the proportion in poverty had risen from 14 per cent to 24 per cent.

The most commonly used measure of poverty, and that normally used by government agencies, is that if a household income is 60 per cent below the average household income for that year (after this has been adjusted to account for the size of household) the household is regarded as in poverty – another reference to a poverty line. In 2004/5 by this measure 11.4 million people in Great Britain were living in households below this 'income threshold'.

Remember!

Levels of relative poverty will vary from society to society and at different times in history.

Income and wealth

Inequalities in society can be measured by comparing differences in the levels of income and wealth by different social groups. 'Income' is a term used to describe the regular flow of money earned from work or income from pensions, benefits or savings, and 'wealth' normally refers to property, shares or other personal possessions that could be sold to generate an income. These terms are difficult to define and also difficult to measure accurately. Reliable data on levels of income and wealth is not easily available. However, data from the Inland Revenue and from the Department of Work and Pensions consistently shows that wealth and income are not evenly distributed through the population. Inland Revenue data published in 2004 showed that the poorest 50 per cent of the population owned only 6 per cent of the wealth and the richest 5 per cent owned 43 per cent. The Department for Work and Pensions data for the same year found that the richest fifth of income earners had 42 per cent of all income.

Unemployment

Closely linked with issues of poverty are the specific issues of unemployment, especially long-term unemployment. State benefits are set at levels linked with Rowntree's concept of the poverty line and kept at very low levels (arguably for political reasons). High taxes are unpopular and state benefits are a direct cost to the tax payer. There is also an ongoing concern that people should not be able to receive more money in benefits than they could earn from paid employment. Low wages can impact directly on the benefit system. In addition, the long-term unemployed potentially suffer the personal consequences of prejudice and discrimination, marginalisation and social exclusion, as well as the continuing impact of poverty.

Take it further

Using government statistics, trace trends in unemployment over the past 10 years. (Key information will be available on the Internet if you do not have paper-based copies in your library)

Identify and discuss the likely impact of long-term unemployment on the children of the unemployed.

The ageing society

In many societies, social status increases with age. Older people, or elders, have a high status and an important role in the family and wider community. In China and many parts of Africa, and on the Indian subcontinent, older people are treated with great respect. In modern Britain, however, older people have a less clear position in society. They may feel they have less of a stake in society. They may even feel that, as they are not at work, they are less important. They may very well be unclear as to what their new role should be.

There is widespread evidence that older people are the subject of discrimination. In 2007, the Age Discrimination Act was passed – a response to the extent of discrimination against older people.

There have also been a number of studies pointing to the higher incidence of poverty amongst older people, compared to the population as a whole. However, recent research supported by the Joseph Rowntree Foundation confirmed that poverty was not evenly spread across the older people in our society. Studies found that the risks of having a low income after the age of 60 were strongly related to occupational group and continuity of employment between the ages of 20 and 60. People who had worked in professional and managerial jobs were far less likely to face a poor retirement than people who had worked in manual or unskilled occupations. The manual workers will typically have earned lower wages, enjoyed less secure employment and are less likely to have a private pension.

Life expectancy at age 65 is 2 years longer for men from social classes 1 and 2, compared to men from the lowest social classes. For women in these groups, it is 2.6 years longer. The causes of death also vary by social class. The incidence of lung cancer and respiratory diseases, coronary heart diseases and strokes cited as a cause of death are lowest in the higher social classes; incidence of these causes of death increases with social disadvantage. In addition, older people from the lower social groups have poorer health than those from the higher groups. Seventy-two per cent of men over the age of 65 who had unskilled manual jobs when working were reported to have long-term ill health compared with 54 per cent from professional groups.

In context

Sarah Cameron is 75 years old. She was born in Jamaica. She and her husband came to live in England in the early 1950s. She was a hospital cleaner and her husband was a London bus driver. He has since left her and their four children have also left home. Sadly, she rarely sees them and has no other relatives in England. Sarah lives in a council house but it is damp and in a poor state of repair. Her only income is her state benefit. She has arthritis, does not get out very much and the shopping is becoming too much for her.

1 **Define the term relative poverty.**

2 **Identify factors in Sarah's life that may have led to her relative poverty in older age.**

3 **Discuss the impact of her circumstances on her health and well-being.**

To compound this, young people who are currently in employment are not making adequate financial provision for their old age (particularly those in unskilled jobs earning relatively low wages). According to figures released by the Trades Union Congress in 2004, 'less than half of those aged 30 years and under have a pension scheme compared to 73 per cent of people born in the 1960's.

Reflect

Why do you think there is a higher rate of long-term ill health among older men from unskilled manual backgrounds compared to their professional contemporaries?

Gender and health

Probably the most noted change in the family since the Second World War has been the changing role of women in wider society. In society, and in the more private sphere of the family, there have been moves towards equality. For example, more women continue in full-time employment after marriage and after the birth of their children, and women are taking a more significant role in public life and within the community. However, despite these changes, there is considerable evidence that inequalities between men and women still exist. Women's hourly rate of pay, despite equality legislation, stubbornly remains lower than men's. The average (median) weekly earning for full time employees in 2006 was £387 for women, compared to £487 for men.

Despite changes in attitudes, and significant evidence that men take a fuller part in childcare and housework than in the past, women are still seen as having the principal responsibility for the home and family.

There are differences between the sexes in life expectancy and health in older age. In 2004, life expectancy at birth was 77 years for males and 81 for females. Since records have been kept, men have died at an earlier age than women but women have experienced longer periods of morbidity, that is, longer periods of ill health. Women

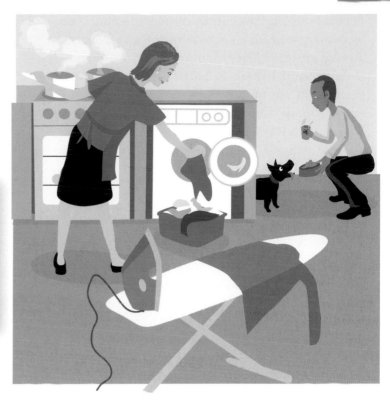

▲ Figure 19.7 Women are still seen as having the principal responsibility for the home!

Theory into practice

In your group, think about a family (either your own or another you know well) which is headed by a man and a woman. Identify who normally takes responsibility for the following domestic tasks:

- making evening meals
- cooking
- washing and ironing
- small repairs around the house
- household cleaning
- household shopping
- looking after sick members of the family.

Collate your information and present it as a bar chart.

Do the results confirm or disprove the view that women take a larger responsibility than men for household tasks?

can expect to live longer than men but they are likely to spend more years in poor health or with a disability. Women are more likely to suffer from arthritis and rheumatism than men. In 2004/5, the prevalence of these conditions for men between 65 and 74 was half that of women. Although the death rate for circulatory diseases (this includes heart disease and strokes) has declined, overall it is still considerably higher for men than women at 2800 per million men and 1800 per million women.

Mental illness and suicide

Mental illness is another term that is difficult to define and therefore difficult to monitor. What is regarded as normal and acceptable behaviour varies from society to society and at different times in history. In addition, the evidence available is derived largely from medical statistics, recording the number of people who present themselves for treatment. However, there may be many reasons why people with mental health problems do not seek professional help. They may not regard themselves as mentally ill, just that they are having 'a hard time at the moment', 'you can't expect to be happy all the time'. They might not want to admit that they have a mental health problem. Some people feel that there is a stigma linked to mental illness that they do not associate with physical illness. They may be frightened to seek medical help, worried that being diagnosed as depressed or phobic would affect their employment prospects. There is some basis for this concern as people with mental health problems have the highest rate of unemployment amongst people with disabilities.

The most common types of mental illness include:
- depression
- anxiety
- panic attacks
- phobias
- obsessive compulsive disorders
- schizophrenia.

Difficulties of definition and diagnosis lead to difficulties in measuring and monitoring levels of mental ill health. An alternative approach to gathering reliable data has been to conduct a 'community survey'. This involves interviewing a sample of the population and, on the basis of their answers to a number of preset questions, identifying whether they have a mental health condition. The most recent survey was carried out by the Office for National Statistics in 2000. At the time of the study, 1 in 6 of the population were deemed to be suffering from mental illness. However, this is not spread evenly across the population.

There is abundant evidence that the incidence of mental illness is concentrated amongst the poorest and most deprived in the community. A statement from MIND claims:

These groups are not only more likely to experience higher infant mortality rates and lower life expectancy but also a higher lifetime prevalence of major mental health problems and relatively poor access to mental health care.

Furthermore, the Social Exclusion Unit report *Rough Sleeping* (1998) estimated that up to half of the people who sleep rough each night have mental health needs but less than half of them are getting treatment. It was estimated that one in two have a serious alcohol problem and one in five misused drugs.

Rates of mental illness and distress also vary between men and women:
- Recorded rates of anxiety and depression are between 1.5 and 2 times higher in women than men.
- Rates of self-harm (including cutting, burning and overdose) are over twice as common in women than men.
- Of the 1.5 million people with eating disorders in the UK, 90 per cent are female.

Lone mothers have particularly high rates of recorded mental distress. Half of all lone parents are on low incomes, twice the proportion of two-parent families.

There is, though, a higher incidence of suicide by men than women and young men from routine and manual backgrounds. They are twice as likely to commit suicide as those with intermediate occupations and three times as likely as those from managerial and professional backgrounds.

Until recently, many people with disabilities were cared for in large institutions or hospitals and were almost invisible to much of society. In recent years, however, there have been significant changes. The Community Care Act 1990 increased the number of people with disabilities being cared for and supported in the community rather than in large institutions. Very importantly, the Disability Discrimination Act 1995 provided legal protection from discrimination in employment, access to public buildings and in the renting of accommodation. However, despite recent progress, disabled people are more likely to:

- be on low incomes
- be without paid employment
- have difficulty in accessing public transport and public buildings
- be without the necessary social support to live full lives.

The poverty rate for disabled adults is twice that for non-disabled adults. The main reason for this, despite the Disability Discrimination Act, is the high unemployment of people with disabilities. Approximately one in five adults with a disability who want to work are unable to find employment. This compares with one in 15 for those without a disability.

Factors affecting life chances

The concept of **life chances** was first introduced by Max Weber, a sociologist in the nineteenth century. He described and discussed the privileged position of the rich and powerful in society and how that privilege provided the opportunity to purchase and enjoy those things regarded as desirable and highly valued in a society. In our society, these 'desirable and highly valued' things include:

- access to good housing
- a good education
- holidays
- satisfying work
- job security
- good health.

The social class system allows for social mobility and may generally be regarded as a **meritocracy**, i.e. people achieve their social position largely on merit. It can be argued there is **equality of opportunity** for all and if people work hard, and achieve good qualifications, opportunities will open up for them.

However, as we have seen, the social class that a child is born into can have an important impact on their life chances. Where many factors linked with poverty and deprivation come together (long-term unemployment, poor housing, pollution, low incomes and poor health) this often leads to a sense of social exclusion, a situation referred to as **multiple deprivation**. This can have serious implications for people's life chances.

Key terms

Meritocracy A society where social position is achieved by ability, skill and effort rather than ascribed at birth. High achievements are open to all.

Equality of opportunity A situation where everybody has the same chance of achieving and acquiring the way of life valued in a society

Multiple deprivation A situation where many factors linked with poverty and deprivation come together, for example, long-term unemployment, poor housing, pollution, low incomes and poor health.

Key terms

Life chances The opportunity to achieve and acquire the way of life and the possessions that are highly valued in a society.

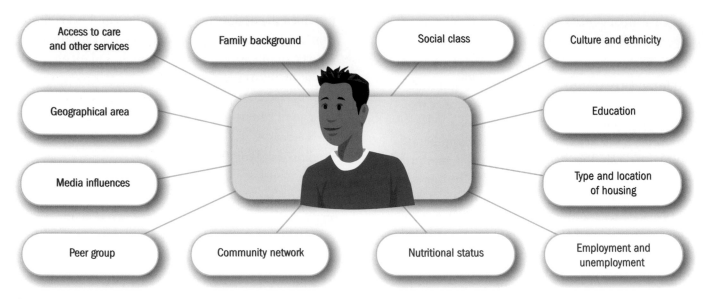

Figure 19.8 Social and environmental factors that affect life chances.

In context

Felicity, aged 13, is the daughter of a merchant banker. Her family lives in a mansion on the south coast. Felicity has a horse of her own, she has piano lessons, a 'nanny' who rides and also speaks French fluently. She has holidays abroad several times each year. Next September she is to attend a prestigious boarding school for girls. Each year over 80 per cent of the girls go to university and many of these go to either Oxford or Cambridge. She hopes to follow a career in banking.

Thomas, also aged 13, is the son of an unemployed miner. His father has not worked regularly since the mine closed and neither have his uncles. The family has relied on state benefits for most of Thomas's life. No one among his family and friends has ever been to university and those who have work are in low-paid, unskilled work. Almost everybody he knows lives in their village. Thomas owns one book. They do not have a computer at home. He has never been on holiday. He imagines he will stay in the village when he leaves school at 16. Nobody has suggested that he stays on at school.

1 **Define and explain the terms equal opportunities and life chances.**

2 **Compare the life chances of Felicity and Thomas.**

3 **Would you say that there are equal opportunities for all in these scenarios?**

Culture and ethnicity

In the UK the majority population is white English. At the time of the 2001 census, the minority ethnic population was 4.6 million or 7.9 per cent of the population. Just over 5 per cent of the population identified themselves as non-white.

Minority ethnic groups are groups within the population who share a particular and distinctive way of life which is seen as different from the majority population. Often this may be linked with nationality or religion. Many ethnic groups have identifiable and different dress codes, diets and music; they may share a different language and celebrate different festivals from the host population.

Evidence from a wide range of sources shows that, on average, ethnic minority groups suffer significant economic hardship. People from minority ethnic groups are more likely to be unemployed or in low-paid manual work, working long hours with limited access to training or promotion.

Evidence for a link between race/ethnicity and inequality, illness and restricted life chances is difficult to systematically study because there are difficulties of definition. In addition, a high proportion of people from minority ethnic groups live in areas of deprivation in inner-city areas with associated poor housing, pollution and relatively high unemployment. It is therefore difficult to know whether the levels of unemployment, low wages and poorer health are due to poverty or race and ethnicity. Nevertheless, compared to the white majority, there is evidence:

- of a higher incidence of unemployment among minority ethnic groups
- of a higher incidence of rickets in children from the Asian subcontinent because of a deficiency of vitamin D in their diet
- of a shorter life expectancy
- of higher infant mortality rates.

In addition to the health implications of higher levels of poverty, there are issues of access to the health services. Full use of them may be limited by language and other cultural barriers. Asian women are often reluctant to see a male doctor. Many of them speak little English and,

despite improvements, translators are in short supply and much important information is not translated into minority languages. In addition, racism (or the fear of racism) is stressful. Unless health and care workers understand the religious and cultural beliefs and practices of minority ethnic groups, their care needs are unlikely to be fully met, leaving them vulnerable to higher levels of ill health.

In context

Mrs Singh speaks very little English. She is 45 years old and has recently come to England to join her husband who is a solicitor. They live in a rural location and are the only Indian family in the neighbourhood. Mrs Singh has developed multiple sclerosis and now uses a wheelchair when she is out of the house. She is feeling very isolated and increasingly depressed. Her GP has suggested that she attends a local day centre for people with disabilities but she doesn't think that this will help.

1 **Describe the reasons why Mrs Singh may be isolated in this community**

2 **Explain why Mrs Singh might be reluctant to try the day centre.**

3 **Discuss the measures that could be taken to help Mrs Singh access this and other care services at this very difficult time.**

Theory into practice

In groups, identify the key cultural patterns of each of the groups below. Briefly describe each group's key religious practices, gender roles, dietary needs, cultural festivals and any important taboos.

- Muslims
- Sikhs
- Jews
- Hindus

Present your information as an A4 handout and distribute it to all members of your class.

Education

There is a wealth of research evidence to show the close link between social class and educational achievement. This is normally measured in terms of examination grades and progression to higher education and associated professional employment. The higher the social class, the higher achievements are recorded.

Economic status

Earlier in the unit we discussed how issues of poverty, social class, income and wealth and unemployment can affect the quality of individual and family life. This includes access to adequate and appropriate housing, good mental and physical health, and to the way of life and possessions valued in our society.

Nutritional status

A balanced diet, appropriate to the individual's age, is central to health and well-being. You might think that what we eat is a matter of personal choice and eating a healthy diet is in our own hands. However, factors that affect our decisions include the cost and convenience of different foods, cultural habits and the preferences and choices made within the family. Sir Donald Acheson in his report (1998) found that people in the poorer social economic groups tended to eat less fruit and vegetables and a lower proportion of high fibre foods than people in the higher social groups. There is evidence that people on low incomes are less likely to be able to afford the balanced diet necessary for health and well-being.

Media and peer group influences

Life chances can be affected by the influence of the media, TV, newspapers and magazines – through advertising and by sustaining strereotypical images of particular social groups. For example, women are too frequently portrayed as concerned with fashion, beauty, childrearing and housework. This is likely to influence their aspirations and ambitions. Young people are often presented as a 'problem' group, involved in anti-social behaviour, often in groups or gangs, negatively influenced by their peers.

Access to services

Despite equality legislation, there is considerable evidence that members of disadvantaged groups derive less benefit from local amenities and services than people from more advantaged groups. Access to many schools and colleges, shops, restaurants and other public buildings, and to many people's homes, is still limited for people with disabilities. Claiming health and social care services and welfare benefits can also be very confusing. Many people, particularly those with literacy problems, or for whom English is not a first language, do not claim the benefits to which they are entitled.

The family and networks of social support

The values, culture and economic circumstances of the family and neighbourhood affect individual attitudes and aspirations. They will also affect life chances. For example, in a family and neighbourhood where education is valued, children are more likely to value achievement at school highly too. Their family and friends are more likely to support a serious attitude to work and hence the possibilities of achievement increase.

Potential effects of social inequalities

Teenage pregnancies

The UK has the highest teenage birth rates in western Europe. One in every 10 babies born in the UK is to a teenage woman. In addition, the infant mortality rate for babies born to teenage mothers is more than 50 per cent higher than the average, accounting for almost 400

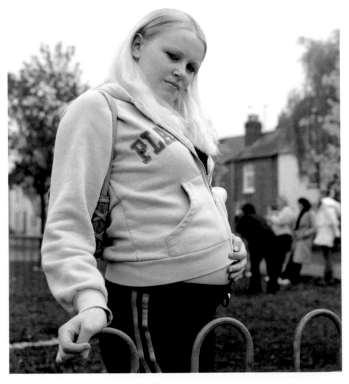

▲ The UK has the highest teenage birth rates in western Europe.

deaths in the year 2000. There is also a higher risk of maternal mortality for young women under the age of 18. However, the incidence of teenage pregnancy varies by social group. Young women from homes with low incomes are four times more likely to become pregnant than those from materially more advantaged homes.

Reflect

Why do you think that there may be a higher incidence of teenage pregnancies in lower income families? Why do you think there is a higher infant mortality rate for these babies?

In context

Emma is 15 years old. She is in the second year of her GCSE courses and has discovered that she is pregnant. She is frightened to tell her parents, frightened of having the responsibility of a child and frightened for her future. She was planning to stay on at school and had hoped to go to university.

1   **What are the possible implications of Emma's unplanned pregnancy for her health and well-being?**

2   **What are the risks for her and her child?**

3   **How can they be addressed?**

Truancy

A study carried out by Ming Zhang (published in *Community Care*, issue 1554, 2004) found that children who come from families with low levels of income are more likely to truant. The study examined truancy statistics from London boroughs between 1997 and 2000, interviewing 90 council education officers and 98 parents on low incomes. They found the social and emotional problems that arose from poverty were very closely linked with the non-attendance of primary school children. Parents who were questioned said they 'sometimes forgot about their younger children's schooling when they hit money troubles'. For secondary school children, especially amongst low achieving pupils, truancy was more linked to peer pressure.

According to official figures, 40 per cent of street crime, 25 per cent of burglaries, 20 per cent of criminal damage and a third of car thefts are carried out by 10 to 16-year-olds when they should be at school.

Ming Zhang found that threatening parents with prison sentences had no long-term impact on improving attendance rates.

Reflect

Have you or your friends ever truanted from school? In your experience, what personal and social factors are linked with truancy?

Crime

Official statistics have consistently pointed to the link between social class, deprivation and offending. The Home Office's *Youth Life Styles Survey 1998/1999* reported that 41 per cent of prisoners were from social classes 4 and 5 which represent only 19 per cent of the population as a whole and 18 per cent from social classes 1, 2 and 3 which make up 45 per cent of the population. Offenders from the higher social classes are less likely to be involved in violent crime and more likely to commit fraud and theft from employers (which is more difficult to detect). Persistent offending is closely linked with social deprivation and is likely to cause continuing financial difficulties as employment prospects are measurably poorer for offenders.

Mental health issues

Earlier in the unit we discussed issues of mental health, the difficulties of definition and of knowing the true levels of mental illness in our society. Persistent mental distress is linked with higher levels of unemployment.

In 2006, the Disability Rights Commission reported that only 20 per cent of people with mental health problems were in employment and with that follow the issues of poverty and deprivation.

Eating disorders

Evidence does not show a clear link between the incidence of eating disorders and deprivation. The Eating Disorders Association has estimated that at least one million people in the UK are affected by an eating disorder and one woman in 20 will have some form of eating disorder, the overwhelming majority of them aged between14 and 25. Eating disorders, particularly anorexia and bulimia, are normally regarded as a mental health condition and are certainly closely associated with persistent mental health problems. The physical and emotional consequences of anorexia or bulimia impact negatively on educational achievements and employment prospects.

Substance abuse

The incidence of drug dependency and other substance abuse (including alcohol) is not linked to particular social groups but the consequences are often more serious for the poor. They do not have the financial resources to fund their habit or savings to help when their addiction leads to ill health, unemployment and debts.

Bullying

Similarly, the impact of persistent bullying is not confined to particular social groups but the consequences can impact very negatively on social, emotional, physical and intellectual development.

Physical health

We have already discussed the links between poor diet, poverty and disadvantage. The challenge of leading a healthy lifestyle, eating well, taking sufficient exercise, keeping safe and warm when living on a low income, and in an area of deprivation, is considerable and may help to explain why there are higher levels of ill health among the poor.

Developing skills and abilities

Increased motivation

In conclusion it is worth considering the possible impact of organising a society that minimises areas of disadvantage and deprivation. If people do not live in poverty, if they have the opportunity for appropriate employment and are paid a just and fair wage with the opportunity to enjoy the financial rewards of their work, then the issues of poor physical and mental health, crime and social exclusion may well be reduced.

Assessment activity 19.3

P4 Describe two examples of social inequalities in your home country.

1 In your own words, using information from this unit and other relevant and reliable evidence to support your work, describe two examples of social inequalities in your own country.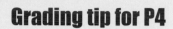

Grading tip for P4

Remember to record accurately the source of any statistical or other evidence that you use to support your answer. This must include accurate references to websites as well as paper-based evidence.

You might find charities and other voluntary organisations a helpful source of up-to-date evidence.

P5 Use six examples to describe potential links between social inequalities and the health of the population.

M4 Use six examples to explain potential links between social inequalities and the health of the population.

2 In your own words, using information from this unit and other relevant and reliable evidence to support your work, use six examples to describe and explain potential links between social inequalities and the health of the nation. **P5**, **M4**

Grading tip for P5 and M4

When considering the health of the population, remember that health can include physical, social, emotional and intellectual well-being.

When referring to statistical and other evidence, remember to give accurate sources for the evidence.

To achieve the merit grade you will need to explain, with examples, the sociological concept of inequality and further explain with up-to-date examples and robust evidence how these inequalities could impact on the health and well-being of individuals and their families in society.

D1 Evaluate the potential links between social inequalities and the health of the population.

3 Discuss the strengths and weaknesses of the evidence presented to explain links between social inequalities and the health of the population. **D1**

Grading tip for D1

You will need to consider the difficulties of defining the terms that are used in these discussions, for example, the difficulties in agreeing a definition of:

- social class
- poverty
- disability
- mental ill health.

If it is difficult to define a term, it is difficult to accurately measure its incidence and the extent of changes and trends.

You will also need to discuss the reliability of data. For example:

- some may be collected by a particular group in order to persuade and gather support
- some may be published in a newspaper to satisfy the views and prejudices of their readers
- even official documents such as death certificates may not give a true picture of the range of causes of death in the population (sometimes a doctor may record a condition that is one of a number of contributory reasons, selecting one that will cause least distress to the deceased's relatives)
- the census is the only record of the whole population
- medical records only record people who have presented themselves for treatment and diagnosis varies.

You will need to point to the fact that statistics must be used with great care.

To achieve the distinction grade you will need to discuss these issues and then weigh the evidence. Despite the limitations, is there sufficient evidence to argue that there are links between social inequalities and the health of the population?

Knowledge check

1 Define the terms:

- *prejudice*
- *discrimination*
- *stereotyping*
- *labelling*
- *marginalisation.*

2 Identify four groups who are often treated unequally in our society.

3 Define the term social stratification.

4 How does classification by social class differ from the caste system or stratification by race?

5 Define the following key terms used by demographers:

- *birth rate*
- *death rate*
- *life expectancy*
- *immigration*
- *emigration.*

6 Why might demographic information of this sort be useful to the health and social care sector?

7 Explain four key reasons for the

- fall in the birth rate
- fall in the death rate.

8 Suggest four reasons why people may choose to emigrate.

9 Briefly discuss the challenges for the health and care sectors of increased immigration to the UK.

10 Define the concept of life chances.

11 Identify four factors that might improve a person's life chances.

12 Identify and briefly explain three types of inequality that might result from:

- poverty
- older age
- disability
- mental ill health
- unemployment.

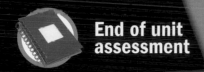
Preparation for assessment

Douglas and his wife Joan live in a multiracial community on the edge of a large northern city. They have lived in the same house for over 50 years. They have seen many changes in their community. The area has become quite run down. There is far more traffic now, which causes pollution and too much noise. There is high unemployment and much poverty. There is, from time to time, considerable racial tension. The houses are rather dilapidated – many of the large houses are now flats. Many of the local shops have closed. A hostel has recently opened for people with mental health problems.

1   When writing about the unequal society, draw on evidence from the case study. Make sure that, where appropriate, you use the formal sociological terminology introduced in this section, for example, social class, marginalisation, social exclusion, culture and ethnicity, stereotyping, prejudice, labelling and discrimination in your answer.   **P1**

2   Consider the changes in population that are referred to in the case study and others that have taken place during Douglas and Joan's lifetime. You may refer to the census or other population data to support your answer. You must refer to the natural changes in the population – changes in birth rates and death rates and also changes in patterns of immigration and emigration.   **P2**

3   Describe how demographic information should be used to address issues to meet the needs of Joan and Douglas and others in their community. You will need to consider how changes in migration and the changes in birth and death rates have affected needs. Ensure that you give accurate references for the data and other evidence that you use and that this appears in the bibliography.   **P3**

4   Describe two examples of social inequality identified in the case study. Again, remember to record accurately the source of any statistical or other evidence that you use to support your answer. You may find that charities and other organisations are a helpful source of information, for example, Age Concern, the Child Poverty Action Group or the Commission for Racial Equality.   **P4**

5   Referring to the groups identified in the case study and other disadvantaged groups, describe the links between inequality and health and well-being. When considering the health of the population, remember that health can include physical, social, emotional and intellectual well-being. You will need to use the sociological terms introduced at the beginning of the chapter, for example, *social class, poverty, minority ethnic groups, discrimination, prejudice* and *marginalisation* in your answer.   **P5**

6   To achieve M1, you will need to provide clear examples to illustrate the sociological concept of inequality and explain how it may impact on the life of Joan and Douglas and other members of the community.   **M1**

7   To achieve M2, you will need to give clear reasons for the recent demographic changes, i.e. the reasons for the natural changes in the population and the patterns of immigration and emigration.   **M2**

8   You will need to explain how the benefits and the value of using accurate and up-to-date demographic data will be felt by the planners, the care providers (paid and unpaid) and also the clients and users of health and care services. Describe how the effective use of this data would improve the quality of life for Joan and Douglas and others in the community.   **M3**

9   To achieve M4, you will need to explain, using evidence, how inequalities and the impact of inequality on specific groups can affect levels of health and well-being. When referring to statistical and other evidence, remember to give accurate

sources of the evidence. Examples of groups where there is ample evidence of inequality include older people, the unemployed, people with disabilities, people with a range of mental health problems, members of minority ethnic groups and the poorest members of society. **M4**

10 To achieve the distinction grade you will need to weigh the evidence for and against the identified potential links between social inequalities and the health of the population. You will need to point to the difficulties of a making a firm judgement because of the difficulty of defining some of the key terms, for example, social class, poverty, disability and mental ill health. You will also need to discuss the issues we raised earlier in the text about the reliability of data. You will need to come to an informed conclusion. Is there sufficient evidence to argue that there are links between social inequalities and the health of the population? **D1**

Resources and further reading

Booth, C. (1889–1903) *Inquiry into the Life and Labour of the People of London* London

Department of Health Press release June 2002 (www. nhsinherts.nhs.uk/hp/health_topics/teenage_ pregnancy/teenage_pregnancy.htm)

Gordon, D. et al (2000) *Poverty and Social Exclusion in Britain* York: Joseph Rowntree Foundation

HM Government (1998) *The Independent Inquiry into Inequalities in Health* London: HMSO

HM Government (1988) *Community Care: An Agenda for Action* London: HMSO

HM Government (1988) *Residential Care: A Positive Choice* (The Wagner Report) London: HMSO

Home Office (2001) *Youth Lifestyles Survey, 1998–1999*, Colchester: UK Data Archive

Mack, J., Lansley, S. (1985) *Poor Britain* London: Allen & Unwin

Mack, J., Lansley, S. (1992) *Breadline Britain 1990s* London Weekend Television

National Centre for Social Research (2007) *Persectives on a Changing Society* London

New Policy Institute (2003) *Monitoring Poverty and Social Exclusion* York: Joseph Rowntree Trust

Office for National Statistics (1999) *Labour Force Survey* London

Office for National Statistics (2006) *Social Trends 2006* London

Office for National Statistics (2007) *Social Trends Volume 36* London

Rowntree, S. (1901) *Poverty*: *A Study of Town Life* London: Macmillan

Social Exclusion Unit (1998) *Rough Sleeping* London: HNSO

Tossell, D., Webb, R. (2000) *Social Issues for Carer*s London: Hodder & Stoughton

Townsend, P. (1962) *The Last Refuge* London: Routledge & Kegan Paul

Townsend, P. (1979) *Poverty in the United Kingdom* Harmondsworth: Penguin

Townsend, P., Davidson, N., Whitehead, M. (eds) (1980) *Inequalities in Health: The Black Report* Harmondsworth: Penguin

Zhang, M. cited on news.bbc.co.uk/hi/ education/2094284.stm

Useful websites

www.archive.official-documents.co.uk

Age Concern
www.ageconcern.org.uk

Centre for Economic & Social Inclusion
www.cesi.org.uk

Child Poverty Action Group
www.cpag.org.uk

Commission for Racial Equality
www.cre.gov.uk

Disability Rights Commission
www.drc-gb.org

Eating Disorders Association
www.edauk.com

MIND
www.mind.org.uk

Office for National Statistics
www.statistics.gov.uk

GRADING CRITERIA

To achieve a pass grade the evidence must show that the learner is able to:	To achieve a merit grade the evidence must show that, in addition to the pass criteria, the learner is able to:	To achieve a distinction grade the evidence must show that, in addition to the pass and merit criteria, the learner is able to:
P1 describe the concept of the unequal society **Assessment activity 19.1 page 250**	**M1** explain the concept of the unequal society **Assessment activity 19.1 page 250**	
P2 describe recent demographic changes in home country **Assessment activity 14.2 page 257**	**M2** explain recent demographic changes in home country **Assessment activity 19.2 page 257**	
P3 use examples to describe the application of demography to health and social care service provision **Assessment activity 19.2 page 258**	**M3** explain the value of the application of demography to health and social care service provision **Assessment activity 19.2 page 258**	
P4 describe two examples of social inequalities in home country **Assessment activity 19.3 page 271**		
P5 use six examples to describe potential links between social inequalities and the health of the population. **Assessment activity 19.3 page 271**	**M4** use six examples to explain potential links between social inequalities and the health of the population. **Assessment activity 19.3 page 271**	**D1** evaluate potential links between social inequalities and the health of the population. **Assessment activity 19.3 page 271**

Health education

Introduction

The government recognised in its White Paper *Choosing Health: Making Healthy Choices Easier* (published by the Department of Health in 2004) that while we now live longer, and the major causes of premature death of the last century are largely under control, the same cannot be said for today's main killers. In this unit we are going to explore how we tackle these modern-day diseases.

The aim of this unit is to introduce the principles of health education, the approaches used and to introduce you to health education campaigns. Health education is a central component of health promotion, which in turn is a major component of public health. This unit therefore links with Unit 12: *Public health*, and aims to extend some of the concepts introduced there.

Health education could be described as any activity that promotes health-related learning and therefore brings about some relatively permanent change in the thinking or behaviour of individuals. You are going to consider a range of different approaches to health education, including the role of the mass media and social marketing. You will then examine different models of behaviour change, relating these to the social and economic context.

Finally, you will gain an understanding of health education campaigns by actively planning, designing, implementing and evaluating a small-scale campaign.

How you will be assessed

Assessment of this unit is largely based on your success in planning, designing and implementing a small-scale health education campaign. This will be assessed by your tutor. You will need to demonstrate that you have taken into consideration recent or current health policy, have gathered the relevant

Thinking points

Most people have some aspect of their life which they would like to change to improve their health – lose weight, be more active, quit smoking, drink less alcohol…

- What health changes have you thought about making in the past?
- Not thought of any?
- Why might that be?
- If you do have a health goal, and you haven't reached it, what has stopped you from achieving it yet?

Try to get a clear understanding of the issue as it relates to you – what made you think about it in the first place? Why haven't you changed yet? What would be your goal? How would you measure success?

This will help you to apply some of the theory in what follows.

information, set clear targets and have described clear aims and objectives of the campaign, outlining the target audience and the choice of approach you have selected. Guidance about the grading for this exercise is included towards the end of this section.

After completing this unit you should be able to achieve the following outcomes:

- Understand different approaches to health education
- Understand models of behaviour change
- Know how health education campaigns are implemented.

Key terms

Health education An aspect of health promotion which largely relates to educating people about good health and how to develop and support it.

Health education is usually defined as the process of giving information and advice and of facilitating the development of knowledge and skills in order to change behaviour that affects health. Health educators come from a wide range of professions including teachers, social workers, practice nurses, health visitors, leisure centre staff, etc. (some of whom we will look at in more detail later). In some cases this is an acknowledged part of their role, for example, in health visiting and practice nursing. However, in others, it might not be so easy to recognise the potential for a health education role. For example, a community beat officer walking the local streets will frequently come across groups of young people who might be smoking and/or drunk – this clearly presents a health promotion opportunity that they may not appreciate or be trained to deal with effectively.

Historical approaches

Hardly a day goes by without some coverage of a health education issue such as the rising levels of obesity and sexually transmitted infections. However, it hasn't always been this way. The current levels of interest have developed over many years of local, regional, national and international activity to raise the profile of health education. The modern-day focus on health education can trace its roots to the mid 1970s and 1980s when a new approach to the public's health began to emerge. In Canada, in 1974, the Lalonde Report was a major influence in identifying four 'fields' in which the factors affecting health can be grouped. These are:

- genetic and biological factors
- lifestyle factors
- environmental factors
- the extent and nature of health services.

This was followed shortly afterwards by a number of other health strategies including the World Health Organisation's (WHO) *Health for All by the Year 2000*, 1977. This approach not only broadened the definition of health but also took a wider view of the major influences on health, particularly behaviour. This was reinforced and extended in 1978 by the Declaration of Alma-Ata at the International Conference on Primary Health Care. This expressed the need for 'urgent action by all governments, all health and development workers and the world community to protect and promote the health of all the people of the world'.

In the UK, the Black Report (1980), and *Inequalities in Health: The Black Report and the Health Divide* (1987), were published. Both clearly identified the relationship between poverty and ill health. This led to a growing recognition of the importance of social and economic influences on health and disease. This began to influence debates in health education and was incorporated into the Ottawa Charter for Health Promotion (WHO, 1986) which defined the role of health promotion as:

- building healthy public policy
- creating supportive environments
- strengthening community action
- developing personal skills
- re-orientating health services.

Models of health education

Health education has many alternative perspectives about how best to support people in adopting healthier behaviours. In this section we explore just two (victim blaming and empowerment). However, it is important to remember there are many others.

Victim blaming

The concept of 'victim blaming' is firmly rooted in the view that people have control and responsibility over their own lives and their health behaviours. In this model the decision to take up smoking is seen as a matter of personal choice, as is the decision to stop.

This is a relatively unsophisticated view and cannot explain, for example, the fact that smoking is not equally distributed within society, with those in lower socio-economic groups smoking more frequently. The *Choosing Health* White Paper (2004) suggested that:

> *On paper, the answers can look deceptively simple – balance exercise and how much you eat, drink sensibly, practice safe sex, don't smoke. But knowing is not the same as doing. For individuals, motivation, opportunity and support all matter … Healthy choices are often difficult for anyone to make, but where people do not feel in control of their environment or their personal circumstances, the task can be more challenging. People who are disabled or suffer from mental ill health, stretched for money, out of work, poorly qualified, or who live in inadequate or temporary accommodation or in an area of high crime, are likely to experience less control over their lives than others.*

The influence of 'control' is seen in a survey quoted in *Choosing Health*, where 46 per cent of respondents agreed that there are too many factors outside of individual control to hold people responsible for their own health. Differences in responses for different groups suggest that people in lower socio-economic, socially excluded or black and minority ethnic groups may feel health is further beyond their individual control than others do. To suggest that a person is responsible for situations outside of their control is termed 'victim blaming'.

Key terms

Victim blaming People frequently simplify health choices by blaming the person who chooses to adopt an unhealthy behaviour for making that choice. In reality things are rarely that simple. For example, people cite lack of time due to work pressures as the major reason why they don't take enough exercise.

Theory into practice

Obese people are often subjected to victim blaming approaches – people suggest that it is their own fault for getting fat and they should simply eat less and take more exercise. To understand just how complex an issue obesity is, tackle the following questions.

- List as many things as possible which contribute to young people being overweight.
- Now try and group these into those issues which are about:
  - the individual's responsibility
  - the local community
  - the nation
  - international issues.
- How did the balance appear between the individual and the wider local, national and international issues?
- Could you identify any international issues?
- Now try to suggest changes which could be made to reduce obesity at each of the levels identified.

The result is what would be called a whole-system approach, one which starts with the individual and works its way out to include national and international actions.

Empowerment

The WHO defined health promotion in the Ottawa Charter as enabling people to take control of their own lives. This approach is based on enabling people to express their own concerns, and to gain the necessary knowledge and skills to address those concerns. It reflects a desire to address the wider determinants which may be influencing the poor health in a person or a community, and not just to focus on medical health concerns. This might mean a community addressing concerns about local traffic, or street violence, or access to nutritious food.

It is important to understand the difference between empowerment of the individual and empowerment of a community.

- Individual or self-empowerment has its roots in non-directive counselling (which aims to help people take control of their own lives).
- Community empowerment develops whole communities who are then able to challenge and change their environment.

Reflect

Have you ever felt strongly about an issue and wanted to do something about it? Perhaps it was something in college or in your local community?

- Did you go on to take action to make things change?
- If you didn't what was it that stopped you?
- What would need to change for you to feel enabled or empowered to make things change?

Approaches to health education

Social marketing

Remember!

Health-related social marketing is the systematic application of marketing concepts and techniques, to achieve specific behavioural goals to improve heath and reduce health inequalities.

In recent years there has been a recognition that health education needs to adopt more sophisticated marketing approaches – the kind which are used so successfully by commercial companies to advertise unhealthy products such as fast food, chocolate and alcohol. This type of marketing is called social marketing and is defined as being:

The systematic application of marketing concepts and techniques to achieve specific behavioural goals, for a social or public good.

It's Our Health! Realising the Potential of Effective Social Marketing, National Social Marketing Centre, 2007

The main features of social marketing are:

- **The customer or consumer is placed at the centre** – social marketing always starts by trying to understand *where the person is at now rather than where someone might think they are or should be.*
- **Clear 'behavioural goals'** – social marketing is driven by a concern to achieve measurable impacts on what people *actually do*, not just on their knowledge, awareness or beliefs about an issue. This approach describes the aim of an intervention in terms of specific behaviours and manageable steps towards a main goal.
- **Developing 'insight'** – social marketing is driven by an understanding of *why* people behave in the way that they do. Particular consideration is given to what people think, feel and believe about the subject.
- **The exchange** – social marketing puts a strong emphasis on understanding what is to be 'offered' (for example, the advantages of being more active). It also requires an appreciation of the 'full cost' of accepting the offer, for example, for being more active, a person might have to invest money, time and effort and sacrifice other social activities, etc. The aim is to maximise the potential 'offer' and its value to the audience, while minimising all the 'costs' of adopting, maintaining or changing a particular behaviour.
- **The competition** – social marketing uses the concept of 'competition' to examine all the factors that compete for people's attention and willingness or ability to adopt a desired behaviour. It looks at both external factors (those outside the individual, for example, competitor advertising) and internal competition (factors within the person, for example, habits, the desire to take risks, etc.).
- **Segmentation** – social marketing uses a 'segmentation' approach. This goes further than traditional 'targeting' by considering alternative ways that people can be understood and profiled. In particular it looks at how different people are responding to an issue and what moves and motivates them; for example,

Diet Coke has traditionally been targeted at women who are known to be more calorie conscious. This feminine association made it hard to directly market this product to men and so the same product was re-badged as Coke Zero and targeted with a different, more masculine, campaign.

- **'Intervention mix' and 'marketing mix'** – social marketing recognises that there are always a range of options or approaches that could be used to achieve a particular goal, and that single approaches are generally less effective than multi-layered approaches. Therefore it uses a 'marketing mix' of different approaches, for example, a campaign aimed at young people to promote safe sex might include:
- radio adverts
- promotional club events
- branded giveaways such as wrist bands, condom packs, etc.

Take it further

Alcohol harm reduction has been identified as a national priority by the government and in 2004 they introduced a national Alcohol Harm Reduction Strategy. Young people's alcohol use is of particular concern with a number of risks to health identified, including alcoholic poisoning, accidents and fires when under the influence, and personal safety.

Choose any one topic relating to alcohol-related harm and design the outline for a local campaign to publicise that specific risk. Think about how you would go about establishing people's views on the subject. What would be suitable behavioural goals to set for your campaign? Think about the 'offer' you are making, i.e. what are the benefits and what might be the costs you have to balance this against? Would you use one approach for everyone or is there market segmentation you could apply to the college population? Consider what might be the relevant mix of marketing approaches.

The role of the mass media

Many people would view the use of the media (newspapers, magazines, billboards, leaflets, radio and television) as the most effective means of reaching the population to promote health. People might assume that because the media reaches a large number of people, its effect will be correspondingly great. However, this is not necessarily the case.

The success of a health message conveyed by the mass media will depend upon the attitudes and viewpoint of the individual who receives the message. Therefore it is not surprising to find that many research studies have shown that the direct persuasive power of the mass media is limited. So how much success can realistically be expected when the mass media is used in health promotion work?

Appropriate aims here might include using the media to:

- raise awareness of health and health issues (for example to raise awareness about the link between over-exposure to the sun and the risk of skin cancer)
- deliver a simple message (for example, that babies should sleep on their backs and not on their tummies; that there is a national advice line for young people wanting information about sexual health)
- change behaviour, if the behaviour is a simple one-off activity (for example, phone for a leaflet) which people are already motivated to carry out.

The use of mass media should be viewed as part of an overall strategy which includes face-to-face discussion, personal help, and attention to social and environmental factors which help or hinder change.

■ What mass media cannot be expected to do

The mass media cannot:

- convey complex information (for example, about transmission routes of HIV)
- teach skills (for example, how to deal assertively with pressure to have sex without a condom or take drugs)
- shift people's attitudes or beliefs. If a message challenges a person's basic beliefs, they are more likely to dismiss the message than change their

belief (for example, 'My grandad smoked 60 a day till he died at 80, so saying I should stop smoking is rubbish')

- change behaviour unless the change requires only a simple action that is easy to do, and people are already motivated to do it. For example, the media may encourage those people who are already motivated to be more active to start walking, because this is an easy and accessible form of exercise. However, it is unlikely to persuade those who are not motivated to do so.

■ Using the local media

While most people are familiar with national and regional media, i.e. the main national newspapers, local evening papers, national radio and television stations, it is far more likely that you will be dealing with local media. The local media can still be a very effective way of reaching people, for example, the local free newspaper will most likely reach every house in your area, but how many people will actually read it? Local media, both radio and print, often have a few key permanent staff members who may be with the paper or station for many years, but the reporters are usually juniors working their way up to the regional and national media. This means they may have little experience

or understanding about the issues you are trying to highlight. The way to overcome this is to provide a press release where you give them the information you want included in the story. In the press release, make sure you give them:

- a title (if it's catchy they may use it directly)
- a brief summary of the main message you are trying to get across (usually three points maximum)
- what is happening, where and when
- the names of any important people who might be attending
- a photo, if possible (or they could send a photographer)
- a quote about the news item from someone the media might be interested in
- some background facts
- the name and details of the person to contact to follow up the news release.

If you write a good press release the paper may largely use it verbatim (word for word), or the radio station may read it directly. If they like your story they might want to interview you. If that happens, make sure you ask to see their questions beforehand. Tell them this will help you prepare the necessary background information and improve the quality of your answers and therefore of the interview.

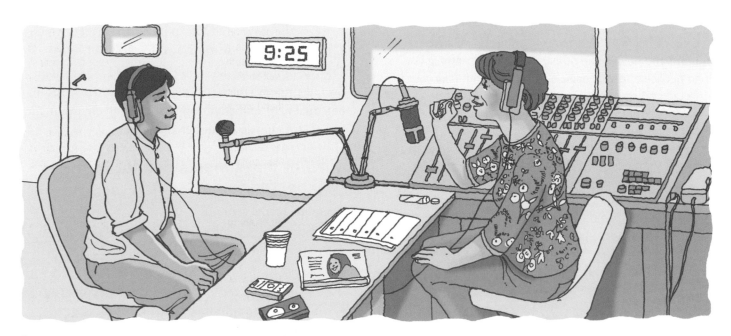

▲ Figure 20.1 Make sure you are well prepared for any interview.

■ Leaflets

Leaflets are the backbone of health education activity. They can serve a wide variety of purposes such as:

- informing people about local services
- providing information about specific health conditions
- giving advice about specific health promotion issues
- engaging people in thought about broader health considerations.

In many cases, leaflets are designed to support specific health campaigns, such as those for immunisation campaigns or for National No Smoking Day. However, it is important to remember that for many people a leaflet will not be an appropriate means of communication. A 2003 national research study for the Department for Education and Skills showed that:

- 5.2 million adults in England could be described as lacking basic literacy (that is, they had failed to reach the standards of reading and writing currently expected for children at age 11)
- more than one third of people with poor or very poor health had literacy skills expected for children at age 11 or below.

Clearly many agencies still do little to take account of people's literacy levels – another survey of readability of patient information produced by hospices and palliative care units showed that 64 per cent of leaflets were readable only by an estimated 40 per cent of the population. (This survey was quoted in the *Choosing Health* White Paper.) Therefore, a leaflet on first appearance is a relatively simple tool, but it requires some thought when designing or using it. Think about:

- Who is this leaflet for? A drugs leaflet that is appropriate for secondary school children will not be appropriate for primary schools.
- Who produced the leaflet? If it is a commercial company, such as a drug company, could this mean they have been selective in their reporting of the information?
- When was the leaflet first produced and is the information still relevant or accurate?
- Is the language level used appropriate to the target audience?

- Is it well designed, i.e. will it grab the attention of the reader from among the other leaflets and posters?
- Will it connect specifically with the target audience?
- Are the key messages clearly identified or are there too many other distractions?
- Where is the best place to display a particular leaflet so that it reaches its target audience?

■ Posters

Posters provide an excellent tool for catching the attention of the target audience. A poster should support the key broad messages which you will then develop in more detail within a leaflet. The factors which draw attention to a poster can be divided into two groups.

Physical characteristics	Motivational characteristics
Size – the whole of the poster as well as the parts within it (like key lettering) need to be large enough to attract attention	**Novelty** – unusual features can help attract attention
Intensity – the use of bold headings	**Interest** – it can be a good idea to make links with items of interest to the target audience, for example, stop smoking posters aimed at young men might feature well-known footballers
Colour – the use of bright colours such as reds, greens and orange, and appropriate use of contrast so that dark text appears on a lighter background and vice versa	**Deeper motivations** – for example, fashion and sex, can also help ensure the target audience looks at your poster
Pictures – using photographs and drawings can help you get your point across as well as making the poster more visually interesting	**Entertainment or humour** – for example, the cartoons can be used to make a serious point

Table 20.1 The characteristics of an eye-catching poster.

The key point of a poster is that it should be eye-catching and big enough to attract attention. It will need to be in colour, or if it is black and white, it should use this for impact or dramatic effect. Wording on posters should be minimal and very bold. Posters need to be placed carefully where the target audience will see them

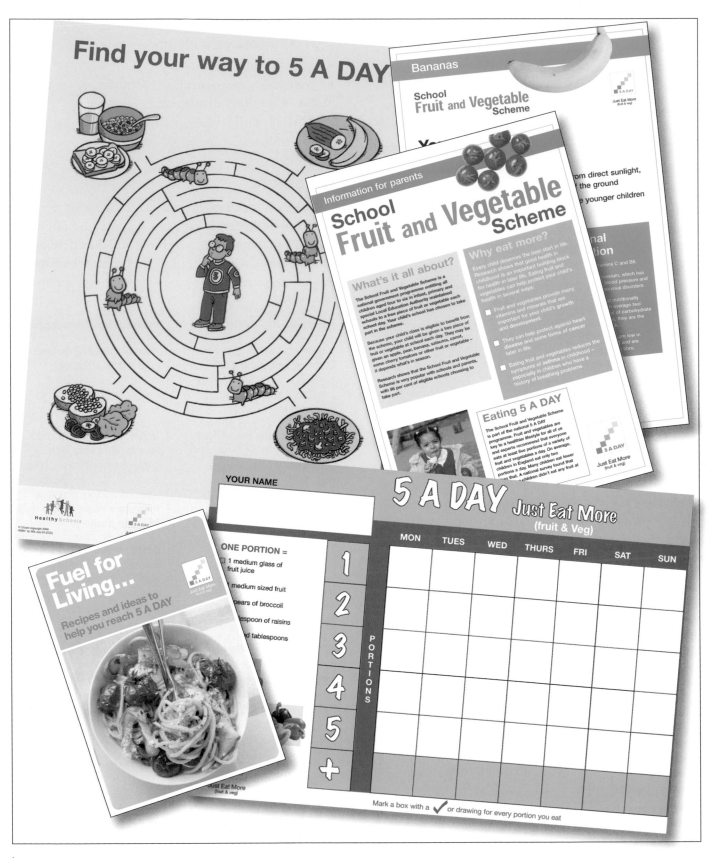

Figure 20.2 Attractive publicity materials from the 5 A DAY campaign.

and they should be changed frequently – after a short period because they become almost 'invisible' once people have seen them a couple of times.

You can find examples of well-designed publicity materials for healthy eating campaigns on the Department of Health website under 5 A DAY. These illustrate two particular points relating to good poster design.

- the use of colour to make the material attractive and draw attention to it
- the simplicity of the message.

Community development

In order to understand where community development for health fits with health education, you first need to understand what is meant by a holistic concept of health.

■ A holistic concept

The word *health* is derived from the Old English term *hael* meaning 'whole'. This suggests that health deals with the whole person – the entirety of their well-being. This brings together a range of aspects of health which together contribute to a person being healthy including:

- **physical health** – this is concerned with body mechanics
- **mental health** – the ability to think clearly and coherently – this is strongly linked to…
- **emotional health** – the ability to recognise emotions and express them appropriately and the ability to cope with potentially damaging aspects of emotional health, for example, stress, depression, anxiety and tension
- **social health** – the ability to make and maintain relationships with others
- **spiritual health** – this can be about personal beliefs, principled behaviour, achieving peace of mind or religious beliefs and practices
- **societal health** – the wider societal impact on our own individual health. For example, this could be the impact of racism on people from a minority ethnic culture, the impact on women of living in a patriarchal society and the impact of living under political oppression.

In this way, any activity which improves any of the aspects of health outlined above will contribute to the promotion of health. This therefore includes community development which Ewles and Simnett defined as:

A process by which a community identifies its needs or objectives, orders or ranks them, develops the confidence and will to work at these needs or objectives, takes action in respect of them, and in so doing develops co-operative and collaborative attitudes and practices in the community.

Community development might include activities which directly influence health as most people understand it, for example, a community food co-op. Other activities might be those which address other aspects of holistic health, for example, a community organising to resist racism could be seen as promoting societal health. In this context, 'community' might be a network of people linked by:

- where they live (such as a housing estate, town, county, country, etc.)
- the work they do (such as the mining community)
- their ethnic background (such as the Muslim community)
- the way they live (such as 'new age' travellers or homeless people)
- or other factors they have in common.

Not all communities will naturally be active; sometimes they require some form of stimulation and encouragement to express their needs and to develop a collective response. A community development approach to health involves working with groups of people to identify their own health concerns, and to take appropriate action. Examples of this type of work might include:

- supporting a group of people with learning difficulties and their carers to consider their sexuality and sexual health needs
- youth and community workers working with young people (outreach work) where they congregate on street corners or in parks to address their substance use issues
- advocacy projects (such as organisations which offer interpreting and/or advocacy for Asian women).

This focus on a holistic view of health, and the principle of challenging inequalities, means community development approaches can really help to tackle health inequalities and to attack the root causes of ill health in some of the most disadvantaged communities.

Remember!

Community development has the following key features:

- A commitment to equality and the breaking down of hierarchies.
- An emphasis on participation and enabling communities to be heard.
- An emphasis on valuing the experiences and lay knowledge of communities.
- The development of a shared view of the problem within the community.
- The empowerment of the community and its individuals through training, skills development and joint action.

■ Advantages and disadvantages of community development activity

Advantages	Disadvantages
It is based in locally identified concerns therefore there is stronger support.	It can take a long time to engage the community and even longer to address the underlying issues.
It focuses on the root causes of ill health.	Results are often not tangible or easily measured.
It builds confidence in the local community.	Therefore evaluation is difficult.
It develops skills in the community – many of which are transferable – for example lobbying, numeracy and literacy skills.	Funding can be difficult to attract and sustain without clear evaluation.
It extends democratic accountability – all participants have equal value – employed workers do not have overall control.	Health promoters can be in a difficult position if the needs of the community conflict with the position of their employer.
	Direct work is often only carried out with a small number of people.
	It tends to draw attention towards small communities and away from larger structural issues.

Table 20.2 The pros and cons of community development.

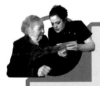

In context

Tom is a local community development worker based in a community centre in the most deprived area of his town. His role is to work with local community and voluntary sector organisations to develop new initiatives which reduce unemployment, increase access to education and training and also reduce the fear of crime. His project is funded by several different sources which explains the mix of objectives he has to work with.

1. **What sort of activities would you suggest Tom offers young people on the estate?**

2. **How could he get the views of young people as to which activities would be best to offer?**

3. **How would you suggest he markets these activities to young people?**

Take it further

1. Can you anticipate any problems Tom might have providing activities which meet his objectives and which are also attractive to young people?

2. How could he evaluate the success of these activities in achieving his key objectives?

Two-way communication

It is hard to quantify the extent to which individual face-to-face interaction can contribute to health campaigning. However, it is clear that the general public holds certain groups within society in high regard; people respect the information they obtain from people such as doctors, nurses and teachers. This creates considerable potential for promoting key health messages simply through the day-to-day work routine. For example, a doctor could suggest to someone attending a health check that they consider giving up smoking, or a district nurse who is visiting an older service user at home could suggest that moderate activity is still possible and potentially beneficial.

It is quite normal for key health campaigns to engage these health promoters when they are trying to communicate a key message. For example, on National No Smoking Day many health practitioners plan specific events to link with the national campaign and offer support to people wishing to quit smoking. Three examples of one-to-one activity are considered in more detail below:

1 **Pre-conceptual care** – for anyone thinking about becoming pregnant, especially for the first time, there may be a number of opportunities for their GP, health visitor, midwife and practice nurse to discuss possible health education issues such as:

- smoking (which is associated with low birth weight and prematurity (early delivery)
- diet (some birth defects such as spina-bifida may be decreased by taking a vitamin called folic acid for some weeks before and during the early months of pregnancy)
- alcohol (consumption of alcohol in large amounts has been associated with abnormalities in new-born babies called foetal alcohol syndrome).

2 **Promoting safe sex** – the UK is currently facing a major sexual health challenge with rates of almost all sexually transmitted infections (STIs) rising. Diagnoses of chlamydia almost doubled during the 1990s, with a marked increase in men and women aged under 20. Other STIs are also increasing – in 2003, syphilis increased by 28 per cent and the number of cases of genital warts increased to 70,883. Alongside this the UK has one of the highest rates of teenage pregnancy in western Europe.

Therefore it is important that safe sex messages (i.e. encouraging correct and consistent condom use) are promoted by all professionals who have the opportunity to do so. This might be a youth worker talking to a young person who they know is having sex with their partner or a GP talking to a woman who wants to start taking the pill.

3 **Immunisation** – as you saw in Unit 12, children are routinely immunised for diphtheria, typhoid, polio, measles, mumps, rubella, etc. However, recent inaccurate publicity about the MMR vaccine has undermined public confidence in it. Therefore, health professionals who work with young families have an important role to play in promoting childhood immunisation. For example, midwives and health visitors can both explain the immunisation programme (i.e. what vaccination at what age) but can also discuss the parents' concerns about immunisation and provide factual information to re-boost public confidence.

■ Theatre in Health Education (TIE)

Theatre in Health Education (TIE) was first developed as a tool for exploring issues of HIV and AIDS within schools in the 1980s and consequently has a particularly strong tradition of work within sex and relationship education (SRE). A number of activities belong under the umbrella term of TIE but the key feature is that projects go beyond a standalone performance and use participatory approaches. This means that performances are often accompanied by:

- preparatory work by actors or teachers
- workshops where issues raised in the performance can be explored
- follow-up activities led by teachers in the weeks after a TIE event.

Activities are often included within performances such as freeze framing (an opportunity to stop the performance and direct the actions of characters) and, commonly, hot seating or truth seating (an opportunity for the audience to question characters about their

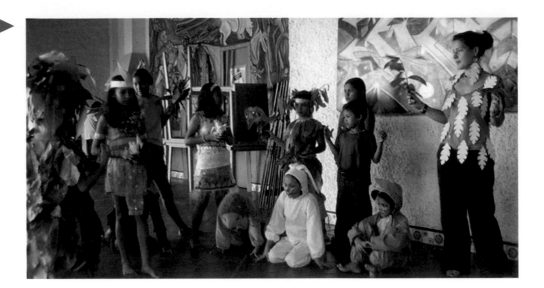

A key feature of theatre in health education is that the performances use participatory approaches.

actions and decisions or to ask them factual questions about issues in the performance).

■ Peer-led approaches

Peer-led approaches aim to use the interactions between peers (usually young people but not in all cases) to promote health-related behaviours. Peer leaders are often seen as having greater credibility than professionals (who are inevitably adults) for young people.

The main method is to use young people (not necessarily the same age as the target audience) who are seen as credible in the eyes of the audience, to provide all or some of the health education input. Defining who might be credible peer leaders must be based on the views of the target audience – this ensures that the peer leaders selected are appropriate and effective. Peer leaders need to be good communicators and unconventional but they also need to demonstrate responsible attitudes.

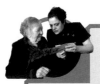

In context

Sally has persuaded her high school to set up a peer mentoring scheme to help tackle bullying. She has read about similar schemes in other schools and knows from her friends that they value them. In her suggestion the role of the mentor would be to support people who are being bullied but also to work with people who are bullying to help them change their behaviour. The school was initially reluctant to admit publicly that it had a problem but have agreed to consider introducing the scheme. However, this is dependent on her providing answers to some of the queries raised by staff and governors:

1 **What criteria would you use to identify suitable peer mentors?**

2 **How would they operate in their role both with the bullied and the bully?**

3 **Would you need a range of different mentors to suit different people's needs?**

Take it further

1 What training or development might these people require to enable them to fulfil their role effectively?

2 How could the school evaluate the success of the project?

3 How could this be linked to work in the curriculum, in particular the *Personal, Social and Health Education* and *Citizenship* aspects of the curriculum?

Figure 20.3 The home page of ▶
www.lookoutalcohol.co.uk

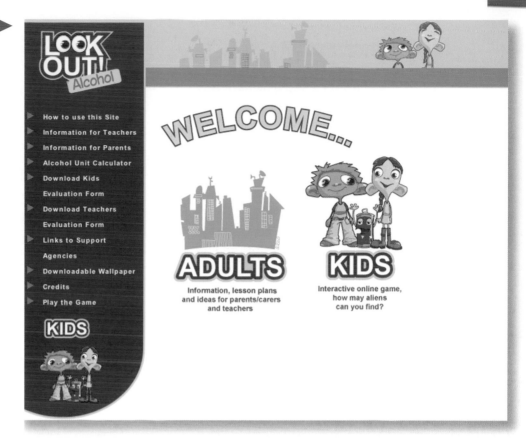

■ Interactive video and computer packages

In the past, health education frequently used videos, workbooks, worksheets and other paper-based media. However, with the widespread use of ICT in schools, there is now an emphasis on using interactive computer packages (either on disk or on websites). These media allow a discovery learning approach for young people, where health education material is often conveyed through a game format – a medium that young people are both familiar and engaged with. A good example here is the online alcohol game for primary age children at www.lookoutalcohol.co.uk, which was designed with the help of primary school children in Lancashire.

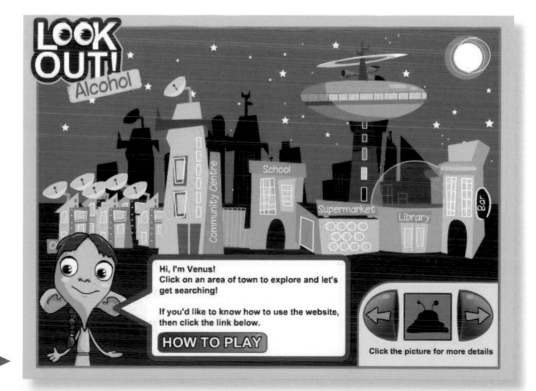

Figure 20.4 Lookoutalcohol's ▶
online game

Assessment activity 20.1

The assessment for this unit will be based on the design, delivery and evaluation of a small-scale health education campaign. Throughout the activities you will be guided through the assessment criteria for your own project and given an opportunity to think about what these mean using a worked example based on the approach taken by the manager of a local chlamydia screening programme.

This programme has a target of testing 15 per cent of the 15–24-year-old population in the PCT district for the STI chlamydia which has seen a dramatic rise in rates in recent years. The introduction of the screening programme is intended to counter the spread of the disease. Carolyn, the manager of the programme, wants to promote the screening service to the students in your college and she needs your help to do this.

First of all you must understand the need for the programme and what chlamydia is. Search out more information on the subject. The background to the programme can be found on the Department of Health website. Find out:

- why people need to be screened
- what a screening test involves
- where your local service operates from.

This might mean searching for local service information on your PCT website. You could even contact the chlamydia team and interview someone from the programme to get a better understanding of how the programme works.

P1 Explain three different approaches to health education.

1 Explain how you could use three of the health education approaches described in the text to promote the service and explain the need for students to be screened. You will need to do the same for your own project.

Grading tip for P1

This activity breaks down into three parts:

- identify the education approaches you intend to adopt from the text
- describe in practical terms what you would do to promote the service using each approach as the basis
- explain how this approach might encourage students to utilise the service.

M1 Compare three different approaches to health education.

2 Which of your ideas do you think is likely to be most successful?

Grading tip for M1

To achieve a merit grade you need to compare three approaches. Your detailed comparison should consider costs, the people involved, advantages and disadvantages of the planned service, and any other practical aspects you can think of.

Models

For a health educator to be effective in their role, they must understand the complex processes which might influence a person to change their behaviour. There are several models of behaviour change which we will explore below.

The health belief model

This was originally developed as a method to explain and predict preventive health behaviour. It originated around 1952 and is generally regarded as the beginning of systematic, theory-based research in health behaviour. The model suggests that an individual is most likely to undertake the recommended preventive health action if they believe:

- a threat to their health is real and serious
- that the benefits of taking the suggested action outweigh the barriers.

In many cases they might also need to be cued to take action.

Key concepts in the model are:

- **perceived susceptibility** – a person's perception of how likely it is that they will get a particular condition that would adversely affect their health
- **perceived seriousness** – a person's beliefs about the effects a disease or condition would have on them, for example, the difficulties that a disease would create including pain and discomfort, loss of work time, financial impact, difficulties with family, etc.
- **perceived benefits of taking action** – once they have accepted their susceptibility to a disease and recognised it is serious, someone may then feel motivated to act and attempt to prevent the disease (but this will also require them to feel there are real benefits from taking action)
- **barriers to taking action** – action may not take place, even though a person believes in the benefits of taking action. This is because of perceived barriers relating to the nature of the treatment or preventive measures (which may be inconvenient, expensive, unpleasant, painful or upsetting)
- **cues to action** – a person may also require a 'cue to action' for the desired behaviour, for example, a call to participate in a screening programme.

Reflect

Is there anything which you might have considered which could improve your health? Do you smoke? Are you less active than you could be? Do you drink more than the recommended guidelines? Think about any aspect of your health where you know you don't conform to recommended advice. What is it that stops you? Think about:

- your perceived susceptibility and seriousness
- barriers to taking action and possible benefits.

Can you explain your current attitude to that health behaviour using this model? What might provide a suitable cue to action for you to make the necessary change?

The theory of reasoned action

This theory provides a framework to study the attitudes which underpin behaviours, suggesting that the most important determinant of a person's behaviour is behaviour intent. This is the individual's intention to perform a behaviour, which is formed from a combination of their attitude toward performing the behaviour and the subjective norm (see below).

If a person believes that the result of adopting a behaviour is positive, they will have a positive attitude toward that behaviour.

If *other people* important to that person also view this action in a positive way, then a *positive subjective norm* is created. Taken together, these two influences would strongly suggest the person would follow the health advice.

For example, if a person thinks that it is important to lose weight and believes that this will make them healthier and happier, and their family and friends support this view, then it is more likely that they will adopt the necessary lifestyle changes to reduce their body weight.

However, if someone is considering quitting smoking, but they are concerned about the impact on their social life because all their friends smoke and these friends are not actively supportive, then it is less likely that this person will choose to quit.

Remember!

According to the theory of reasoned action, the most important determinant of a person's behaviour is *behaviour intent*, i.e. the individual's intention to perform a behaviour. This is a combination of attitude towards performing the behaviour and the subjective norm.

The theory of planned behaviour

This is actually a development of the theory of reasoned action, based on a recognition that behaviour is not 100 per cent under an individual's control. This led to the addition of a third influence, *perceived behavioural control*, which is defined as our perception of the difficulty of performing a behaviour.

The theory suggests that people view the control they have on their behaviour on a continuum which ranges from behaviours that are easily performed to those requiring considerable effort, resources, etc. The difficulties which might influence the perception of control could include:

- the time needed to do something, for example, to prepare fresh food as opposed to using ready meals
- the financial cost, for example, to go swimming regularly
- the difficulty, for example, the skills needed to negotiate condom use, etc.

However, if the person has a positive behaviour intent and a strong positive subjective norm towards a

behaviour, then it is also highly likely that they will view the perceived control favourably. Thus, they will feel they have few barriers to deal with and a high degree of control over the behaviour change.

The theory of social learning

Social learning theory (SLT) is a category of learning theories grounded in the belief that human behaviour is determined by interaction between three sets of factors:

- cognitive (knowledge and attitudes)
- behavioural (for example, personal skills)
- environmental (services in the community, attitudes of peers).

This three-way relationship can be seen in the diagram below:

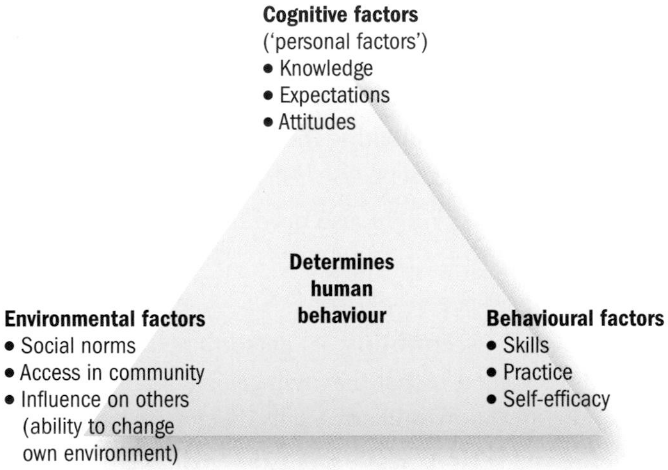

Cognitive factors
('personal factors')
- Knowledge
- Expectations
- Attitudes

Determines human behaviour

Environmental factors
- Social norms
- Access in community
- Influence on others (ability to change own environment)

Behavioural factors
- Skills
- Practice
- Self-efficacy

 Figure 20.5 The three-way relationship between cognitive, environmental and behavioural factors.

There are three main aspects to social learning theory:

1 The likelihood that a person will perform a particular behaviour again in a given situation is strongly influenced by their perception of the likely consequences (for example, the previous rewards or punishments which they experienced when performing the behaviour).

2 People can learn by observing others (called vicarious learning), in addition to learning by participating in an act personally.

3 Individuals are most likely to adopt behaviour observed in others they identify with (this has obvious links to peer education approaches).

If social learning theory is applied to condom use among young men, the cognitive factors might include:

- the understanding of the risks associated with unprotected sex
- attitudes to teen parenthood
- their expectations of sex.

The environmental factors might include:

- the views about condom use among their peer group
- the ability to access condoms from local services
- their ability to change their own views on the subject (perhaps after a class discussion at college).

The skills might include:

- how to put a condom on correctly
- how to negotiate its use with their partner.

Theory into practice

Now consider again the chlamydia screening programme for the under 25s.

1 State some examples of possible cognitive factors.

2 What environmental factors might influence people's likelihood of taking the test?

3 What skills might be required here?

The Stages of Change model

This model is now widely accepted and routinely used in substance use services, for smoking, alcohol and many illegal substances. It suggests there are five stages within the process of behaviour change:

- **pre-contemplation** – there is no intention to change behavior in the foreseeable future (many individuals in this stage are unaware or under aware of their problems)
- **contemplation** – people are aware that a problem exists and are seriously thinking about overcoming it but have not yet made a commitment to take action

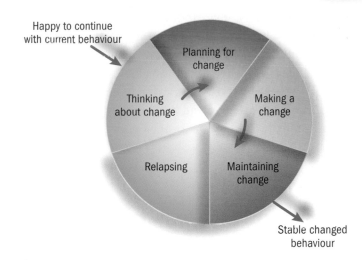

▲ **Figure 20.6 The Stages of Change model.**

- **preparation** – individuals in this stage are intending to take action in the next month and have unsuccessfully taken action in the past year
- **action** – individuals modify their behaviour, experiences or environment in order to overcome their problems. It requires considerable commitment of time and energy
- **maintenance** – people work to prevent relapse and consolidate the gains attained during action.

While the model is frequently illustrated as a wheel, it is known that in many cases a person will have to repeat the process several times to successfully leave the cycle and achieve a stable changed behaviour. For example, think about the people you know who may have tried to quit smoking on several occasions – each of these attempts is part of the learning process which builds their chances of achieving the desired behaviour change. For this reason the process is often portrayed as a spiral with the person gradually moving up the spiral to the desired change.

The importance of social and economic context

It is important to remember that not everyone has the same ability to bring about change in their health behaviours (as discussed in the section on victim blaming on pages 278–9). If you think back to Unit 12:

Public health, you were introduced to the importance of social factors which influence health status and the importance of income in particular. Therefore, while we can consider the theoretical approaches to behaviour change, we have to take account of people's social and economic circumstances and the way they affect their success in making a change for the better.

Peer pressure

Peer pressure may happen in the workplace, at school or within the general community. It can affect people of all ages and backgrounds. Peer pressure occurs when we are influenced to do something we usually would not do or are stopped from doing something we would like to do because we want to be accepted by our peers. A peer can be anyone we look up to or someone who we think of as an equal in age or ability. A peer could be a friend, someone in the community or even someone on TV. We may experience peer pressure as we live up to either the individual's or group's expectations or follow a particular fashion or trend. Peer pressure may be a positive influence and help to challenge or motivate us to do our best, but it may also result in someone doing something that may not fit with their sense of what is right and wrong. It can influence us in a number of ways, including:

- fashion choice
- alcohol and other drugs use
- the decision to have a boyfriend or girlfriend
- our choice of friends
- academic performance.

Reflect

Have you ever felt subjected to peer pressure? What was the pressure about? How did you respond to it? Would you react differently now? Can you see peer pressure at work among your peers?

Peer pressure can be:

- **direct** – for example, someone telling you what you should be doing
- **indirect** – a group of friends may have particular habits or activities that they do together (for example, a person may only smoke when they are with certain friends or may be more likely to study when they are with other friends)
- **individual** – sometimes the pressure comes from within. Feeling different from the group may be hard and, to avoid this, we sometimes do things to make sure we feel like the rest of the group.

It may be hard to resist peer pressure and remain individual but part of being an individual involves making decisions based on what is best for us. It can mean we take ownership and responsibility for what we do and how we think. Being an individual can still mean that we are a valued part of a group.

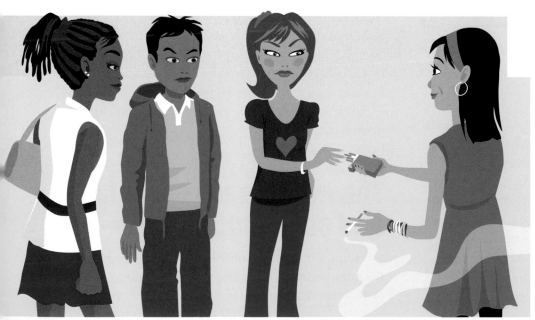

◀ Figure 20.7 Smoking when you don't really want to is often a result of peer pressure.

Assessment activity 20.2

A key part of the chlamydia screening programme is the prevention of possible future sexually transmitted infections. This involves encouraging students to use condoms if they are going to have sex, which might require a change in behaviour to either carry condoms or negotiate their use.

P2 Describe two different models of behaviour change and the importance of the social and economic context.

1 Describe how you might set up a peer education project to increase condom use amongst sexually active students. The first things you need to consider are the social or economic factors that might affect students' condom use. Your peer educators will need to be aware of these before they try to discuss the issues with their friends and colleagues.

2 Look at the social learning theory described earlier in the unit. Describe how peer education relies on this model for its effect. Some people may not be ready to change their behaviour. Explain how the Stages of Change model will enable your peer educators to work effectively in promoting condom use. **P2**

Grading tip fo P2

To achieve P2 you must describe the key parts of the two models and the factors which affect condom use. When you are considering your own project you will also need to consider the social or economic factors which might affect the behaviour you are trying to change as well as considering how two models of behaviour change could be applied to your project design.

P3 Describe the design and implementation of your own small-scale health education campaign.

3 Start by developing an outline plan for a poster and radio campaign. Draft out a project outline using the template in section 3 (page 299) for your campaign and define the following for the project:
 - a clear aim
 - three key objectives which are SMART
 - the main actions (in the order in which you need to tackle them).

4 Describe how you would go about putting the plan into practice, i.e. describe the process of delivering the campaign. **P3**

Grading tip for P3

'Design' means planning the campaign while 'implementation' means delivering it, so to achieve this you must do both, i.e. when you plan your own campaign you must show evidence of your planning as well as describing what you did.

M2 Explain the approaches and methods used in own health education campaign relating them to models of behaviour change.

5 How have you used the social learning theory and the Stages of Change Model as the basis for the design of your campaign?

Grading tip for M2

This requires you to demonstrate how you use theory to influence practice. For example, show how your knowledge of social learning theory has been used in the design of your peer education project.

D1 Evaluate the approaches and methods used in your own health education campaign relating them to models of behaviour change.

6 This is difficult for this theoretical exercise but for your own project you must assess what worked well and discuss the theoretical approaches on which successful aspects were based. **D1**

Grading tip for D1

In this context 'evaluate' means that you should assess the different approaches and explain why you have chosen those models. Explain why these link best to the social learning theory and the Stages of Change model.

Health educators

A holistic model of health would suggest that almost any agency can act as a potential health promoter. However, some are acknowledged as leaders or key players in the field of health education. We are going to touch on the role of a few below.

The World Health Organisation (WHO)

The WHO has been instrumental in shaping and influencing health policy across many nations through its *Health For All by the Year 2000* programme. This has been crucial in a move away from medically dominated models of health promotion to a broader based approach which encompasses social and environmental influences. The key feature of this programme was the introduction of the first targets for improving health.

The WHO's constitution defines it as 'a directing and co-ordinating authority on international health work', with its aim being 'the attainment by all peoples of the highest possible level of health'.

National organisations – the government

Government action to make improvements in health takes place across all departments, as was seen in the first health strategy, *The Health of the Nation* (1992). The government department which has the lead role for health is the Department of Health. This might equally be called The Department of Health *Services* since its main role is to manage the delivery of health services through the National Health Service (NHS). However, in recent years its role in improving health has been increased through white papers like *Choosing Health*.

The Health Protection Agency (HPA)

We saw in Unit 12 that the role of the HPA is to provide support and advice on preventing and reducing the impact of infectious diseases, chemical and radiation hazards, and major emergencies on human health.

This includes a health education role, for example, to inform people about the role of vaccination in reducing the spread of infectious diseases as well as providing information about other communicable diseases such as food poisoning and water-borne infections.

Local agencies – Primary Care Trust (PCT)

When national policy is put into practice at the local level, it relies on a range of local agencies working together effectively on health issues with a common purpose. A key local partner is the Primary Care Trust (PCT), which has the following responsibilities:

- to improve the health of the local population
- to develop local primary health care services
- to commission other local health services in line with local health needs.

The primary function of the NHS is to treat sick people. Although health education activity could and should be a feature of many health service roles, in practice this aspect of health activity has often been seen as secondary to the primary goal of treating the sick. However, *Choosing Health* has a specific target for all NHS staff (both clinical and administrative) to become health promoters. The PCT has a key role in local health promotion programmes with several key staff groups who can be involved with projects, including health

Theory into practice

Find out where your local health promotion team are based – start with your PCT website.

What health information can they provide about your local area or about young people in particular? What resource materials can they provide which might help you with your project?

Find out if there is anyone in their team with a remit to work with schools and colleges who might help you.

promotion staff, the public health team and community nurses such as health visitors and school nurses.

Health strategies

Legislation

Examples of health promoting legislation would include:

- the factory acts of the nineteenth century which limited the hours that children, women and men could work
- the public health legislation which required towns to take steps to improve sanitary conditions
- the clean air acts of the 1950s which significantly reduced city 'smogs' (pollution-laden fogs)
- the Water (Fluoridation) Act of 1985 which enabled health authorities to ask water companies to add fluoride to drinking water to cut dental decay.

Another often quoted example of public health policy was the introduction of seatbelt legislation for drivers and front seat passengers in 1981. This led to a reduction in fatal and serious accidents of about 30 per cent for passengers and 25 per cent for drivers over the next three years.

National health strategy

We looked at the key government health strategies of recent years in Unit 12: *Public health. Choosing Health: Making Healthy Choices Easier, Saving Lives: Our Healthier Nation*, the Acheson Report and other key policy documents are considered in detail in that unit.

Links to national priorities and policy

There are certain accepted principles which guide effective planning for health education activity. The starting point for any activity should be an identified need for the activity. This could be due to a national priority or target. For example, a current priority is to reduce the waiting time for access to GUM (Genito-Urinary Medicine) services (i.e. sexual health clinics which deal with the treatment of sexually transmitted infections). To support this aim, a major national TV campaign was launched to promote the adoption of safe sexual practices (using a condom) and therefore reduce the demand on GUM services, an equally effective means of achieving the national target.

Planning and implementing a health education activity

In order to plan effectively, you need a clear understanding of what you are trying to achieve. As a health promoter you need to define clear aims and objectives before you do anything else. Planning should provide you with the answers to three questions:

- What am I trying to achieve?
- What am I going to do?
- How will I know whether I have succeeded?

Identifying your target audience and need

As a health promoter, your first action in undertaking any campaign will be to identify the source of the need you are considering. This will identify who you are targeting. Identifying your target audience for a campaign starts with the question: 'What is the health need which I should be addressing?' The need for a campaign will usually come from one of four sources:

1 **Normative need** – defined by an expert or professional according to their own standards. For example, a person with a body mass index above 30 is classed as obese.

2 **Felt need** – the needs which people feel, i.e. the things we want. For example, people might want their food to be free of genetically modified (GM) products.

3 **Expressed need** – a felt need which is voiced. For example, the felt need to have GM-free food may become a public debate, with pressure groups focusing on the issue.

4 **Comparative need** – this arises from comparisons between similar groups of people, where one group has access to a health promotion activity and the other does not. For example, one college might employ a student counsellor where another might not.

The evidence of need for your own project can be established from national regional and/or local health information. There are many sources for this type of information including:

- your local Primary Care Trust (the health promotion unit or public health department in particular)
- the local authority
- key websites where you can access data, in some cases for areas as small as individual electoral wards. These include the Public Health Observatories (one for each regional health authority area), the Office for National Statistics, the Department of Health and, in the case of drug and alcohol use, the Home Office.

Having established the target audience and needs for your health promotion project, you will start to translate the idea of how to meet these needs into aims and objectives.

Theory into practice

If you were to carry out a health promotion activity locally, how would you start to identify local needs which would frame the aims and objectives of your work? What felt or expressed needs are you aware of within the student body of your college?

List possible sources of useful information for the needs you may be aware of. How can you add substance to the expressed need with some normative information? How would you decide whether this information is a reliable basis for your decision making?

Aims and objectives

An *aim* is a broad overall goal for the whole project. It is often a very broad statement of the underlying intention and will be hard to use to assess the success of a project. An *objective* is a specific goal to be achieved as part of delivering the aim. This may well be useful for evaluating the effectiveness of a health promotion activity. However, an objective should not be confused

with an *outcome measure* which is explained in more detail later.

Any one aim may have several supplementary objectives within it. Objectives are usually defined as being SMART:

- **S**pecific – defined in terms which are clear and precise
- **M**easurable – when the work is finished we can see whether the objective has been achieved or not
- **A**chievable – realistic, i.e. within our power to achieve
- **R**elevant – focused on addressing an appropriate issue within our broad aim
- **T**imed – we have agreed a timescale by which we expect to have delivered this objective.

Objectives must be SMART to be effective aids to planning. They may be aims which require breaking down further into specific objectives. Without this level of detail, an objective becomes immeasurable and therefore evaluation of the work is undermined.

Remember!

An *aim* is the broad overall goal for a piece of work. Usually a project has only one or two aims. An *objective* is a specific goal to be achieved as part of delivering a stated aim or outcome.

A planned approach to a Theatre in Health Education project ▶

Objective

State your objective here (use a separate sheet for each objective).

Use a TIE approach to engage young people in an accessible, fun but rigorous discussion about the legal, health, personal and social consequences of decisions made in relation to drugs, sex and crime. Plan and deliver this activity within the next school term.

Key tasks/activities

Briefly describe what service or activity you will provide and evaluate to achieve this objective.

- Interactive theatre performances by a team of actors with groups of 60–90 students, lasting 90 minutes.
- Students will receive preparatory and follow-up work in the school.
- Some preparatory and follow-up work will be done with school staff.

Results

What do you hope will change as a result of this activity?

- Students will show a greater repertoire of behaviours enabling them to make informed and safe decisions.
- Students and staff will feel more confident and informed when discussing the issues raised in the performances.
- Staff will feel able and confident to follow up this work.
- Students and staff will feel that the interactive theatre experience can make this learning enjoyable and memorable.

Measures

How will you measure the described change?

- Assess student attitudes before and after the performances.
- Assess staff attitudes and confidence before and after the performances.
- Observe and evaluate the performances.
- Follow up after 6 months to review progress.

Standards
Define the levels of success for your project.

What will be the best you could hope for? (a great result!)	*What will you be happy with? (a satisfactory result)*	*What will you be unhappy with? (a disappointing result)*
• A highly enjoyable experience with high levels of satisfaction. • Students have much more confidence when discussing and giving feedback. • Staff very pleased and happy to continue and develop the work. • The school uses some interactive techniques in its PSHE curriculum. • We get to do more work with them!	• The students and staff enjoy the day. • There is evidence of some change in student knowledge and attitudes, and some staff express interest in continuing the work. • Some follow-up takes place in school and there is evidence of links to the PSHE curriculum.	• Preparatory work is not done or done badly. • Feedback from students and staff is only satisfactory. • There is little evidence of increased knowledge or changed attitudes in the students. • Staff don't attend the performances and show little interest in following up the work or using or developing the techniques as part of their curriculum.

Establishing clear objectives for your own work

While we might be trying to improve the health of individuals and society as a whole, this is at best an aim and not easily measurable or attributable to our work. Therefore, when you are trying to define objectives for your project, you might think about objectives like the ones in the table below.

Objective type	A possible example
Health-related learning	To improve the knowledge of parents who are attending a workshop to learn how to discuss drug use with their children
Exploring values and attitudes	Provide an opportunity for a group of members from a local community to explore attitudes to racism in their locality
Promoting self-esteem and self-empowerment	To increase self-awareness and self-belief in a group of people from a local community in order to encourage them to be active in decision-making in that community
Providing knowledge and skills for change	To develop the necessary knowledge and skills of a group of people to enable them to stop smoking for a period of at least four weeks
Changing beliefs	To reduce the proportion of parents holding negative views about the MMR vaccine through a health visitor-led awareness event at a local surgery
Changing attitudes	To increase the numbers of people who are contemplating stopping smoking after an awareness-raising session in a local workplace
Changing behaviours	To increase the numbers of young people who are using a condom when having sex
Changing lifestyle	Increasing the numbers of people who report they are using active forms of transport to get to and from work on a local industrial estate

Table 20.3 Different types of objectives.

Other planning issues for consideration

- **Choice of approach** – if you have selected the topic and the audience, you must now make a crucial decision– what approach will you use to deliver the message? Is this a media-driven campaign, or one which would work best through a one-to-one approach (for example, using peer educators), or a community development project? Whatever approach you adopt, you will need to be able to explain it and justify why it has been selected.
- **The approach 'starts where the client is at'** – as you will already have seen in the discussion of social marketing principles, successful health education has to seek to understand *where the person is at now* rather than *where someone might think they should be.*
- **The information you are using is accurate and up to date** – this can be particularly problematic for printed materials. Information can become outdated but it is still available because people don't regularly check the content and remove them from circulation.
- **The medium for conveying the message is appropriate to the target audience** – newspapers, radio, TV – the right media could be crucial. Radio stations tend to have very specific target audience age ranges so selecting the wrong radio station for your campaign could mean that a campaign about drug use is targeted at the over 60s!
- **Prejudice and misinformation are challenged** – in the section on immunisation you saw that one person's views can distort the perception of a large part of the population. In that case, it has reduced immunisation levels for measles, mumps and rubella to dangerously low levels. This illustrates the responsibility of health educators to make sure the information they are giving out is both accurate and free from prejudice. This can be particularly difficult in an environment where education materials can often be sponsored by commercial companies leading to a conflict of interests. For example, snack food manufacturers might provide school PE equipment in return for large numbers of wrappers from their products.

- **Liaison with other agencies** – health education is rarely effective when the activity is focused within one organisation. The causes of ill health are so broad that it requires a wide range of agencies to work together to have a positive influence on health. When you are working with other agencies, it is important to know who you need to work with and at what stages. You need to make sure you don't miss them out of your planning and then find that they are either unable or unwilling to support the work or can't fit in with your timescale.

Ethics

To act ethically is to act in a principled way. Health promotion is founded on a set of principles which define an ethical approach. These principles include:

- a respect for autonomy, i.e. the right of the individual to make their own choices and determine their own life
- not doing harm
- doing good
- a commitment to justice, i.e. being fair and equitable.

Health education can present serious challenges to the educator. For example, if a health promoter works with a person, gradually exploring their health needs and supporting them towards making an informed choice, the individual might still decide not to follow the health promoter's advice and choose to adopt a health-damaging behaviour. The educator has respected the individual's right to autonomy but can they accept and respect that decision and not coerce or persuade the person to adopt a different choice because of their concerns about the impact on their health?

The danger with health education activity is that health promoters become fixed on the goal of improved medical or physical health, to the detriment of other aspects of holistic health. It is all too easy for professionals to adopt a victim blaming approach, deciding what is best for the individual to the exclusion of that person's right to self-autonomy. It is important to remember that empowering people is an integral part of effective and ethical health promotion work.

Evaluation and outcome measures – have I succeeded?

Evaluation is something we actively engage in on a daily basis, when we ask ourselves questions such as:

Do I enjoy my job or should I apply for another one?

Will I go to that club again?

Or, on a professional footing:

How did that session go?

Did I achieve what I set out to do?

Did that service user really understand what I was explaining to her or was she just being polite when she said she did?

In other words, evaluation is about assessing the value or worth of something, which includes an element of subjectivity, i.e. our own appreciation of it.

Key terms

Evaluation A judgement of the worth of something.

In the context of evaluating health promotion activity, we are probably considering a more formal approach to evaluation. The evaluation may be more public or open to scrutiny by outsiders. In this type of evaluation there are two key aspects:

- defining what we hope to achieve, i.e. aims and objectives
- gathering information to assess whether we have met these aims and objectives.

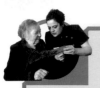

In context

Grace is a midwife who has worked her patch of the district for the last seven years. She has just finished her first visit (the induction visit) to Alison, a 19-year-old woman who already has a two-year-old called Sean. Grace was also Alison's midwife throughout her pregnancy with Sean. Alison is pregnant and is currently smoking 25 cigarettes a day, and on initial enquiries doesn't want to consider quitting. Most of her family smoke and Alison's mum says she smoked through her pregnancy with Alison and she is OK, isn't she? Alison was smoking a similar amount throughout her pregnancy with Sean, who was born a month premature weighing only 4½ pounds and has subsequently had problems with asthma and repeated chest infections.

1   **Should Grace be telling Alison to quit smoking?**

2   **What would the appropriate messages be for her to convey to Alison?**

3   **Is she failing in her role as a midwife if she accepts Alison's wish to continue smoking?**

Take it further

1   In this situation, who is better placed to judge what is right for Alison and her family, and how do you justify that opinion?

2   If Grace was very directive, how might this affect her relationship with Alison and what might the implications of any change in the relationship be?

3   Should health behaviour be a matter of personal choice, or is too important to leave to the individual?

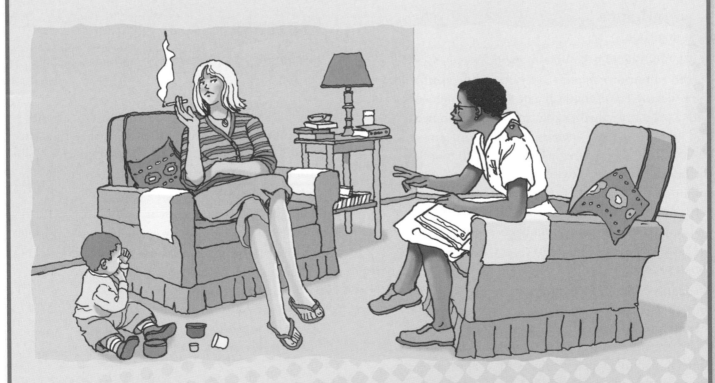

▲   **Figure 20.8 Health professionals have to consider ethical issues when discussing health-damaging behaviours such as smoking.**

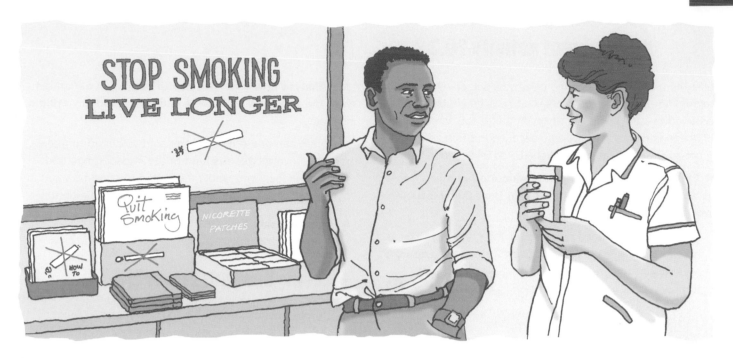

▲ Figure 20.9 The success of 'stop smoking' services is measured by the number of ex-smokers who don't take up smoking again.

Forms of evaluation

In your assessment of your own project, you will need to reflect upon its strengths, weaknesses and areas where it could have been improved upon. This is part of an **outcome evaluation** which tries to establish the worth of work when it is finished. Or is it an ongoing appraisal of the progress made? Evaluation that involves feedback during the course of a project, when things are still taking shape, is termed **formative evaluation**, or an *evaluation of process*.

An **outcome measure** is the end point of the piece of work a health promoter undertakes. This can be a target as challenging as those seen in *Saving Lives* (which refer to reductions in disease) or something quite small scale, such as improving the knowledge and skills of people from a specific geographical community about healthy cooking. There will be considerable overlap between outcome measures and objectives here but it is important not to confuse the two.

Key terms

Outcome evaluation This seeks to establish the worth of work when it is finished.

Formative evaluation This evaluates a project as it progresses.

Outcome measure An indicator of success for a health promotion activity.

So for your assessment activity you need to ask yourself, 'How will I know that this has been a worthwhile activity?' You will need to identify the information that enables you to state categorically that your aim has been achieved. You might want to scale down some of your objectives and outcomes when you begin to do this as you might realise how ambitious you have been!

Assessment activity 20.3

Let's return one last time to the chlamydia screening programme. The manager wants you to design a radio and poster advertising campaign which promotes the screening service to students in the college because this is a key setting for accessing her target population (15- to 24-year-olds).

P4 Explain how your own health education campaign met the aims and objectives, and explain the ethical issues involved.

1   How would you define success for the campaign, i.e. how would you know you had been successful and most importantly what evidence would you collect to prove that to someone else?

Grading tip for P4

In this example you are working with a theoretical example of a health education campaign. In this case you need to show you can come up with clear success criteria and some sensible ideas for how you will demonstrate you have achieved them. You will have to do this for real for your course work.

Go back to the section on ethical practice in health education on pages 301–02; any health education activity based on the issue of sexual health is likely to raise ethical issues, so think about the ones this project might raise for you. It is likely that some of your friends are putting themselves at risk of contracting chlamydia by not regularly using condoms.

- What ethical issues might be raised by a group of students designing a campaign for such a sensitive subject for their peers? The line between drunken consensual sex and rape can be difficult to judge – have any of your friends been in a situation where rape might have occurred? Who would you tell?
- How might your relationship with your friends at college be compromised by this work? What would your friends' reaction be if you suggested they had engaged in risky sexual behaviour?

These are important issues for you to consider in your own work, particularly if your campaign is aimed at people with whom you have close links.

M3 Analyse how your own health education campaign met the aims and objectives and addressed any ethical issues.

2   When carrying out your campaign you need to make some overall assessment of the impact it has had. For this level you would also need to show how you will address the possible ethical issues you identify above.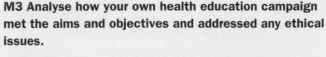

Grading tip for M3

In this context 'analyse' is used to mean 'consider', i.e. to discuss it but not necessarily assess its success. (That is what you need to do to achieve a distinction grade.)

P5 Explain how your own small-scale health education campaign links to local/national/international targets and strategies for health.

3   Summarise the local, national and international targets and strategies which support the chlamydia screening programme.

Grading tip for P5

Any project proposal usually starts by showing its importance through links to local, national and, if possible, international health strategy. That might sound daunting but this exercise is usually a simple piece of desk-based research using the Internet. Try searching your local PCT site for references to chlamydia then look for national and international references to it using, for example, the Department of Health and the World Health Organisation websites. Identify which documents it is mentioned in and what targets (if any) are set against it. This will be an important starting point for your own project as well.

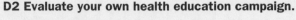

M4 Analyse the role of your own small-scale health education campaign in terms of local/national/international targets and strategies for health.

4   What might your project's contribution be to the reduction in chlamydia rates? Look again at the current trends and make an assessment of how your project might contribute to the local achievement of the chlamydia screening target and in turn to the national target.   **M4**

Grading tip for M4

This assessment activity is asking you to think about the part each small-scale intervention can play in achieving the national target. Your own project might seem small and insignificant but you need to think about the way in which the sum total of all activity can add up to make a real difference.

D2 Evaluate your own health education campaign.

5   How will you evaluate the success of the project? What process and outcome measures will you use to measure this success? How well did it go against these measures?   **D2**

Grading tip for D2

This is the final drawing together of many of the earlier points to compile an overall statement of evaluation, i.e. an overall assessment of your project.

Knowledge check

1   Why might a 'victim blaming' approach to health education be described as being over simplistic?

2   List two advantages and two disadvantages of a community development approach to health education.

3   What are the seven main features of a social marketing approach?

4   When designing a leaflet, what are the key questions you would need to consider?

5   What are the stages described in the Stages of Change model? Why is it sometimes represented as a spiral as opposed to a circle?

6   What were the underpinning principles for the *Choosing Health* white paper?

7   If you were to undertake a health promotion project to reduce the unsafe level of alcohol consumption

in a particular estate in your locality, you would first need to identify the need for this project. Describe a possible example of:

• a normative need
• a comparative need
• a felt need
• an expressed need.

8   What does SMART stand for when defining objectives?

9   What is the difference between an outcome evaluation measure and a formative evaluation measure?

10 A friend of yours has had unprotected sex on several occasions, usually while under the influence of alcohol. You are worried that they are regularly putting themselves at risk of catching a sexually transmitted infection and also that they are making themselves vulnerable when they are intoxicated. What are the ethical considerations you need to think about if you wish to discuss this with them?

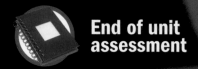
Preparation for assessment

Assessment of this unit is largely based on your success in planning, designing and implementing a small-scale health education campaign. The easiest way of drawing together the necessary information is in a campaign report which would have to deal with the following aspects of your work.

In the **methodology** you must include an explanation of the approach you have adopted in the planning and implementation of the campaign. It will be important to have a sound understanding of at least three health education approaches before you attempt any detailed planning. You must describe these three possible different approaches **P1** and compare them, weighing up the advantages and disadvantages **M1** as well as demonstrating a good understanding of the applied approach. You will need to have described two different models of behaviour change and shown some consideration of the importance of social and economic context in which a health education campaign takes place **P2**. This section will need to include a clear description of your design and implementation of the health education campaign **P3**.

You need to explain the approaches and methods you used, relating them to models of behaviour change **M2**. You could go further and *evaluate* these approaches and methods, i.e. assess which are likely to be most effective for your campaign **D1**.

The objectives of the campaign will link directly to the different stages and tasks which need to be completed, to ensure the campaign takes place as efficiently as possible. You also need to consider the intended outcomes of the campaign so that effectiveness can be measured accurately. Try to identify the skills you use, for example, practical, organisational and communication skills. This would be the **aims and objectives** section of your report.

You would usually include here your **project plan** based on the planning template in the last section.

At this point you would usually include a specific section explaining any **ethical issues** presented by the project **P4** as well as some comments on how you intend to address them **M3**.

In the final section of your report (the **evaluation**) you must explain how the health education campaign met the aims and objectives **P4**. Analysis of success against the aims and objectives **M3** would require some assessment of how well it performed against the objectives, while an evaluation **D2** would include a more rounded assessment. For example, you would provide evidence of reflective practice where you make judgements about your performance and the success of the campaign against the pre-set criteria stated.

You will need to demonstrate that you have taken into consideration recent or current health policy, **P5** and having gathered this background together, made some judgement as to how well your campaign has supported the achievement of policy targets and strategies **M4**. This would usually form the **background and context** section of any campaign report.

To organise your report you could either follow the order set out in the assessment guidance or you could use an authentic project report format which would follow this pattern:

- background and context
- aims and objectives
- methodology
- ethical issues
- project plan
- implementation
- evaluation.

Resources and further reading

Benzeval, M., Judge, K., Whitehead, M. (1995) *Tackling Inequalities in Health: An Agenda for Action* London: Kings Fund Publishing

Downie, R.S., Tannahill, C., Tannahil, A. (1996) *Health Promotion Models and Values* Oxford: Oxford University Press

Draper, P. (ed) (1991) *Health Through Public Policy*: Green Print

Ewles, L. Simnett, I. (1992) *Promoting Health: A Practical Guide* London: Scutari Press

HM Government (2004) *At Least Five a Week: Evidence on the Impact of Physical Activity and its Relationship to Health* London: HMSO

HM Government (2004) *Choosing Health: Making Healthy Choices Easier* London: HMSO

HM Government (1992) *The Health of the Nation* London: HMSO

HM Government (1998) *Independent Inquiry into Inequalities in Health* London: HMSO

HM Government (2006) *It's Our Health! Realising the Potential of Effective Social Marketing* London: HMSO

HM Government (2001) *National Strategy for HIV and Sexual Health* London: HMSO

HM Government (1997) *The New NHS: Modern, Dependable* London: HMSO

HM Government (1997) *Saving Lives: Our Healthier Nation* London: HMSO

Jones, L., Sidell, M. (1997) *The Challenge of Promoting Health: Exploration and Action* Milton Keynes: Open University

Katz, J., Peberdy, A. (1997) *Promoting Health: Knowledge and Practice* Buckingham: Macmillan/OU Press

Moonie, N. (2000) *Advanced Health and Social Care* Oxford: Heinemann

Naidoo, J., Wills, J. (1996) *Health Promotion: Foundations for Practice* London: Baillière Tindall

Townsend, P., Whitehead, M., Davidson, N., Davidsen, N. (1987) *Inequalities in Health: The Black Report and the Health Divide* Harmondsworth: Penguin Books

Useful websites

British Heart Foundation
www.bhf.org.uk

Calculate your Body Mass Index
www.nhlbisupport.com/bmi/bmicalc.htm

Department of Health: www.doh.gov.uk

Food in Schools
www.foodinschools.org

Give up Smoking
www.givingupsmoking.co.uk

Healthy School Lunches
www.healthyschoollunches.org

Mind, Body & Soul
www.mindbodysoul.gov.uk

National Drugs Strategy
www.homeoffice.gov.uk/drugs/index.html

National Institute for Clinical Excellence (NICE)
www.publichealth.nice.org.uk/

NHS in England: www.nhs.uk/england

NHS immunisation information
www.mmrthefacts.nhs.uk

National Social Marketing Centre
www.schoolfoodtrust.org.uk

School Food Trust
www.nsms.org.uk

The quick guide to checking information quality on the Internet: www.quick.org.uk

Wired for Health
www.wiredforhealth.gov.uk

World Health Organisation
www.who.int/en/

GRADING CRITERIA

To achieve a pass grade the evidence must show that the learner is able to:	To achieve a merit grade the evidence must show that, in addition to the pass criteria, the learner is able to:	To achieve a distinction grade the evidence must show that, in addition to the pass and merit criteria, the learner is able to:
P1 explain three different approaches to health education **Assessment activity 20.1 page 290**	**M1** compare three different approaches to health education **Assessment activity 20.1 page 290**	
P2 describe two different models of behaviour change, and the importance of the social and economic context **Assessment activity 20.2 page 295**		
P3 describe the design and implementation of your own small scale health education campaign **Assessment activity 20.2 page 295**	**M2** explain the approaches and methods used in your own health education campaign, relating them to models of behaviour change **Assessment activity 20.2 page 295**	**D1** evaluate the approaches and methods used in your own health education campaign relating them to models of behaviour change **Assessment activity 20.2 page 295**
P4 explain how your own health education campaign met the aims and objectives, and explain the ethical issues involved **Assessment activity 20.3 page 304**	**M3** analyse how your own health education campaign met the aims and objectives and addressed any ethical issues **Assessment activity 20.3 page 304**	
P5 explain how your own small scale health education campaign links to local/national/international targets and strategies for health. **Assessment activity 20.3 page 304**	**M4** analyse the role of your own small scale health education campaign in terms of local/ national/international targets and strategies for health. **Assessment activity 20.3 page 305**	**D2** evaluate your own health education campaign. **Assessment activity 20.3 page 305**

Applied psychological perspectives

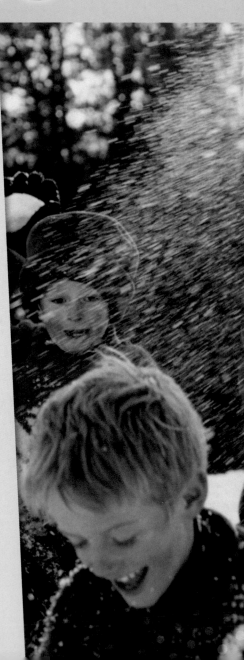

Introduction

Psychology involves the scientific study of mind, behaviour and emotions. The study of psychological perspectives and the application of these theories will enable you to gain enormous insight into human growth and development. Human beings are complex and multi-faceted with many influences on their behaviour. Understanding a particular behaviour in a number of ways will be deepened by studying a variety of perspectives.

How you will be assessed

This unit will be assessed by a written assignment internally marked by your tutor. You will be given opportunities throughout the unit to work on assessments and check your knowledge and understanding. By the end of this unit you will be able to achieve the following outcomes:

- Understand the contribution of psychological perspectives to the understanding of the development of individuals
- Understand the contribution of psychological perspectives to the understanding of specific behaviours
- Understand the contribution of psychological perspectives to the management and treatment of specific behaviours
- Understand the contribution of psychological perspectives to residential care provision.

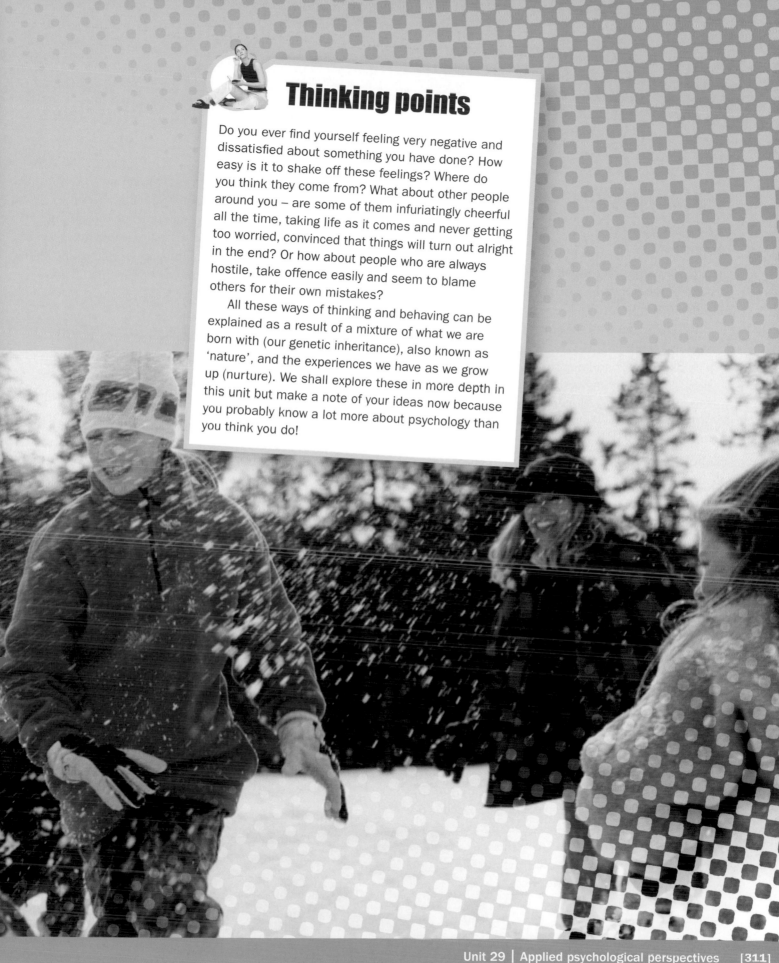

Thinking points

Do you ever find yourself feeling very negative and dissatisfied about something you have done? How easy is it to shake off these feelings? Where do you think they come from? What about other people around you – are some of them infuriatingly cheerful all the time, taking life as it comes and never getting too worried, convinced that things will turn out alright in the end? Or how about people who are always hostile, take offence easily and seem to blame others for their own mistakes?

All these ways of thinking and behaving can be explained as a result of a mixture of what we are born with (our genetic inheritance), also known as 'nature', and the experiences we have as we grow up (nurture). We shall explore these in more depth in this unit but make a note of your ideas now because you probably know a lot more about psychology than you think you do!

Debates in developmental psychology

Nature v nurture

This debate centres on the extent to which our personality, development, intelligence and behaviours are genetically inherited (**nature**) or acquired as a result of interaction with the environment (**nurture**). Behavioural psychologists take the view that we are born as 'blank slates' and our behaviour and personality develop as a result of interactions with the environment (nurture). Biological psychologists believe that many of the influences on our development come from our genes and the influence of biochemistry on our behaviour (nature). Others believe that there is an interaction between the two factors.

Key terms

Nature All aspects of a person that are inherited or coded for in the genes.

Nurture Influences from the environment which shape development and behaviour.

■ Nature

A nature account of development, personality and behaviours focuses on what is innate (what we are born with) such as left-handedness, the genes we have inherited, etc. Issues such as temperament (are you shy and withdrawn or outgoing and confident), intelligence and susceptibility to developing certain illnesses or diseases bring this debate into focus; there are arguments in favour of the nature perspective, stating that our inheritance has a very large influence on who we become.

■ Nurture

Nurture refers to all that happens within the environment (even in the womb) that influences the growing child. It involves the way someone is brought up (socialisation) and the way they are treated by important others such as parents, teachers and peers. All of this influences behaviour and development and goes towards building a personality.

One way of illustrating the nature v nurture debate is by looking at intelligence. If intelligence is an inborn quality that merely develops, then the influences of the environment should have no effect. This seems unlikely, though, since children who are exposed to enriching environments, where they get the opportunity to develop their talents to the full, seem to do better than those who have less fortunate educational opportunities.

A second example is the development of gender. While sex refers to the biological characteristics of being male or female, gender is the word used to describe behaviours, beliefs, expectations and attitudes commonly associated with the two genders. A boy might be born with a tendency to be more boisterous than a girl, but if he is brought up in an environment where quietness and restraint are valued and encouraged, these boisterous tendencies may reduce over time.

Continuity v discontinuity

This debate is about whether development is a smooth process with no distinct changes taking place (**continuity**) or a discontinuous process where development takes place in stages (**discontinuity**).

■ Continuity

A continuity account of development looks at quantitative rather than qualitative change. Change involves smooth growth, for example, skull size grows, the number of words in a child's vocabulary increases. The analogy of a sponge is sometimes used to explain this, where growth simply drips in just as water soaks

Key terms

Continuity A view of development which sees growth and development occurring slowly and continuously, for example, growth in height.

into a sponge (which gets heavier and more laden with water but does not change shape).

■ Discontinuity

In this characterisation of development, the differences between stages are qualitative rather than quantitative. A good way to illustrate this is to imagine the development of a butterfly. This moves from the caterpillar stage to the chrysalis stage to the final emergence of a butterfly – all very distinct stages involving qualitative change. This can be seen in children in the development of walking rather than crawling, the emergence of social smiling, etc. Stage theories in psychology as suggested by Freud, Piaget and Erikson are examples of discontinuity.

Key terms

Discontinuity A view of development which involves stages. Each stage is qualitatively different from the preceding and the next stage.

Nomothetic v idiographic

Nomothetic, as applied to psychology, is concerned with the study of features that are common to a group or class of individuals. The cognitive psychologists (for example, Piaget) researched into why all children made similar errors in logic, problem solving and reasoning at a certain age.

Idiographic refers to the study of an individual and those unique characteristics that distinguish them from others. Case studies in psychology take an idiographic approach as they are concerned to find out why a particular individual developed in the way they did. The case of Genie, described on page 335, is a good example of an idiographic approach.

Key terms

Nomothetic This approach is concerned with investigating a group of individuals to see what traits and behaviours they have in common.

Idiographic This approach to development involves the study of all the unique characteristics of one particular individual.

Assessment activity 29.1

P1 Describe three debates in developmental psychology.

1. List the key aspects of the nature–nurture debate in psychology.

2. Explain what is meant by the continuity v discontinuity hypothesis, giving one example of each.

3. Describe the difference between a nomothetic and an idiographic approach to psychology. **P1**

Grading tip for P1

To achieve P1.1 you could create a table with columns for nature and nurture and include aspects of development that are considered to *fit into these* categories. For example, our genes play a part in our physical development, but environmental factors such as diet also influence this.

To achieve P1.2 you could describe a stage theory of development, such as those proposed by Piaget, Freud or Erikson, and explain how the child moves from one stage to the other (discontinuity). For the continuity hypothesis, you could explain Bowlby's theory of attachments.

To achieve P1.3 you could explain Piaget's way of studying individuals with a case study, such as Genie.

M1 Analyse one debate in developmental psychology.

4   Critically consider the contributions made by the nature v nurture debate in psychology. Give examples to illustrate your answer.

Grading tip for M1

You can use your work for P1.1 as a basis for this. Describe aspects of nature that apply to development, and discuss the extent to which nurture helps us to understand the way the two go together and affect each other.

of that behaviour. If the consequence is **reinforcing** (i.e. it provides something the individual wants or values) it will be repeated. Over time the behaviour is strengthened and becomes a typical pattern of behaviour. If the consequence is unpleasant (**punishment**) there is a possibility that this unpleasant consequence will lead to a lessening of the behaviour. However, in operant conditioning it has been found that punishment is much less effective than reinforcement.

A very simple example can be shown by a child having a tantrum in a supermarket. If this behaviour leads to the consequence of dad buying her a bag of sweets to keep her quiet, she will learn to repeat the behaviour in order to receive this consequence. The bag of sweets (consequence) is experienced as reinforcing.

Principal psychological perspectives

Behaviourist

This perspective is widely used to understand the development of human behaviour. The basic assumption is that all human behaviour can be understood as the result of learning. There are two types of learning: classical and operant conditioning.

■ Classical conditioning

This refers to an association being made between two events. The first event is called a stimulus and the second is a response. Suppose, for example, a young child runs up to a large dog and puts out her hand to pat the dog. The dog barks loudly (the stimulus) causing the child to have an automatic physiological reaction of being startled and afraid (the response). The pairing of these two events creates an association leading the child to fear dogs in the future. (For more detail on the process of classical conditioning see Book 1, Unit 8).

■ Operant conditioning

This theory of explaining behaviour believes that behaviour is learnt according to the **consequence**

Key terms

Consequence Something that happens as a result of your behaviour.

Reinforcement When a consequence is experienced as desirable or pleasurable.

Reinforcer Something that acts to reinforce behaviour. This could be a treat, praise or thanks or a simple smile.

Punishment An undesired consequence of behaviour.

Social learning theory

Social learning theory is sometimes called a theory of **observational learning**. It was developed by Albert Bandura who states (in Haralambos, M., 2002) that behaviour can develop as a result of observing and imitating others. When we observe others behaving, dressing or speaking in a particular way, we notice what kind of response they get. If a school child is disruptive in class, others are likely to observe whether this behaviour is reinforced, and this will influence their decision whether or not to imitate this behaviour – if not now then at a later stage. When behaviour is learnt but not performed until a later date, this is called **latent learning**.

Key terms

Observational learning A type of learning where we do not experience a consequence directly but learn from watching others perform a behaviour and noting the consequence they receive.

Latent learning This refers to the situation where a new behaviour has been learnt by being observed, but is not necessarily performed.

Key terms

Motivation This is the key factor that determines whether someone will put what they have learnt into practice. Motivation is mostly governed by the individual's own emotions, thought processes, wishes, etc.

For performance of the learnt behaviour to take place we need to be **motivated** to perform the behaviour. Motivation depends on a number of factors including how attractive or prestigious the model is. We are more likely to imitate behaviour performed by someone we admire and want to be like than someone we dismiss as not being important. The consequences for the model also influence motivation. If the model gets punished, we are less likely to imitate behaviour. However, if the

model gets a reinforcing consequence, we are more likely to imitate behaviour.

Sometimes there can be more than one consequence. In the example of the disruptive school child the teacher is likely to offer punishment in the form of words or another sanction of some sort. On the other hand, if the rest of the class roars with laughter or encourages the child, the consequence that he or she pays attention to is likely to be this reinforcing response from his classmates.

In context

Hassan has been brought up quite strictly by his parents. He believes, as they do, that alcohol, drugs and all forms of tobacco should be avoided. He watches his friends going out on a Friday night to a local park where they drink beer and smoke cigarettes.

1 **Has Hassan learnt the behaviour of drinking and smoking?**

2 **What might motivate Hassan either to imitate or not to imitate this behaviour?**

3 **Consider how important models are in motivating Hassan to imitate this behaviour.**

Psychodynamic psychology

This perspective looks at underlying unconscious processes in individuals. It is covered in detail in the section below.

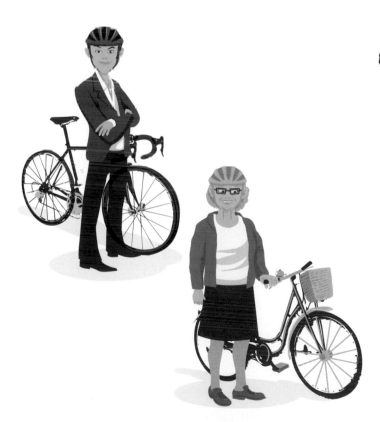

▲ **Figure 29.1 Our motivation to imitate behaviour is influenced by characteristics of the model.**

Humanistic psychology

This perspective understands human development according to how the self develops. From a very early age children develop a sense of self in terms of self-concept and self-esteem. Self-concept refers to how we see ourselves. It includes:

- physical and biological characteristics such as being female, tall, blue-eyed
- skills and competencies, such as being good at sport or swimming, being a scout leader
- psychological aspects such as being kind, shy, outgoing, lively, thoughtful, carefree
- relational aspects such as being a daughter, sister, mother, uncle
- occupational aspects such as being a firefighter, a care-worker, a solicitor, a baker, etc.

Self-esteem refers to how we feel about ourselves: how much value we give to ourselves and how lovable and likeable we believe ourselves to be. When we are very small we believe everything grown-ups tell us. If they say a particular object is a tomato, we believe them. If they say 'you're a waste of space' we also believe them! We have no capacity to sift between what is factual and what is someone's opinion. Self-esteem develops from the way we are loved, listened to, respected, valued, responded to, etc. by others. A child who is neglected, ridiculed, criticised, told he is unwanted or ignored will develop very low self-esteem. He will feel himself to be unworthy of love, to be unwanted by everyone else. He may respond by being subdued and lacking confidence or, alternatively, he may become very angry and behave destructively. There is a close link between self-esteem and self-concept.

Cognitive psychology

Cognosco is the Latin word for 'I know'. Cognitive comes from this verb and refers to all aspects of an individual's cognitive processes that are involved with learning, thinking, knowing about, reflecting on and understanding the world. Cognitive psychologists study the following aspects of human cognitive processes:

- thinking
- memory
- intelligence
- perception
- problem-solving
- reasoning.

Developmental psychology

Developmental psychology is a perspective that looks at development over the life course – from the foetus in the womb to old age and death. Subjects of interest to developmental psychologists include:

- the development of the physical self including the brain and the body
- social and emotional development
- sex differences and the development of gender roles
- moral development
- the development of language and communication skills
- the development of intelligence
- cognitive development (all aspects of thinking, learning, memory, attentional processes, visual perception, problem solving, etc.).

Assessment activity 29.2

P2 Explain the principal psychological perspectives as applied to the understanding of the development of individuals.

1　Read the case studies below and show how the psychological perspectives of social learning theory and the humanistic approach can be applied to understanding the behaviour of these two children. **P2**

> Ruby is 5 years old and is a popular, outgoing little girl. She likes helping others, has a sunny nature and is easy-going and friendly. Her brother, Eric, who is 9, is withdrawn and shy by contrast. He seldom has friends to play and spends most of his time alone. He often refuses to attempt new things because he says he is certain to fail.

Grading tip for P2

To achieve P2, explain how Ruby's development could be understood using the principles of social learning theory. Describe Eric's self-esteem and use the humanistic perspective to explain this.

Application of theories to development

Cognitive developmental perspective

■ Piaget's views

Jean Piaget held the view that children develop intellectually as a result of informal experiences with the environment – instruction from others is relatively unimportant. The interactions with the environment need to provide intellectual challenges for development to take place.

Piaget spent many years researching the way in which children seemed to move forward in stages in terms of their ability to use knowledge and to process and organise information. He was especially interested in the development of the following three skills:

- the ability to think logically
- the ability to reason
- the ability to solve problems.

His was a 'nomothetic' approach to the study of children. Rather than being concerned with what was unique about each child, he was interested in what was common to all children of a certain age. He thus developed a stage theory of cognitive development.

Piaget believed that children develop schemata for both physical and mental actions. A **schema** (schemata or schemas, is the plural) is an internal representation of an action. He sees the reflex responses of the newborn as innate (i.e. inborn) schemata, for example, a schema for sucking, grasping, etc.

Key terms

Schema A type of mental shortcut to understanding physical and mental objects, thoughts, situations and events in the world. It is built up from previous experience. For example, an interview schema contains information about what to wear and how to behave at an interview.

As the child grows and develops cognitively, these schemata become more elaborate and they develop and change using the process of **assimilation** and **accommodation.** The process of assimilation involves using an existing schema to make sense of a new object or phenomenon. Suppose, for example, a child has an existing schema of a bird – an object that flies through the sky. If the child sees a kite on a string flying through the sky it may well say 'Look, daddy, a bird!'. The child has assimilated the kite into its schema for 'objects that fly through the sky'. When the child's father corrects him, and explains that kites are a different category to birds, the child is able to create a new schema for 'other objects that fly through the sky but are not birds': this is accommodation. The original schema has thus been used to understand the object but modified to allow for a clearer and more detailed understanding of the environment.

Key terms

Assimilation The process of adapting to new situations and problems by using existing schemata to make sense of incoming knowledge.

Accommodation A process that goes alongside assimilation and allows an individual to modify their understanding of concepts in order to create a new type of understanding.

■ Developmental stages

Piaget's theory postulates four developmental stages. The child cannot move from one stage to the next until a biological **maturation** point has been reached. Although some children may move through the stages rather more quickly or slowly than others, this is due to maturational processes rather than stimulation in the environment.

Key terms

Maturation The biological changes that take place as the child develops. Intellectual growth and change cannot take place until this maturational process reaches a stage where the child is ready to move on.

Stage 1: the sensori–motor stage (birth to about 2 years)

This stage is called sensori–motor because the child interacts with the world through:

- its senses – seeing, touching, hearing, smelling and tasting
- physical (motor) activity such as kicking, punching the air, touching, moving around, hitting objects, etc.

The child is not capable at this stage of thought as we would understand it. It cannot think abstractly.

An interesting feature of this stage is that the child can only focus on the here and now. This is demonstrated by what is known as lack of object permanence. What this means is that the child appears to believe that if an object they have been playing with vanishes from sight, it has literally disappeared, giving new meaning to the phrase 'out of sight out of mind'! Suppose, for example, you are playing peek-a-boo with a child. A very young child who lacks object permanence will lose interest the minute you move out of sight. It is as if you never existed. As the maturation process moves forward, the developing ability to use language and memory means that the child can now think about the past and the future. The concept of object permanence is one feature that marks the end of this stage.

Theory into practice

If you are in contact with a young baby, you could try the following activity. Show the baby an object of some kind (for example, a fluffy toy). When the child is interested and playing with the toy, cover it up with a towel. A child in the early part of this stage will simply lose interest.

If the baby is a relative you may want to ask permission to videotape this activity to show to the rest of your classmates.

Stage 2: the pre-operational stage (about 2–7 years)

This stage involves the development of thinking and the ability to use language, thought and memory to represent objects mentally. There is still a large focus on the child's own perceptions and there are two major features of mature cognition that are absent in a child of this age.

1 An inability to see the world from the perspective of others.

   Piaget termed this **egocentrism**. It means that the child is, both literally and metaphorically, unable to imagine that anyone has a viewpoint which is different from their own.

   This egocentrism is illustrated in Piaget's famous 'Three mountains' experiment. The child is asked to sit in a particular place in front of a model landscape of three mountains, all of different shapes and sizes. The child is asked what another person seated in a different position (for example, at the back of the landscape) would see. The child at this stage, however, is only able to describe what they see themselves.

2 An inability to **de-centre**.

   The term **centration** refers to a tendency to focus on only one property of a situation and ignore all others. Piaget tested this by means of other famous experiments called **conservation** tasks.

- **Conservation of volume**
  In the first part of this experiment the child is shown a short, 'fat' beaker containing water and asked to pour water into a second beaker, exactly the same as the first, until they are satisfied that the amount in both beakers is the same.

  The child is then asked to pour the water from one of the beakers into a tall 'thin' beaker. This part of the

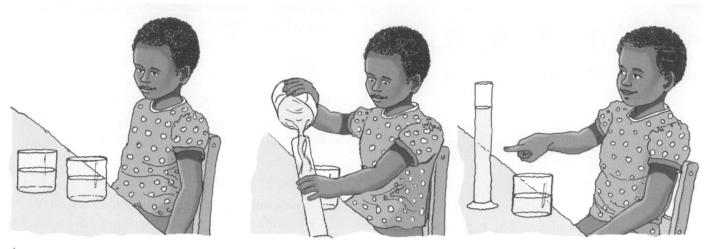

▲ Figure 29.2 The child pays attention to appearance only. She cannot conserve volume yet.

procedure is called the transformation – when the water is transformed to appear to be a different shape (tall and thin versus short and fat). When asked again if there is the same in both beakers, the answer comes: there is more in the tall beaker. The child is unable to focus on the aspect of height and cannot **conserve** volume. They cannot reason logically that there must be the same amount of water, as they cannot understand the concept of volume, but pay attention instead to the appearance of the water (an example of centration).

Piaget explains this inability to de-centre with reference to the child's immature intellectual state. They have not yet learnt to perform **operations**. An operation is a high level skill which involves being able to grasp complex skills and knowledge about how things work in the environment. An operation

is **reversible**. This means that an operation that can be carried out mentally can also be reversed. A good example of this is mathematics. Mathematical operations include addition, division, subtraction and multiplication. Children of around five are able to perform the operation $3 + 1 = 4$ with relative ease. This is mastered earlier than the reversible mathematical operation of subtraction (for example, $4 - 1 = 3$) which is a more cognitively demanding task.

Key terms

Reversibility An ability to reverse, in one's mind, something that has just happened. For example, knowing that if water is poured into a new beaker it can be poured back and stay the same.

Key terms

Conservation An ability to recognise that objects do not change when they are moved into different positions or their shape is changed.

Operation The process of working things out. In the early stages of life this is by touching objects or using fingers to count. In later stages it is being able to do this in your head.

- **Conservation of substance**
  In this experiment, two identical balls of plasticine are shown in the form of 'cakes'. The child recognises that they contain equal amounts. Then one of the two 'cakes' is rolled into a sausage shape. The child, lacking the mental capacity to reverse this operation and imagine the newly shaped sausage back as a 'cake', judges the sausage to contain more plasticine than the cake.

Phase 1

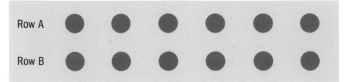

Phase 2

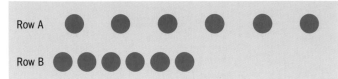

 Figure 29.3 An experiment to examine conservation of number.

- **Conservation of number**

    In this experiment, Piaget showed children two identically spaced lines of counters. Each child was asked, 'Are there the same number of counters in each row?' Children agreed they were the same.

In the second part of the experiment, the experimenter changes the arrangement of the counters (in full view of the child) and then asks the same question, 'Do the rows still contain the same number of counters?'

At this point, most children believe there are more counters in row A than in row B. Once again, the child is paying attention to one feature only and is unable to conserve or perform the operation of reversibility (i.e. imagine back to when the counters where first shown to him, before the experimenter moved them).

Stage 3: the concrete operational stage (about 7–11 years)

The child now becomes capable of a level of abstract thinking that enables him or her to handle the concept of reversal. They know now that you can do something and then reverse it.

If presented with the conservation task involving the plasticine, the child will now recognise that the plasticine is the same, however it is shaped. However, the child still needs to deal with concrete (real, actual) objects and cannot represent problems in abstract form. Thus, for example, 'the child at this stage will have difficulty dealing with the verbal problem 'Joan is taller than Susan; Joan is smaller than Mary; who is the smallest?' in his or her head but would have no difficulty if given

three dolls to represent Joan, Susan and Mary.' (Cited in Birch & Malim, 1988.)

Stage 4: the formal operational stage (about 11 years onwards)

The child can now think in the abstract in the same way as an adult, and doesn't need concrete objects to manipulate in order to reason and solve problems.

■ Critics of Piaget

Despite his influence on psychologists and educators working with children, Piaget is not without his critics.

Margaret Donaldson

Margaret Donaldson suggested that children might understand more than they showed. The experimenter was quite a powerful person and the children may have been confused by the second question asking whether there was the same number/amount when the experimenter repeated the question. They may have thought that they had got it wrong and that the experimenter was hinting to them to change their mind!

A colleague of Donaldson's set up an experiment to investigate children's ability to conserve number, this time using a toy ('naughty teddy') to make the transformation instead of the experimenter. When the naughty teddy intentionally moved the counters for the second part of the experiment, 34 per cent of children got the correct answer. This is equivalent to the Piagetian task with a teddy moving the counters instead of the experimenter.

In a variation on this, however, when the naughty teddy *accidentally* moved the counters, 72 per cent of children were able to state that there was the same number of counters after the transformation as there was before! It

 Remember!

Piaget believes cognitive development takes place in stages. Until the child has reached the right point of maturation it cannot proceed to the next stage. Each stage involves qualitative differences in problem-solving, thinking and logic.

seems as though there is something about the deliberate nature of the transformation that confuses the children and encourages them to give the wrong answer – maybe in order to please the experimenter. (McGarrigle, cited in Donaldson, 1978.)

Lev Vygotsky

Vygotsky was a Russian psychologist with a strong sociological influence on his study of psychology. He suggests a more social model than Piaget, believing that we need social interaction with more mature, skilled people in order to develop our own skills. He believed that children need to acquire language in order to develop new concepts. Language enables a child to talk about or label objects or concepts. Language is seen as a tool which allows the child to develop abstract thought. As we learn language, the structure of language becomes internalised.

Vygotsky further disagreed with Piaget on the need for social interaction. Whereas Piaget believed that the child was rather like a mini-scientist, working things out on his own by experimenting with objects and ideas in the environment, Vygotsky believed that social interaction and language drive cognitive development. For example, a child who breaks a crayon while drawing might be distressed that they can no longer complete the drawing. Upon being told by another that 'you can use either piece of crayon to continue the drawing' the child learns that a crayon still performs the same functions, whether it is whole or broken into pieces. This cognitive development has been driven by language.

Although Piaget and Vygotsky agree that, at the age of about 4, the child changes cognitively, the reasons for such cognitive changes are explained differently. Vygotsky refers to the 'zone of proximal development' by which he means that a child who is nearly ready to grasp something can be speeded up in this process by working with a slightly more advanced child.

In summary, whereas Vygotsky saw language as driving cognitive development, Piaget believed that cognitive development leads to language acquisition.

Jerome Bruner

Like Vygotsky, Bruner emphasised the role of language and interaction with others in enhancing cognitive development. He believed that by teaching children to use symbols they could speed up their cognitive development.

He agreed with Piaget on the following points.

- Children are born with basic cognitive structures which mature over time enabling more complex organisation of information.
- Children are intrinsically motivated to explore their environment and adapt by interacting with it.

However, rather than seeing development as a series of stages, he focused on underlying internal representations (ways of understanding the world) called modes.

- **Enactive mode** – here, thinking develops as a result of physical actions. When a baby plays with a toy, it develops an internal representation of that toy. This learning operates throughout life, for example, riding a bike, throwing a ball and swimming.
- **Iconic mode** – in this mode, the child is able to form mental images in all senses – visual, tactile, olfactory and auditory. These help the child to build a 'picture' of the environment although as yet unable to represent this verbally. A range of images are stored in the memory which are not suited to enactive representation (for example, remembering someone's face).
- **Symbolic mode** – once the child develops language it can use the symbolic mode. It develops systems for language, number, music, etc. The capacity for abstract, flexible thought is enhanced and the child can begin to manipulate and transform ideas.

■ Information processing approach

This approach is part of the cognitive perspective which focuses on the way we take in and interpret information. An example of this is the use of schemas. These can be viewed as packets of information based on previous experience which enable us to process information quickly. Schemata (plural for schema) are generally shared, as can be seen in the activity below.

We build up schemata over the course of our lives, including those about ourselves and others. If I think I am a failure I am likely to have a fairly large range of explanations for why I am a failure, including other people's judgements of me, my comparison of

Theory into practice

Ask five or six students to describe a librarian. They can use as many details as they like, for example, is the librarian male or female? Describe clothing, hobbies, favourite TV programmes, holiday destinations, etc.

Then ask them to describe a waitress. Again, elicit as much detail as possible. This is a fun activity and people normally enjoy doing it.

Look at the descriptions and see how much similarity there is between each person's description of the librarian. This similarity demonstrates the power of schemata and the shared nature of them.

myself with others and past experiences of failure. The following two theorists have developed a method of helping people to break down these negative schemata which inevitably lead to depression, anxiety, unhappiness and low self-esteem.

The views of Aaron Beck

Aaron Beck is sometimes known as the 'father of cognitive therapy'. He has developed and widely used a form of cognitive behavioural therapy (see page 326) which can be used with all age groups, even children as young as eight. Beck views all emotional distress as originating from negative or irrational thoughts. Thoughts influence feelings, which in turn influence behaviour. So an individual who believes themselves unpopular may well feel unwanted and take steps to avoid social company. This in turn confirms the view of the self as being unwanted. Beck believes that by breaking this cycle, by changing thoughts, people can be helped to develop more positive views of themselves and raise their emotional spirits.

The views of Aaron Ellis

Aaron Ellis founded a form of cognitive therapy called Rational Emotive Behaviour Therapy. Rather like Beck, Ellis believes that if we can reach an understanding of how our thinking may be irrational or unhelpful, then we can challenge these thoughts and replace them with thoughts that are more beneficial to our emotional well-being and personal growth. If an individual can be helped to think more rationally and view life in a more balanced perspective, their emotions don't get out of control and they are less likely to fly into rages and suffer from depression and other powerful but negative emotions. The underlying philosophy of this therapy can be summed up in the following extract from the Serenity Prayer, written by Karl Paul Reinhold Niebuhr (1892–1971) and used by Alcoholics Anonymous:

Grant me the courage to change the things I can change, the serenity to accept those that I cannot change and the wisdom to know the difference.

■ Encoding

This is the term given for the way in which we receive information from the outside world and 'represent' it in our minds. For example, if I see a beautiful sunset I will encode this as a visual image which I can then re-create when I want to remember it. Some people have trouble encoding information securely. This means they may find it difficult to know which parts of incoming information to pay attention to and how to co-ordinate this activity with what is happening within their mind. This sheds some insight on what it is like to have attention deficit hyperactivity disorder (otherwise known as ADHD).

■ Attention deficit hyperactivity disorder

ADHD consists of three main symptom clusters:

- an inability to sustain attention
- hyperactive behaviour
- a tendency to be impulsive.

The symptoms of inattention (attention deficit) are detailed in the *Diagnostic and Statistical Manual of Mental Disorders* (latest version *DSM-IV-TR*), published by the American Psychiatric Association. They are reproduced below:

- Often becoming easily distracted by irrelevant sights and sounds
- Often failing to pay attention to details, and making careless mistakes

- Rarely following instructions carefully and completely losing or forgetting things like toys, or pencils, books, and tools needed for a task
- Often skipping from one uncompleted activity to another

It should be remembered that children with just an inability to sustain attention may not be hyperactive or impulsive.

Hyperactive children are often fidgety, unable to sit still, constantly 'on the go' and have a tendency to move around and touch things or, when sitting, tap their feet or a pencil. In adolescence and adulthood this manifests itself as an internal restlessness.

Impulsive children tend to say whatever is on their mind without consideration of the consequences. They act on the spur of the moment and are quite likely to hit another child if they get in the way or have something the impulsive child wants.

Theory into practice

Using a source of your choice, research into the prevalence of ADHD in the UK. Find out if the numbers of children being diagnosed with this disorder have changed over time. Suggest reasons why.

Language development

Spoken language is learnt easily and rapidly and doesn't need explicit teaching. It is almost impossible to prevent children learning language and they acquire a large vocabulary with ease. By contrast, written language is quite slow and difficult to acquire – some children can find it extremely difficult. Explicit teaching is needed for written language. So how does language develop?

■ Behaviourist perspective: the views of Skinner

As with his theory of other types of learning, B.F. Skinner proposed that children learn as a result of reinforcement. There are three key principles to this:

1 The child initially imitates a sound made by others (this is called an **echoic** response). Those hearing the sound then react with pleasure which in turn increases the probability of the child repeating the word.

2 When the child produces a request word or gesture, called a **mand** (for example, 'banana', 'open'), people around respond by fulfilling the request (for example, bringing a banana, opening a box). This response reinforces the child in its use of requests.

3 When a child imitates a word in the presence of an object this is again met with approval (called a **tact response**.) This increases the likelihood of the word being produced in the correct circumstances in future.

In this manner, through trial and error, reinforcement and imitation, the child develops a repertoire of language which matches that of an adult.

Key terms

Echoic A sound made in imitation of a sound that has been heard (a bit like an echo).

Mand A verbal or non-verbal request or command that is regularly reinforced with a predictable consequence. For example, when a child gestures to a parent with their arms open, it is reinforced by the parent picking the child up.

Tact response Reinforcement of a child when it recognises that a word (the tact) is being used to name a given object.

■ Nativist perspective: the views of Chomsky

A nativist perspective is one where humans are seen as biologically programmed with a particular skill or competence. Noam Chomsky disagreed with Skinner's explanation of language development, arguing that the complexity of the structure of language is too great to be learnt through trial and error learning and simple reinforcement. Chomsky proposed that we are born with an innate structure that enables us to understand not just language but the rules of grammar, syntax, etc. He called this a **language acquisition device**. As long as children are exposed to language, this innate device will be available to make sense of the language usage around and to internalise new rules of language. For example, children who are able to use the word *feet* as a plural for *foot* may begin to say 'foots' instead of 'feet'. This suggests that they have understood that the rule to make a word plural is to add an *s* to the end (for example, *sock* becomes *socks*) and are over-applying this rule. They are definitely not imitating others since adults do not say *feets*! This phenomenon certainly supports Chomsky and the nativist approach rather than Skinner.

ey terms

Language acquisition device A device believed by Chomsky to be an innate, pre-programmed system that prepares us to develop language. The device is thought to be located somewhere within the brain.

■ Prelinguistic language development

Up until the age of between 10 and 13 months a child is said to be in the **prelinguistic** period of language development. This means they cannot yet use meaningful words but they are still very responsive to language.

ey terms

Prelinguistic Literally meaning 'before language', this refers to all types of communication used before language takes over. It includes things like pointing and turn taking.

The prelinguistic child communicates using sounds. The first of these is a cry. Different types of cry signal different needs (for example, hunger, pain, discomfort) and they vary from infant to infant. Crying thus reflects the infant's state both psychologically and physiologically.

This is followed by vocalisations such as chuckling, burbling, etc. When you watch a mother and baby

together you will find that this takes on a language-type quality. The infant makes a vocalisation which is then repeated by the mother, and thus the communication skills are developed. These vocalisations are probably not of an imitative nature because deaf children also make them.

■ Phonological language development

Babbling eventually develops into **phonemes**. Phonemes are the basic units of sound, of which there are about 45 in English but no more than 60 in any language. Every language has a set of rules for combining phonemes. For example, we put together *st* for *street, start, station,* etc. but we do not use the combinations *sg* or *sb*. It seems we are born with an innate capacity to develop any language. For example, in the English language we can hear the difference between *z* and *s*, but in some languages listeners cannot differentiate between *sip* and *zip*. It seems we 'tune in' to the language of our culture and, during the first year of life, 'tune out' phonemes and sounds we do not encounter.

Key terms

Phonemes Units of sound used within a language.

■ Syntax

Syntax refers to a system of grammar which governs how one sign is related to another. For example, in the statement 'John hit Richard' John is the agent who did the hitting whereas Richard is the object who was hit. The meaning of the sentence would be completely altered if it were expressed as 'Richard hit John'. We all know these rules implicitly and can use them effortlessly but cannot explain them verbally as we are unaware that we know them!

■ Semantic language development

Semantic language development refers to understanding the expressed meaning of words and sentences. Using words to name objects is fairly easy – we associate the sound with the object. However, words such as *in, on, under,* are more abstract.

■ Humanistic psychology

Carl Rogers and Abraham Maslow are both associated with humanistic psychology. This is not strictly speaking a perspective or approach in psychology, but refers to a core set of beliefs about the self which are shared by humanistic psychologists. They are primarily concerned with aspects of the self, such as the development of self-concept and self-esteem. The starting point of this concept of self is that people are fundamentally whole, healthy and basically good. The development of self is concerned with concepts such as love, creativity and the development of autonomy. Humanistic psychologists also take an optimistic view of the development of the self and personality as they have a strong belief in the ability of the self to develop throughout life and to make choices that will help us grow as individuals.

Carl Rogers

Rogers believed strongly in the **actualising tendency** within people. This refers to a desire to grow as people, to develop all our capabilities and creativity. He focused on the importance of the way people perceive the world, believing that this gave a far greater insight into the individual than an investigation of their real, external reality. This reflects his belief that we construct our own reality and, in doing so, we also construct our sense of self. This includes what is known as the **ideal self** – a view of ourselves as we should be and which we try to live up to. Personal distress can occur when our ideal self is unrealistic or too idealistic. We then judge ourselves as constantly failing.

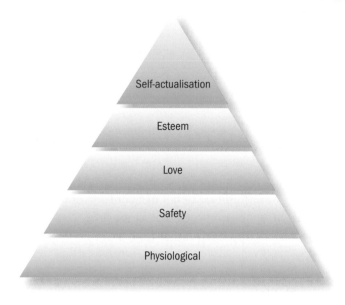

▲ Figure 29.4 Maslow believed our needs at the bottom of the pyramid must be satisfied before we can move up towards the top of the pyramid.

Abraham Maslow

Maslow saw individuals as seeking **self-actualisation**. This refers to an innate desire to be all that one can be – physically, intellectually, spiritually and creatively (in other words to develop all capacities to the full). When self-actualisation is achieved, the individual is able to be warm and giving, autonomous, non-judgemental, realistic and accepting of both self and others.

Maslow saw people as progressing towards self-actualisation through a series of stages, represented in Figure 29.4 as a pyramid.

(For more information on self-actualisation, see Book 1, Unit 8: *Psychological perspectives*.)

Key terms

Actualising tendency An innate (inborn) tendency to become all that we can be. To use all skills and qualities both psychological and physical, to the full.

Ideal self An internal view of ourselves as we would like to be. This provides a standard against which we can judge ourselves.

Key terms

Self-actualisation The achievement of the actualising tendency. People who have achieved self-actualisation include Albert Einstein.

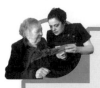

In context

Svetlana is a refugee from Kosova. She arrived in the UK at the age of 16 having been given a place on a lorry after both her parents were killed. When she reached the UK she applied for asylum. She was housed in temporary accommodation for the first 18 months and then was granted leave to remain and given a bedsit. She spent this time studying English. Having applied to her local college of further education, she was offered a place on an A level course to study law, history and business studies. She worked very hard to gain her A levels and gained a grade B in law and business studies and a grade C in history. She was offered a place at the local university to study law. By the time she was 22, Svetlana had obtained a degree in law and met her future husband, Roland. The two of them plan to buy a house and begin a family. Svetlana has ambitions to become a civil rights lawyer.

1 **At what stage of Maslow's hierarchy of needs was Svetlana when she first arrived in England?**

2 **What needs was she satisfying by pursuing her studies?**

3 **What stage of the pyramid is Svetlana moving towards by planning to marry, buy a house, start a family and work towards her ambition of being a civil rights lawyer? Explain your reasoning with reference to the stages of Maslow's pyramid.**

■ The cognitive–developmental approach

Robert Selman examined the developing ability of children to take the perspective of others. He suggested that this occurs as a result of role-taking and becomes more sophisticated over time. The following stages have been identified.

As their ability to understand perspective-taking becomes more sophisticated, children similarly develop a more complex view of friendship. Children move from seeing friends as people who give them things or do nice things for them, to a recognition that friendship involves give and take and a fair amount of forgiveness of one

another's foibles and mistakes. The ability to role-take is associated with sociability and popularity. It seems that children who are able to infer the needs, feelings and emotions of others are more socially skilled than their peers who lag behind with such expertise.

Egocentric or undifferentiated perspective (3–6 years)	Children are unable to imagine any perspective other than their own.
Social–informational role-taking (6–8 years)	Children know that other people have different perspectives but believe this is because others have been given different information.
Self-reflective role-taking 8–10 years	Children recognise that other people can have the same information as they do and still take a different perspective.
Mutual role-taking 10–12 years	By now a child is able to form their own views, and place themselves 'in the shoes' of another person. They are also aware that other people can do this too.
Social and conventional system role-taking 12–15 years +	The adolescent is able to consider their own and others' perspectives, and also to compare them with the perspective an average person in their society would take. Perspective-taking is thus very complex.

Table 29.1 A child's ability to take the perspective of others develops over approximately five stages.

■ Environmental psychology

This type of psychology investigates the way the individual's environment affects behaviour. There is a particular focus on the roles that people take within different social settings. For example, the roles to be adopted in church or school are fixed and known by all and thus determine behaviour while in that setting. However, on a beach or in a party we have more freedom to express other aspects of ourselves.

Learning theory

The views of Bandura, outlined above (on page 316), suggest that we develop a sense of self via observation and imitation of others as well as direct reinforcement and punishment. Our sense of self is largely influenced by the degree of self-efficacy we believe ourselves to have. Self-efficacy is built upon mastering experiences, and influences how motivated we will be to take on new challenges and how we feel about ourselves if we succeed or fail. Someone with a high sense of self-efficacy is likely to have a strong belief that if they try something they will probably succeed – if not at first, then after making adjustments to their efforts. They will show perseverance, motivation and a confidence in the likelihood of success. Unfortunately, the reverse is the case for someone with a low sense of self-efficacy. You have probably all known someone at school who gives up before they start. They are convinced they will fail at whatever they do and so are reluctant to try anything new.

Interpersonal theory

The views of two sociologists, Charles Cooley and George Herbert Mead, have been influential within the study of aspects of the development of the self. A fundamental principle was that the self develops out of social interactions with others.

Charles Cooley

Cooley used the term the 'looking-glass self' to explain the development of the self. Other people's judgements of our behaviour, our appearance and other aspects of ourselves give us information about who we are and what we should think about ourselves. However, we do not just receive one 'reflection' as everyone we encounter acts as a looking glass.

George Herbert Mead

Mead has a different interpretation of the development of self. He sees the self as lying within the individual. We can communicate within ourselves as well as with others around us. So we have beliefs about ourselves to begin with. The influence of others is incorporated into this sense of self largely through the taking on of roles. For example, a child playing teacher does more than just copy what a teacher does. They actually take on the role of a teacher and in their pretend play will develop aspects of themselves to do with authority, values, manners of speech and so forth. This constant taking on of roles allows us to reflect upon who we are and thus develop a sense of a multi-faceted self.

Acquisition of behaviour

Reflect

Ask a friend to describe you, using as many adjectives as possible (for example, friendly, moody, outgoing, shy, daring, nervous, kind, etc).

Now consider how similar you are in these respects to a sibling (if you have one) or to a parent. How could you explain this?

Do you think you inherited these characteristics, or do you think they developed as a result of your environment?

Make notes on which aspects of your personality you believe are innate and which you have developed as you have grown up.

The behaviourist approach

The American behaviourist John Watson famously stated:

> *Give me a dozen healthy infants, well formed, and my own specified world to bring them up in and I'll guarantee to take any one at random and train him to become any type of specialist I might select – doctor, lawyer, artist, merchant, chief, and yes, even beggar-man and thief, regardless of his talents, penchants, tendencies, abilities, vocations and race of his ancestors. There is no such thing as an inheritance of capacity, talent, temperament, mental constitution, and behavioural characteristics.*

Watson, 1925, cited in Shaffer (1993)

What Watson is referring to here is the importance of environmental experiences in development. For example, a child who grows up in a loving, caring environment may develop into an optimistic, confident individual. If the same child, however, were to grow up in an environment where they are neglected, they may become withdrawn and quiet.

Classical conditioning

This theory of learning explains behaviour as arising out of a series of learning experiences. It is concerned with reflex responses (involuntary responses such as the eye blink or the startle response). The founder of this theory of learning, Ivan Pavlov, investigated the basic principles when working with dogs. He discovered that a dog was salivating not just when it saw or smelt food (a natural reflex) but when it saw the white coat of the lab assistant or an empty food bowl.

He then conducted a series of experiments to investigate this type of learning. His aim was to see if he could train a dog to have a reflexive response to a stimulus (an object presented to create a response) that does not by itself cause a response.

- Before conditioning – the stimulus initially is called an unconditioned stimulus or UCS. It is unconditioned because no learning has taken place and it automatically leads to an unconditioned response of salivation.
  A bell is then rung (the conditioned stimulus) and this leads to no response.

- During conditioning – every time food is presented a bell is rung. The food + bell lead to an unconditioned (unlearnt, reflex) response of salivation.
- After conditioning – the dog has now learnt to associate the bell with the response of salivation. When the bell is rung the dog will now salivate. Salivation has thus become a conditioned response.

Pavlov believed that a number of behaviours, especially anxiety and fear responses, can be learnt in this way.

Take it further

Research into Watson and Raynor's experiment with Little Albert. This involved using the principles of classical conditioning to teach a small boy to learn to fear a previously loved object, a white rat.

The following website contains an interactive activity where you can train your own dog!

http://nobelprize.org/medicine/educational/pavlov/index.html

Operant conditioning

According to B.F. Skinner, behaviour is acquired as a result of a series of learning experiences in which the consequences of behaviour (reinforcement or punishment) provide the building blocks of the development of behaviour (and personality). So a child who is shy may have been punished for being noisy and boisterous ('Oh for goodness sake, Sally, nobody wants to listen to you singing now!') and reinforced for being quiet and retiring ('Well done, Sally, you were so good we hardly noticed you were there. Good girl').

The social learning theory perspective

The social learning theory of personality development relies heavily on external, environmental factors. It is associated with two theorists, Albert Bandura and Walter Mischel. The learning experiences acquired as an individual grows up will determine personality. Behaviour that is reinforced will be produced more often, behaviour that is punished less often. In this way a whole range of personality traits can develop over time. So if a

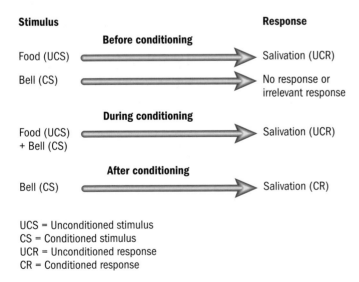

UCS = Unconditioned stimulus
CS = Conditioned stimulus
UCR = Unconditioned response
CR = Conditioned response

▲ Figure 29.5 The process of classical conditioning.

child is consistently punished for behaving aggressively but, equally consistently, is positively reinforced for being polite and helpful, the aggressive behaviours will gradually drop away while the behaviours associated with being polite and helpful will increase.

Remember!

Punishment can consist of disapproval, reprimands or removal of attention. This type of punishment is far more effective than the harsher form which involves smacking or shouting.

■ The psychodynamic perspective

Sigmund Freud developed an internal model of personality where unconscious structures influence development. Development is seen as a dynamic process which proceeds in stages.

It is a rather pessimistic account of personality where there is perpetual conflict between the urges of the **id** and the ruthless civilising influences of the **ego** and **superego**. Personality is thought to be relatively fixed by the age of 5.

Key terms

Id The part of the psyche that is determined to get its own way. It contains all the drives without knowing any bounds – aggression, sexuality, happiness. It operates on the pleasure principle.

Ego The part of the psyche that attempts to mediate between the demands of the id for instant gratification and the superego for restraint. The ego operates on the reality principle and tries to steer a course that will keep the person on an even keel.

Superego The part of the psyche that develops last (at about 3–5 years of age). It is composed of all the morals and requirements of socialisation. Resembling a conscience, the superego is the part of the psyche that governs reason and restraint.

■ Psychodynamic approaches to personality development

Sigmund Freud

There are three strands to Freud's theory of personality development. These are:

- forces within the psyche
- progression through psychosexual stages
- ego defences.

1 The psyche

This is a hypothetical structure roughly equivalent to the mind. There are three parts to the psyche which are continually in conflict. The id, which is present at birth, operates on the **pleasure principle**. This means that it is devoted entirely to satisfying instincts and needs. It is insatiable (meaning it can never be satisfied) and has no sense of reality – the focus of this part of the psyche is simply to get its own way when it wants something.

The second structure of the psyche, the ego, develops around the age of 2. This operates on the **reality principle**: its purpose is to negotiate between the id and the superego and to find a rational course to follow.

The id is in conflict with the superego, the third structure of the psyche which develops last. Roughly equivalent to a conscience, the superego contains all the moral values and the socialisation practices which have taught us right from wrong, all of which are internalised. The superego also contains our 'ideal self'. It develops around the age of 5.

A healthy personality is characterised by a balance between the id and the superego. Too much id energy will create a personality that is reckless, selfish,

Key terms

Pleasure principle A drive towards self-gratification. It has to be kept in check by the ego and superego.

Reality principle An awareness of what is socially acceptable and necessary for the individual to negotiate safely through life. This is the prime function of the ego.

unconcerned with others or aggressive. Too much superego energy will lead to a personality type who is shy, unassertive, guilty and maybe over-moralistic. If the ego can balance these energies then a personality will emerge that is able to be assertive rather than aggressive and able to enjoy themselves without going over the top or feeling guilty. A strong ego is needed to create this balanced personality.

If the id dominates, an erotic personality type will emerge. This person will be most concerned with sex, love and the pursuit of pleasure. A dominant ego with a weak superego results in a narcissistic personality where the individual is only concerned with meeting his or her needs and indifferent to their effect on others. In extreme cases this may be connected with criminal behaviour. An individual with a very strong superego is likely to be guilty with a tendency towards being obsessional.

2 **Psychosexual stages**

- The oral stage – this stage begins at birth. The infant's libido is centred around the mouth, preoccupied with feeding and using the mouth to explore objects. Fixation can occur at this stage if the child is under-gratified or over-gratified.

  Under-gratification may occur because of early weaning before the child is emotionally and psychologically ready, or feeding by the clock, leaving the child frustrated and hungry. The infant is unable to move adequately through the later stages of development and becomes an oral personality characterised by envy, impatience, greed and a tendency to become addicted (for example, to smoking).

  A child who is over-gratified at this stage (too much feeding, maybe when the child doesn't want to feed or a child who is weaned very late) is optimistic, gullible and full of admiration for others around him. They are symbolically sucking for the rest of their lives.

- The anal stage – at 1–1½ years, the child moves from the oral to the anal stage. The key focus here is on potty training. If parents are too harsh in their potty training, the child may resist pressure to excrete. There is some suggestion that the child may experience a pleasurable sensation from faeces

building up in the intestine. This retention results in the development of an **anal retentive** personality characterised by obsessive tendencies, a desire for order and maybe passive–aggressive tendencies.

The other possible outcome of the anal stage is the development of an **anal expulsive** personality. This occurs when the child enjoys resisting his parents by excreting other than on the potty – maybe just before or just after he is placed on it. Personality characteristics associated with anal expulsives include being defiant, reckless and disorganised.

Key terms

Anal retentive A child in the anal stage who feels pressured by their parents into being potty trained may rebel by 'refusing to go'. This is associated with later personality traits such as obstinacy and miserliness.

Anal expulsive A personality type originating in the anal stage when the infant rebelliously expels their faeces anywhere. Adults fixated at this stage tend to be messy and creative.

During the phallic stage (between the ages of 3 and 5 years) the child's sense of gender is developed as they identify with the same-sex parent (boys with their fathers and girls with their mothers). The superego is also developed at this stage. Fixation at the phallic stage develops a phallic character, which is reckless, resolute, self-assured, excessively vain and proud.

The latency period (ages 5–11) is not a psychosexual stage of development, but a period in which the sexual drive lies dormant. Energy is focused mostly on friends and the outside world.

In the genital stage (from puberty onwards) the child's energy once again focuses on his or her genitals, and they become interested in heterosexual relationships.

3 **Ego defences**

Ego defences are strategies used by the mind when something happens which is so threatening and painful that it cannot be dealt with. It is pushed into unconsciousness so the individual isn't aware of it. Common ego defences are denial, when the individual refuses to recognise something painful (for example, a diagnosis of a terminal illness) and repression, when the person buries painful memories so they do not have to be aware of them (for example, following a traumatic event).

Eric Erickson

Erikson's theory sees development occurring in a series of stages which continue throughout life. He called these the Eight Stages of Man.

Stage 1: Trust versus basic mistrust (ages 0–1) – at this stage the infant is totally helpless and relies entirely on others to meet its needs and provide good quality emotional and physical care. If the main parenting figure is able to meet the infant's needs in a satisfactory, responsive and caring way, the infant learns a sense of *trust*. Self-confidence grows and the world is believed to be a dependable and predictable place. He learns that he has some influence over others and this will transfer to later stages.

If, by contrast, the carer is unresponsive, lacks warmth and affection and doesn't meet the infant's needs or is inconsistent (maybe leaving the baby to cry alone for long periods of time coupled with being over-indulgent) the infant will develop a basic *mistrust* of others. It will feel a fundamental sense of not being able to influence others. In terms of later personality development this child will be filled with fear and suspicion. It may be withdrawn or apathetic.

Stage 2: Autonomy versus shame and doubt (ages 1–3) – the child is now more mobile. They are beginning to think more and are also developing a sense of being separate from parents. They want to be independent and to do things for themselves. Toilet training is an important crisis to work through. If this is begun too early, or is very harsh, the child may feel a sense of shame at lack of control over its bowels.

- Autonomy – the child is allowed to experience things without being controlled. They are supported, not criticised, through failure/accidents, etc. They feel competent and have a sense of self-belief.

- Shame and doubt – the child is controlled and this induces doubt about their own abilities. The child fails frequently (perhaps they are being expected to do too much too soon) and/or criticised (which induces shame). The child feels powerless and may revert to thumb sucking and is likely to become

attention seeking. The child rejects others and becomes closed off.

Stage 3: Initiative versus guilt (ages 3–6) – there is rapid social, emotional, physical and intellectual growth and development at this stage. The child is acquiring new skills through interaction with the world and others. If development is impeded at this stage, the child may lose its sense of initiative and become passive and unwilling to try new things.

Initiative can be fostered when the child's curiosity about life is welcomed and met with interest and encouragement to explore new ideas and learn new skills. When play of all varieties is encouraged, this enhances the development of initiative, as does physical activity which helps the child to develop skills. The negative potential outcome of the crisis at this stage is *guilt*. This may occur if parents dampen their child's curiosity about the world – perhaps by ignoring their questions or telling them not to be silly. Similarly if fantasy play is discouraged and physical activities are banned as 'too dangerous' the child's sense of growing competence and their ability to take initiative will dwindle. They will be left with a sense of guilt and a belief in their own lack of competence.

Stage 4: Industry versus inferiority (ages 6–12)

The child is concerned at this stage with understanding how things are made and how they work (including making things by themselves).

Significant others now begin to include teachers and other adults as well as parents.

The peer group begins to be important – children compare themselves in order to assess their own achievements. This is influential in the child's development of the self. A sense of *industry* is developed when the individual is encouraged to take on realistic tasks where there is a high degree of success and being supported and encouraged to try things out. This results in high self-esteem and a sense of competence. *Inferiority* results if the child is pushed to do things they are not ready for without enough guidance and encouragement and then criticised for failure.

If unfavourable comparisons are made with others (either by the child or by others), a sense of inferiority will develop, leading to a negative self-concept and low self-esteem.

Stage 5: Identity versus role confusion (ages 12–18)

Erikson saw adolescence as a time of *storm and stress* – a period of psychological turmoil which has a far-reaching effect on the self-concept. The self-concept is affected by the following factors.

- Physical changes bring about an altered body image which affects one's sense of self.
- Intellectual development allows the adolescent to become aware of what is potentially possible as well as what currently exists.
- Emotional development involves increasing emotional independence.
- The individual is also involved in making decisions about careers, values and sexual behaviour.

The main goal of the individual at this stage is to achieve a lasting and secure sense of self, or *ego identity*. This has three parts:

- a sense of consistency in the ways they see themselves
- a sense of continuity of the self over time
- a sense of mutuality (i.e. agreement between one's own perceptions of self and the perceptions of others).

The peer group is very important in this process and the developmental task of the adolescent is to establish a vocational and social identity so that they see themselves as a consistent and integrated person. If this does not happen, they will not develop a sense of their role in life and will be unable to be faithful to people, work or a set of values. In extreme cases, they may develop a negative identity, particularly if they feel they cannot live up to the demands being made of them. (For the final three stages, see Ewen 1993.)

Theories of attachment

Reflect

When something unpleasant or alarming happens to you, do you feel a need to go to one special person for a hug? We all have attachment figures in our lives who provide support, safety and comfort at times of need. Why are they so important to us?

■ Stages in the development of attachments

In 1964, Rudolph Schaffer and Peggy Emerson carried out research into how attachments developed. They observed infants over a period of time and developed a stage theory of attachments, as outlined below (cited in Shaffer 2002).

The asocial stage: birth to around 6 weeks

Asocial means non-social. Schaffer and Emerson believe that during this period babies don't act in a social way. They don't seem to respond differently to people from the way they do to any inanimate stimulus. Individual people (for example, mum, grandad) are not recognised – all people seem to be responded to in the same way.

Indiscriminate attachment: 6 weeks to around 7 months

Indiscriminate means making no distinction, seeing no difference. According to Schaffer and Emerson, infants can now distinguish between people and objects and they are becoming more sociable with people – for example, they begin to smile at around six weeks. They have not yet formed attachments and are happy to be held by anyone without showing signs of distress.

Specific attachment: from 7 months

At this stage the infant shows signs of having formed a strong emotional bond with a particular person (usually, but not necessarily, the mother).

Signs that attachment has taken place include:

- **Separation anxiety**
  Infants protest against being separated from their attachment figure, often showing acute distress. They are, however, easily comforted when reunited with their attachment figure.

- **Stranger anxiety**
  This is shown when infants are left with a person they are unfamiliar with. Whereas previously they were happy to be held, fed and comforted by anyone, they now show distress with strangers and are unhappy until they are reunited with their attachment figure.

■ Multiple attachments

The infants in this study were not only attached to their mothers. By 18 months of age, some infants were attached to five or more people, including grandparents, fathers, siblings or even babysitters. It appears that each attachment figure serves a particular purpose. For example, in 1978, Lamb and Stevenson found that infants seek out their mother when they are upset, frightened or hurt whereas fathers are preferred attachment figures for other activities such as playing (research cited in Shaffer, 2002).

■ The effects of separation

Robertson and Robertson

James Robertson was a social worker who, together with his wife Joyce, conducted the first observational studies

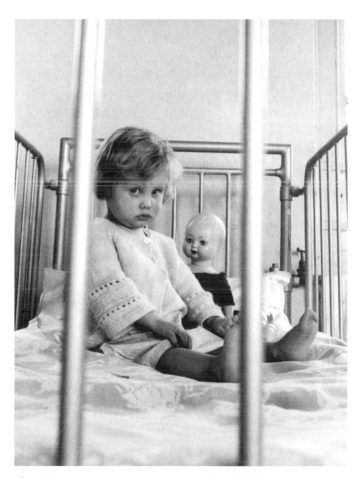

▲ Figure 29.6 This still from James Robertson's film shows clearly the distress experienced by two-year-old Laura when separated from her mother during a hospital visit.

into the distress shown by children when admitted to hospital. In the 1950s it was customary to admit children to hospital alone, with parents only allowed to visit every few days. When Joyce Robertson's own daughter was admitted to hospital, she saw the intense distress experienced by her little girl and this fuelled her desire to make a film to convince hospital authorities that separation could have damaging effects on young children.

Robertson identified three stages of emotional distress suffered by children in this situation.

- Protest – the children showed great distress, calling and crying for the absent care giver and some appeared panic stricken. Anger and fear were evident.

- Despair – the children became calmer but apathetic as they showed little interest in anything. Self-comforting behaviours were observed such as thumb sucking and rocking.

- Detachment – the children appeared to be coping with the separation as they showed more interest in their surroundings but they were emotionally unresponsive. They avoided forming new attachments and showed no interest when the care giver returned. However, most children re-established the relationship over time.

■ The effects of deprivation

The views of Bowlby

John Bowlby worked in a child guidance clinic where he encountered children and adolescents who showed delinquent and disturbed behaviour. He developed a theory known as the **maternal deprivation hypothesis**.

Key terms

Maternal deprivation hypothesis A belief that deprivation results from long periods of separation or many short periods of separation from the mother, particularly in the early years of life. Bowlby believed this would inevitably lead to damage to later personality.

This states that if a child is deprived of his or her mother between 6 months and 5 years of age then this would lead to difficulties in later life. They would be unable to form attachments with others and would be likely to turn to crime. Bowlby suggested that separation experiences in early childhood caused **affectionless psychopathy**. This is the inability to have deep feelings for other people and leads, therefore, to a lack of meaningful personal relationships. Bowlby pointed out the need for continuous care giving for healthy development.

Key terms

Affectionless psychopathy A serious psychological condition where the individual shows no conscience and is unable to form intimate relationships with others.

Bowlby's hypothesis was developed from his work in the clinic where he conducted a famous study known as the '44 thieves'.

Bowlby interviewed 44 children who had been referred to a child guidance clinic because they were stealing and 44 children who had emotional problems but had not committed any crimes. He found that the thieves lacked a social conscience, while the other group of children showed signs of disturbance, but otherwise functioned reasonably well emotionally.

32 per cent of the thieves were diagnosed as affectionless psychopaths and 86 per cent of the thieves diagnosed in this way had experienced separation for at least a week before the age of 5.

From these findings, Bowlby concluded that maternal deprivation can seriously disrupt healthy emotional development.

Later research, however, has suggested that the importance of the mother may have been overstated. While an infant certainly needs an attachment figure, this does not necessarily have to be the mother.

Schaffer and Emerson

Rudolph Schaffer and Peggy Emerson developed their theory of attachments by conducting observational studies of infants interacting with mothers, fathers and other family members. Their observations led them to conclude that attachments were more dependent on the quality of interaction than the quantity. A child who was mostly looked after by a mother could, in certain circumstances, show the strongest attachment to another family member, including the father. The fact that infants could form multiple attachments also suggested that the effects of deprivation could be minimised for such children in the event of separation from a main care giver.

Rutter

Michael Rutter suggested that anti-social behaviour may be the result of discord in the family and that the development of an affectionless personality may be a result of a failure initially to form an attachment. He called this **privation**.

Key terms

Privation This occurs when a child forms no bond at all with a care giver. Children in orphanages where there is a very low staff-to-child ratio have been found to suffer from privation because they have no interaction with others.

In 1976 he carried out a large-scale study on the Isle of Wight. He found that when children from good to fair homes were separated, this did not lead to delinquency. Similarly, if a separation was associated with illness it was not associated with delinquency. However, where separation was associated with stress, children were four times as likely to become delinquent.

Rutter concluded that Bowlby's thieves had probably suffered from **privation** not deprivation. Privation involves a situation where no bond is formed in the first place. This is much more serious than deprivation where a bond is disrupted but can, with care, be re-formed.

In some cases, privation can lead to a complete inability to form attachments in later life. This is called *reactive attachment disorder* and is illustrated in the *In context* case study opposite.

In context

Adam was adopted at the age of 19 months by a couple who were extremely sensitive and caring. He was a much longed-for child. The mother, Serena, gave up work so she could devote herself to his care. Serena and her husband James were aware that Adam might have difficulties in settling as he had already been fostered by two different sets of parents. He was taken into foster care initially because his mother, a single parent, didn't want him. She had given him no physical contact and fed him by holding a bottle at a distance. When observed interacting with Adam, it was noted that the birth mother never smiled, talked to or made eye contact with the child.

Adam was, indeed, difficult to look after. He showed no emotions at all, neither happiness nor unhappiness

and he was completely unable to accept affection from his adoptive parents. He appeared to be frozen inside. As he grew older, however, a huge amount of anger began to show itself. He was prone to violent rages when he would smash and throw things. Eventually, Serena and James were unable to cope with Adam, who was also terrorising their other children. Adam was eventually taken into care.

1   **List two factors that influence attachment.**

2   **Explain why the lack of maternal sensitivity could have affected Adam so dramatically.**

3   **Discuss the kind of care giving that would be needed to help someone, not quite as badly damaged as Adam, to recover from privation.**

■ Case studies of isolation

The following two case studies report on children who were isolated from human contact during the early part of their lives. According to the maternal deprivation hypothesis, they should not be able to form attachments later in life. As we shall see, some interesting findings emerged.

The Koluchova twins

In 1972, a researcher called Koluchova reported the case of two identical twins who had been beaten, locked up and cruelly treated until the age of 7. When rescued they only communicated using gestures and were terrified of the outside world.

However, the two boys were fostered by a devoted foster mother and they developed both language and social and cognitive skills. By the age of 20 both were in employment and maintained good relationships with their foster mother.

This study shows that the effects of early privation can be overcome if the care provided is of sufficient quality. It may also be that these two boys used one another as attachment figures, which would have mitigated the damage of privation.

Genie

Genie was aged 13 when she was rescued from her home. She had been held in a locked, darkened room, tied to a potty-chair during the day and in a sleeping bag at night. No one spoke to her and her father used to beat her if she made a sound. When he came to give her food he grunted at her and scratched her. She had had no social interaction at all.

When found, Genie could not stand upright, had no social skills, did not understand language and could not speak. She developed few social skills and although she acquired a large vocabulary she was unable to learn the rules of grammar and so could not construct sentences properly.

The development of attachment

There are a number of explanations for why attachments develop. The following section outlines some of these.

■ Feeding

An early theory of why attachments develop was proposed by the behaviourist perspective. Infants become attached to those who satisfy their need for nourishment and tend to their physiological needs. Infants associate their care givers with the feeling of gratification that comes with relief from hunger and discomfort. The infant learns to approach his or her care giver in order to have their needs satisfied. Eventually this generalises into a feeling of security whenever the care giver is present. Sometimes known as the cupboard love theory, this theory is contradicted by the findings of Henry Harlow.

■ Physical contact

Harlow devised an experiment using rhesus monkeys to examine whether infant monkeys would choose food over physical comfort. He separated infants from their mothers and placed them in a special housing unit with two 'surrogate' mothers. One was covered with terry toweling, was soft to the touch but provided no milk. The other was a wire monkey which provided milk but no comfort. The infant monkeys spent almost all their time clinging to the cloth monkey and, when able, leant across to obtain milk from the wire monkey while still clinging on to the cloth monkey. He concluded from this that contact comfort is much more important than feeding. This appears to be the main basis for attachment.

Bowlby's theory was influenced by the work Harlow carried out, and also by research by Konrad Lorenz, into imprinting (cited in Gross, 2001). Lorenz found that a duck or goose would imprint (form an unbreakable bond) on the first object it saw when it hatched. Normally this would be the biological mother but cases occurred where imprinting took place to a human. You may have seen the film *Fly Away Home* which illustrates this phenomenon.

Bowlby believed that infants are born with an innate fear of the unknown which drives them to seek **proximity** (closeness) with a care giver. Both mother and infant are biologically predisposed to form an attachment bond. The infant produces **social releasers** such as crying, vocalising, making eye-contact, smiling, etc. which produce a response in the mother who is drawn closer to her baby.

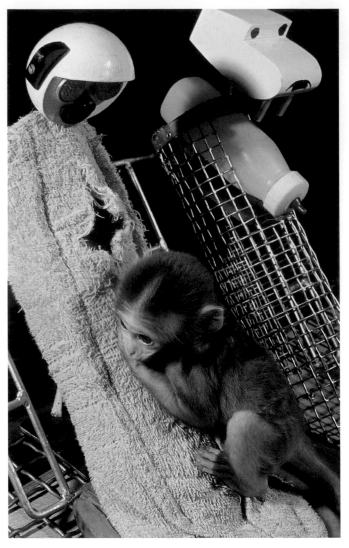

▲ Figure 29.7 The infant monkey shows a strong preference for the contact comfort offered by the cloth monkey.

Key terms

Proximity A state of being close. In terms of attachment, proximity is very important to give the infant a sense of security. When proximity is broken, and the infant is farther away from their care giver than they are able to bear, they will show signs of acute distress.

Social releasers These are things an infant does that cause others to react instinctively with care giving behaviour.

■ Time and care giving

As we have seen above, children form attachments to those who play with them and are sensitive to their needs but not necessarily to those who feed and change them. The following section gives some reasons for differences in attachment.

■ Individual differences in attachment

The quality of attachment a child has with his or her primary care giver is of great importance to the development of personality and to his or her own parenting in turn. When an infant has formed an attachment, they are beginning to be capable of symbolic thought, which means they can think about the parent when they are absent. The infant begins to build what Bowlby calls an internal mental model of their own experiences. This arises from interaction with the primary care giver. This becomes like a template which the child uses to predict the behaviour of others. An internal mental model that is negative can arise if the child is ignored or responded to harshly. Such a child is likely to grow up with poor self-esteem and to believe they will be met by rejection or inconsistency from others. If the model is positive, with the care giver being sensitive and responsive to the infant's needs, the child will predict that others will treat them in a similar way. Consequently, they are more likely to be confident and have a strong sense of self-esteem and competence in later life.

Ainsworth

Mary Ainsworth developed a procedure designed to measure the differences in attachment shown by different children. The procedure, called the strange situation, involves a sequence of events carried out in a laboratory designed to assess infant attachment style. The procedure consists of the following eight episodes.

1 Parent and infant are introduced to the experimental room.

2 Parent and infant are alone. Parent does not participate while the infant explores. (Exploration behaviour is a sign of secure attachment.)

3 Stranger enters, converses with parent, then approaches infant. Parent leaves inconspicuously.

4 First separation episode: stranger's behaviour is geared to that of infant.

5 First reunion episode: parent greets and comforts infant, then leaves again.

6 Second separation episode: infant is alone.

7 Continuation of second separation episode: stranger enters and gears behaviour to that of infant.

8 Second reunion episode: parent enters, greets infant and picks up infant; stranger leaves inconspicuously.

The infant's behaviour upon the parent's return is the basis for classifying the infant into one of three attachment categories.

1 **Secure**
   The infant shows a moderate level of proximity-seeking to the care giver and is comfortable to explore the environment. Although upset by the care giver's departure, they greet them positively on their return. They may find the situation stressful but can be easily calmed by the care giver.

2 **Insecure/avoidant**
   The infant tends to avoid contact with the care giver especially at reunion after separation, although not unduly upset when left with the stranger. Generally these infants do not find the situation very stressful – other than when left alone

3 **Insecure/ambivalent**
   The infant is highly distressed by separation from the care giver and tends to be wary of the stranger. However, when the care giver returns, they are difficult to console, one minute seeking contact, the next wriggling away.

Remember!

Attachment types (secure, insecure, disorganised) are highly significant for later development including social, emotional, cognitive and even physical development. Securely attached children can be predicted to be more confident and self-assured in later life than other attachment types.

A fourth attachment type was later identified by Main and Solomon in 1986 (cited in Haralambos 2002).

4 **Insecure/disoriented**

This attachment type is characteristic of children with unusual and often dysfunctional combinations of behaviour, for example, avoidant and resistant.

■ Responsiveness and sensitivity

Why do some infants have a secure attachment with their care giver, whereas others do not? According to Ainsworth's care-giving hypothesis, the sensitivity of the care giver is of crucial importance. (Ainsworth, 1979, cited in Shaffer 2002.)

Ainsworth found that most of the care givers of securely attached infants were very sensitive to their needs and responded to their infants in an emotionally expressive way. In contrast, the care givers of resistant infants were interested in them but often misunderstood their infants' behaviour. Of particular importance, these care givers tended to vary in the way they treated their infants. As a result, the infant could not rely on the care giver's emotional support.

Finally, there are the care givers of avoidant infants. Many of these care givers were uninterested in their infants, often rejecting them and tending to be self-centred and rigid in their behaviour. However, some care givers of avoidant infants behaved rather differently. These care givers acted in a suffocating way, always interacting with their infants even when the infants did not want any interaction; almost as though the infant were satisfying their own needs. What these two types of care givers have in common is that they are not very sensitive or appropriately responsive to the needs of their infants.

■ The child's temperament.

Critics of the care giving sensitivity hypothesis suggest that that some differences are innate and that the infant's behaviour also shapes the parent's response. (For example, an infant who is easily soothed, who snuggles and stops crying when picked up, increases the mother's sense of competency and attachment. The infant who stiffens and continues to cry, despite efforts to comfort

it, makes the mother feel inadequate and rejected.) The type of attachment formed may therefore come from the child.

Kagan (1984) calls this the temperament hypothesis (cited in Shaffer, 2002). Evidence to support this comes from research by Belsky and Rovine, 1987 (cited in Cardwell & Flanagan 2002). They found that newborns who showed signs of behavioural instability (for example, tremors or shaking) were less likely to become securely attached to their mother than newborns who did not. In other words, it was their innate personality that was the key factor in the formation of an attachment.

■ Continuity hypothesis

Bowlby's theory that early attachment relationships form the basis of an internal working model of relationships would imply that a securely attached infant will develop to become a socially competent child and later adult. There is a considerable body of research which supports this prediction but it has also been found that attachment types can change according to factors influencing the family and the care giver.

Belsky and Fearon (2002) used data from the National Institute of Child Health and Development (NICHD) to examine attachment patterns at the age of 15 months and, later, to measure social and emotional development. Children classified as securely attached at the age of 15 months who continued to receive sensitive mothering scored highly on the following measures of development:

- low levels of problem behaviour
- high social competence
- use of expressive language
- use of receptive language
- school readiness.

Those infants classified as insecure at 15 months, but who subsequently received sensitive mothering, scored significantly higher on these measures of competence than those classified as secure at 15 months but who later received low-sensitive mothering. Sensitivity of mothering was associated with maternal and family stress.

Take it further

Find research that has investigated the following aspects of attachment and behaviour acquisition:

- attachment and parental sensitivity

- attachment and personality development
- attachment and romantic love
- the long-term effects of maternal deprivation.

Assessment activity 29.3

P3 Describe four key pieces of research into the role of attachment in behaviour acquisition.

1   Most good psychology textbooks cover the following key pieces of research into this topic. Suggested studies and sources are:

- Hazan & Shaver (1987) – The influence of early attachments on romantic relationships later in life (included in Haralambos et al, 2000)
- Holmes (1993) – Follow-up studies of children classified as infants as securely or insecurely attached (included in Moxon, Brewer & Emerson, 2003)
- Bowlby – The effects of deprivation on personality development (included in Moxon, Brewer & Emerson, 2003)
- Hodges & Tizard (1975), Tizard & Hodges (1978), Hodges & Tizard (1989) – Three studies following up children brought up initially in an institution (included in Moxon, Brewer & Emerson, 2003)

Grading tip for P3

When you describe research it is a good idea to give details of the sample and method used if this information is given. Particularly important, though, are the findings and conclusions of the research as they give most information on how attachment affects later behaviour.

You could include Bowlby's study of the 44 thieves. The recommended reading given at the end of this unit will be invaluable in finding other research studies.

M2 Analyse the contribution made by the four pieces of research to the understanding of the role of attachment in behaviour acquisition.

2   To what extent do you think these four pieces of research are useful in explaining the role of attachment in behaviour acquisition?

Grading tip for M2

To analyse you need to assess the strengths and weaknesses of the four pieces of research you have selected. You could do this by looking at the methodology used and making a judgement about whether it produced valid findings. You could also consider the possibility of alternative explanations that may 'break' the cause and effect chain between attachment and later behaviour (for example, family discord, parental depression or stress, improved family circumstances, etc.)

D1 Evaluate the contribution made by the four pieces of research to the understanding of the role of attachment in behaviour acquisition.

3   Summarise the strengths and weaknesses of the four pieces of work you have chosen in terms of how well they help us understand the role of attachment in behaviour acquisition. State your views about the most useful aspects of each piece of research and draw a conclusion about the one you think offers the greatest contribution. **D1**

Grading tip for D1

Remember that evaluation involves weighing up the strengths and weaknesses of something. If you find weaknesses, it is a good idea to find an alternative explanation that would fill any 'gaps' in the explanation.

Perspectives

The perspectives you have learnt about in this unit are:

- behaviourist (classical conditioning and operant conditioning)
- social learning theory
- psychodynamic
- humanistic
- cognitive
- developmental
- biological.

All these perspectives have different assumptions about causes of particular behaviours. Some can be used together and complement one another, others have quite a different way of understanding behaviour. Let's look at some specific behaviours to illustrate this, starting with depression.

Specific behaviours

■ Depression

The cognitive perspective sees depression as originating with negative thoughts. An individual who sees him or herself as worthless and unlovable will feel sad as a result of such feelings and may well withdraw from social interaction because of these beliefs and feelings.

The social learning theory account would explain that depression results from too much punishment, leading to sadness, guilt and loss of self-esteem. This punishment could take the form of any negative life events including criticism, failure of a marriage, redundancy or too many stressful life events. If the depressed individual is then reinforced for their depression – for example by being given extra attention, kindness and support – this may lead to a continuation of the depressive behaviour since it is bringing such positive rewards!

These two perspectives are in stark contrast to the biological perspective which would look to genetic inheritance for the cause of depression. If there is a family history of the illness, this would indicate that the individual may have a faulty gene. Additionally, brain chemistry and the functioning of the endocrine system would be seen as a possible cause. Low levels of the neurotransmitter (brain chemical) serotonin are associated with depression, as are high levels of the hormone cortisol which is secreted by the endocrine system at times of stress.

■ Anxiety

Anxiety ranges from mild feelings of discomfort and apprehension to full-blown anxiety attacks with sweating, rapid heart and pulse rate, feelings of dizziness and nausea and a terrible sense of dread. Although psychological perspectives would emphasise the causes of anxiety (for example, apprehension about taking a driving test, fear of going to the dentist or a generalised sense of anxiety which is often associated with depression), the biological perspective explains this with reference to physiological processes. Anxiety is associated with arousal of the 'fight or flight response'. This is an automatic response, left over from our Stone Age days, which arises when we are faced with a threat. The following physiological changes take place:

- the heart rate and strength increase
- lung capacity increases
- sugars are released from the liver into the body for use by the muscles
- pupils dilate (to enable better vision)
- blood clotting capacity is increased.

All these changes prime the body for a fight (for example, with a wild boar) or to run away (for example, to flee a sabre-toothed tiger).

On occasions when we can respond in a physiological way to this response (for example, if there is a car speeding towards us and we need to run away at high speed) this response is short-lived. It dies away once the danger has passed. However, anxiety about sitting an exam arouses the same response but we are not able to take immediate physical action and so the effects of increased heart rate, etc. leave us feeling uncomfortable and agitated. (For more information on the fight or flight response, see Book 1, Unit 8.)

■ Separation and loss

Humanistic psychology would approach this type of emotional hurt from the viewpoint of how the individual perceives the meaning to the self of separation and loss. For example, a parent might experience a child leaving home as a devastating experience if a large part of their self-concept is associated with being a parent. From the viewpoint of attachment theory, separation in early life can weaken the bond of attachment while loss actually breaks it. Children who have experienced the loss of a parent in early life are significantly more likely to be troubled by a further loss in later life than someone who has not had such an experience.

■ Stress and coping

This is a good example of where two perspectives come together to provide a better explanation than just one alone. From the biological perspective, stress causes the release of two neurotransmitters, adrenaline and noradrenaline, together with the hormone cortisol. Adrenaline and noradrenaline make us feel agitated and uncomfortable, while prolonged secretion of cortisol can impair immune system functioning and is associated with depression.

However, two people can be exposed to the same stressful events and react quite differently. This can be explained by the cognitive approach. If a negative event happens (for example, you lose your job) the stress response is mild for someone whose thoughts are along the lines of 'this is an opportunity, or a challenge, rather than a threat' and much more severe for someone who thinks 'this is the end of the line for me'.

■ Self-harm

Self-harming takes many shapes and forms, from cutting oneself with a bottle, razor or other sharp object, to self-inflicted bruises and tissue damage from other causes. Self-harming behaviour is a complex phenomenon with almost exclusively psychological causes. People who self-

harm frequently explain this as the only way they know to rid themselves of overwhelming feelings of anxiety, self-loathing, fear or shame. Sufferers often report the intense relief from psychological pain that is achieved by causing physical pain. It is as though the physical pain is much more manageable because it is visible and in some way controlled, whereas psychological distress is huge and uncontrolled.

An alternative reason for self-harming is when a person feels numb psychologically. In this situation, physical pain reminds them that they are alive. The desire to self-harm seems out of one's control. A person may think obsessively about it and it takes massive self-control to resist the urge. Although reasons for self-harming are many and varied, risk factors include intense emotional pain, perhaps originating earlier on in life, coupled with the absence of a supportive emotional environment in which to explore difficult feelings.

■ Prejudice and discrimination

Reflect

How often have you encountered people making negative comments about certain groups within society (for example, asylum seekers or Muslims)? We all have prejudices but we don't have to act upon them. Where do you think prejudice originates?

Prejudice refers to a negative attitude towards a group or object. The prejudiced person has negative feelings (which may involve dislike and/or fear). Negative beliefs and attitudes (often involving stereotypes) may be used to justify the prejudiced attitude. By contrast, discrimination refers to behaviours. These may be behaviours designed to avoid, belittle, or even get rid of members of the group one is prejudiced against.

An influential psychological theory of prejudice is known as the realistic conflict theory and was proposed by psychologist Muzafer Sherif in 1966 (cited in Eysenck & Flanagan 2001). This theory proposes that we view ourselves and our friends and family as members of in-groups and others as belonging to out-groups. On the basis of this we develop the belief that in-group members can only do well at the expense of an out-group: in other words, one group only can be dominant. A second assumption of this theory is that if there is a situation where competition arises between groups, this inevitably leads to prejudice.

Reduction of inter-group prejudice can only be achieved by involving both groups in working towards a goal where they have to co-operate in order to succeed in achieving an important task.

A second explanation for prejudice and discrimination is the theory known as social identity theory, proposed by the French psychologist Henri Tajfel in 1982 (cited in Eysenck & Flanagan, 2001).

According to this theory, merely seeing ourselves as members of a group will lead to favouritism for one's own group and prejudice against another. The reason for this is that we all desire a positive social identity to maintain self-esteem. This is achieved by seeing ourselves as members of an 'in-group' which we favour and seeing other people as members of an 'out-group' which we automatically perceive as inferior to us in all respects.

While Sherif's theory of prejudice sees this as developing within a social context, other explanations focus on the upbringing and experience of individuals. In 1950 Adorno et al (cited in Eysenck & Flanagan, 2001) saw childhood experiences as forming the origins of prejudice. A child who is treated harshly by parents is unable to express hostility or anger towards them, but instead adopts similar harsh and rigid views towards, and expectations of, others. The hostility they unconsciously feel towards the original object of their anger (their parents) is displaced onto other people or groups, particularly those who are powerless or are existing targets for hostility in society.

In order to test this theory, Adorno created a questionnaire to find out about prejudice against different cultural groups such as travellers, Jews and Muslims. He also asked questions about the extent to which people have certain personality traits such as being rigid and inflexible, having unquestioning respect for authority and holding very conventional values. High scores on these questionnaires are good at predicting prejudiced attitudes towards others.

Theory into practice

How authoritarian are you in your attitudes? Complete an online questionnaire by going to the website below.

www.anesi.com/fscale.htm

■ Child abuse

Child abuse includes neglect, psychological abuse and physical abuse. A neglected child does not have their basic needs met and may be ignored or deprived of conversation and other forms of stimulation. Psychological abuse could consist of criticism, ridicule or being told they are unwanted. Physical abuse unfortunately is all too common and consists of anything from being bruised to being starved or even tortured.

It is difficult to find a common explanation for child abuse. However, in 1980 Belsky (cited in Shaffer 2002) did find that an unduly high proportion of parents who abused children had themselves been abused, neglected or unloved by their own parents. However, it seems that abuse is not inevitable but is triggered by stressful life experiences.

From an attachment theory point of view, it is likely that those parents who themselves received insecure parenting are more at risk of abusing their own children than those who were securely attached.

■ Addiction

Addiction to cocaine and/or amphetamines can be explained very clearly by the biological approach. These two drugs produce feelings of well-being and heightened pleasure because they cause increased amounts of the neurotransmitter dopamine to be available within the brain. This increased dopamine is responsible for the pleasurable feelings induced by these drugs. However, over-stimulation of dopamine also causes levels to drop dramatically resulting in feelings of depression. The quickest and easiest way to overcome these unpleasant depressed feelings is to take more of the drugs. In this way, an addiction is formed.

Theory into practice

Research into the effects of nicotine and marijuana on the brain. What effects do they have on the brain and other physiological systems that lead to addiction?

■ Violence and aggression

Once again we have two perspectives that can work together to explain violence and aggression. From the biological perspective, the role of the hormone testosterone can, in part, explain a tendency towards aggressive behaviour. Evolutionary biology would explain this as a necessary characteristic for males who need to compete for resources and to secure the best mates in order to ensure that their genes are passed on.

However, hormones alone do not necessarily *cause* violence and aggression. What is more likely is that there is an interplay between the hormonal secretion of testosterone and environmental factors. For example, social learning theory explains aggression as being capable of being triggered by observing aggressive behaviour which is seen to provide some sort of gains (reinforcement) for the individual being aggressive. These two perspectives can thus come together to explain why some people may react in an aggressive and violent way; they have learnt that this will somehow benefit them, while others have learnt that such behaviour will be met with punishment (for example, in the form of disapproval).

Assessment activity 29.4

P4 Explain two specific behaviours using psychological perspectives.

1 Explain depression using the cognitive perspective and aggression using the biological perspective in psychology. **P4**

M3 Analyse the role of psychological perspectives in understanding the two specific behaviours.

2 To what extent is the cognitive perspective good at explaining depression? Are there any aspects of this illness that could be better explained by another perspective? How good is the biological explanation of aggression? **M3**

Grading tip for P4

One fairly straightforward way of meeting this criterion is to choose one behaviour which can be explained from competing perspectives (for example, biological and cognitive) and one which can be explained from fairly similar perspectives (for example, cognitive and social learning theory). You may find it helpful to draw up a table with the perspectives in columns and the behaviours in the rows. Summarise the explanations of two to three perspectives before you decide which ones you will choose to write about.

Grading tip for M3

To achieve M3 you need to be aware of the strengths and weaknesses of the two perspectives in the way they can adequately explain the two behaviours you choose. It is usual in psychology that one perspective offers a range of explanations but leaves some aspects unexplained. These can often be explained better by another perspective. If you adopt the advice given for P4 you could draw up a similar table but add information on what is well explained and what is missed out. Then look through the explanations of other perspectives to see if they can 'fill the gaps'.

Contribution of psychological perspectives

Just as different psychological perspectives can shed light on the causes of specific behaviours, they can also offer different types of management and treatment of such behaviours. Sometimes these are used in combination, sometimes alone.

Cognitive behavioural therapy (CBT)

This type of therapy was designed by Beck and Ellis (see page 322) and has become a much used and very effective form of therapy over the past 30 or so years. We shall examine its use in the management and treatment of phobias, depression and post-traumatic stress disorder, as well as its use in managing challenging behaviour and monitoring and improving behaviour.

■ Phobias

Phobias involve fear of an object or situation which is excessive in relation to the real danger of this object or situation. They tend to disrupt a person's life quite significantly because the person makes changes to their lifestyle in order to continue avoiding the fear.

Cognitive behavioural therapy would be used to help the patient recognise all their thoughts associated with the object of fear. For example, they may be asked to write down all their fears. These could include thoughts and beliefs such as, 'I will die if I have to walk past a dog.' The physical sensations that occur for a person with a phobia of dogs are indeed extreme. They include rapid heart rate, dizziness, difficulty breathing, a dry mouth and knots in the stomach.

The goal of cognitive behavioural therapy in the treatment of phobias is to help the individual recognise that their thoughts are irrational and to replace them with more assertive and positive thoughts (this is the cognitive part). So, for example, an individual will be encouraged to think of all the alternative possible

thoughts to replace the original one, 'I will die if I have to walk past a dog.' These may include: 'I shall feel extremely uncomfortable, but this will pass.' 'The more I confront my fears, the less they will rule my life.' 'If I approach this in small stages, I will succeed.'

The second aspect of this therapy involves trying out new behaviour and confronting, rather than avoiding, the feared situation. The person will be taught how to use relaxation techniques to reduce the physiological response and will then confront the feared situation in small stages. For example, they may walk past a dog 50 metres away which is held firmly on a leash. This behaviour can then confirm the new thoughts and make them stronger. It also begins to teach the brain to reduce its activity and produce less extreme fear reactions. Over time, with repeated examination of thoughts, the individual continues to face the feared object until they are able to at least walk past a dog, if not actually pat it!

■ Depression

Reflect

How often have you criticised yourself for hurting someone or doing something you are not proud of? Do you tend to think about your shortcomings a lot? The cognitive perspective believes that negative thinking is at the root of depression. Once you have read the following section you will be able to help not only yourself, but others.

This therapy has been extremely successful in treating depression. Unlike other talking cures (counselling, psychotherapy, group therapy, etc.) it does not seek to discover the cause of emotional distress but rather to examine how thoughts, beliefs and behaviours in the here and now are creating or maintaining depression.

- **Recognising negative thoughts**

  The first stage of the process is to recognise our thoughts. We sometimes have a sort of running commentary in our heads focusing on what we are doing wrong or ways in which we may be falling short. Identifying these automatic thoughts is one goal of the therapy and patients are often asked to write down all the negative thoughts they encounter during the course of each day. As the process of recognising such thoughts becomes easier, the patient will be asked to identify triggers – events that lead to such thoughts. In this way they begin to recognise what they are actually thinking and there is a chance to begin to break down a huge, overwhelming feeling of gloom into more manageable parts.

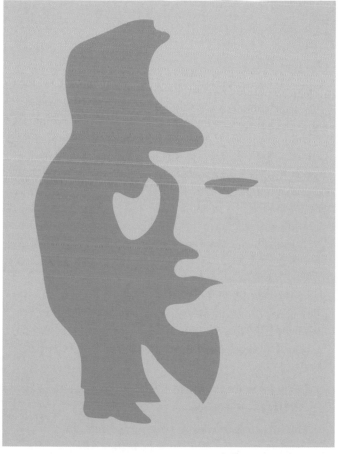

▲ Figure 29.8 This illustration shows how two completely different things can be seen in the same drawing. You need to 'shift' perspective to move from one picture to another. This is what we do when we challenge negative thoughts and consider alternative ones.

- **Challenging negative thoughts**

  With the help of a therapist, **negative** or **irrational thoughts** can then be challenged. Alternative explanations for an event which has prompted a negative thought can be sought. For example, a student who sees her best friend and another person she is not too keen on talking together in low voices may think, 'My friend has turned against me. She's going to go off with that other person!' If the two of them laugh, the thoughts may be even worse, 'They're making fun of me. My friend is giving away all my secrets.'

  Alternative explanations can then be sought. The client may generate a list such as:

  - They are both studying performing arts. They might have been talking about an assignment.
  - When they laughed, it could have been about something that happened last week on a trip to the theatre.

  Although it can be very difficult when we are in the midst of gloom to think of alternative explanations for events, it can be done, but we may need help to do it. Figure 29.8 above shows how the same object can be seen from two different perspectives leading to two quite different outcomes – not always an easy task!

Key terms

Negative thoughts Thoughts which are self-critical.

Irrational thoughts Thoughts which have no real basis in fact or which do not accurately reflect reality.

- **Changing behaviour**

  When we are depressed, or thinking negatively about ourselves or the world, there is a tendency to become socially isolated. The more the world seems an unsafe or unfriendly place, the less we are inclined to explore it. The behavioural element of this therapy involves taking small steps to change behaviour and monitoring the effect these changes have on us. This could be as simple as going for a short walk to buy a pint of milk, weeding the garden or visiting a friend. Once again, a diary is often used to monitor this, in order to recognise changes. A common technique is to keep an activity diary and record each activity, along with the amount of pleasure or enjoyment this brings plus the sense of achievement felt at completing the activity. It is not uncommon in the early stages to feel a great sense of achievement but very little pleasure. Over time, however, as we recover from deep depression, enjoyment can return and this can be seen visually from the diary record.

- **Solving problems**
  Cognitive behavioural therapy may also include an element devoted to solving future problems. For example, if a particular situation is always difficult for us to face and we tend to avoid it, we can work out with a therapist ways we can deal with this more effectively in the future. Having strategies planned in advance can be very supportive and helpful in dealing with situations that have in the past been (or are likely to be) a trigger for negative thoughts.

■ Post traumatic stress disorder (PTSD)

Post traumatic stress disorder is a very distressing disorder which can follow a traumatic event, such as rape or being involved in a horrific car crash. It was first recognised among soldiers returning from war where they had experienced unimaginable horrors. Symptoms include terrible, ongoing fear of some aspect of life that is in some way associated with the original event together with vivid flashbacks which make the person keep reliving the event. CBT is used to help sufferers from this disorder recognise their thoughts and beliefs and the feelings and behaviours they subsequently lead to (see the case study below). Having established what is actually happening to the sufferer, it is then possible to begin to challenge these thoughts. Over time, and with help in thinking of alternative explanations for events, the individual can begin to challenge these thoughts and become aware that there are other, equally valid, explanations. In turn, these new thoughts influence feelings, which then become less negative. The more positive feelings also change behaviour. People with PTSD are often

very anxious about facing situations that resemble the original traumatic situation. However, having changed their beliefs and feelings about the source of the trauma, they are then better equipped to change their behaviour.

When we approach a feared object or situation with a clear agenda to really confront our thoughts, it is much easier to change our feelings when a dreaded or feared outcome does not, in fact, happen. We may feel relieved, proud, energised and so on from having tested out our usual beliefs or thoughts and found them to be incorrect. We actually experience quite a sense of freedom. This encourages us to change our behaviour which in turn allows for new thoughts, new feelings and new positive behaviour.

In context

Liam, an army officer stationed in Northern Ireland, was involved in an operation where the soldiers he was supervising were killed by a bomb hitting the jeep they were travelling in. He was convinced that he was somehow responsible. This is sometimes called *survivor's guilt*. It is clearly an irrational belief since the people responsible were those who planted the bomb, not Liam. Nevertheless, he was haunted by the memory and after leaving the army, suffered from uncontrollable rages and periods of deep depression. His marriage broke up because of his altered behaviour upon returning home and he was almost unable to leave the house because any loud sound (such as a car backfiring) would fill him with such terror that he was almost unable to function. He truly believed he was back in Northern Ireland and would experience the same terror he had felt at the time

1 **Explain what is meant by identifying negative or irrational thoughts.**

2 **Identify the irrational or negative thoughts shown by Liam and show how they affected his emotions and behaviour.**

3 **Devise a programme for treating Liam, using the principles of cognitive behavioural therapy.**

Approaches to challenging behaviour

It is not uncommon for individuals who feel hurt, frustrated, misunderstood or simply not listened to, to show challenging behaviour. This can range from merely irritating behaviours, such as butting in to other people's conversations or showing negative attention-seeking behaviour, through to prolonged bouts of screaming or self-harming. The fundamental principles of CBT can be put to good use with this type of behaviour. Once again, the key is to understand the thought processes that lead to the behaviour. This can be extremely difficult when working with individuals who find it difficult to communicate with others (for example, those with autism or other severe learning difficulties). If this is the case, it may be necessary for care workers to carry out detailed observation of behaviour and to identify triggers for challenging behaviour. In this way, following full discussion with colleagues, it may be possible to infer the thoughts of the individual. For example, they may feel left out, ignored or believe they have been treated unfairly.

Having identified negative thoughts, the same procedure can be used as with all forms of CBT: alternative explanations can be explored and proposed and suggestions for behaviour change made as appropriate.

Monitoring and improving behaviour

We have already touched upon the monitoring of behaviour in the section on the use of CBT as a therapy for depression. Similar methods can be used by individuals or their carers to monitor behaviour. If the individual is not able to keep their own log of behaviour, this can be done on their behalf, with small targets set for behavioural changes. The individual is asked to give feedback on positive actions or activities they have undertaken, together with the sense of achievement and pleasure they gain from these. For an individual with learning disabilities this could be done visually in the form of stars or charts used to monitor progress and show, visually, how improvements have been made.

Social learning theory

This theory helps us to understand how to change behaviour through the use of the principles of observational learning and reinforcement and punishment. The fundamental principle of this theory is that behaviour is learnt and therefore can be unlearnt, or changed.

Reflect

Have you ever felt encouraged by finding out that someone competent and famous has overcome the same difficulties in life that you are facing? For example, Christopher Reeve, the actor famous for playing the part of Superman, refused to give up when he became paralysed after a riding accident.

Use of positive role models

Positive role models can be used to portray desirable behaviour which offers an alternative to the unhelpful behaviour being performed by an individual. Social learning theory sees the model (i.e. the person performing a particular behaviour) as being especially important in influencing how much attention we pay to the behaviour being modelled and how motivated we are to imitate it. To use the example of depression, there is an increasing tendency for public figures to acknowledge that they have suffered from this disorder. The fact that they are in the public eye means that they usually have high status, are admired and are perceived as having more special qualities than ourselves. For example, a successful business woman or politician who tells us about their experience of depression can make us feel less alone in our own experience. We feel we are in 'good company' and that it does not make us 'feeble and worthless' because the person on television or in the paper is clearly worth a lot! This can be a very motivating factor towards getting help.

Treatment of addictions

Once again, the principles of observational learning can be used in treating addictions. By observing an individual modelling non-addictive behaviour, an individual can learn strategies to achieve this. Being exposed to someone else receiving punishment for addiction (for example, debt, illness, prison sentences, etc.) enables the individual to take a step back from their own situation and learn from others some of the negative consequences of addictions. Equally, positive consequences can be observed (for example, interviews with husbands or other family members who express pleasure at having their loved one free of the tyranny of addiction) which can be experienced as reinforcing by the observer.

■ Treatment of eating disorders

One of the symptoms of eating disorders is a distorted view of one's physical body. Being able to observe another individual with a similar eating disorder (particularly anorexia nervosa) may bring it home to the individual just how thin and ill they look. We can also learn through observing another person being positively reinforced for changing their behaviour. So if an individual suffering from anorexia is exposed to a role model who is reinforced for recovery from this illness, this can motivate them to also work towards recovery. As with all aspects of social learning theory, reinforcement is highly subjective and so the treatment would have to focus on showing reinforcement that would be appealing to the patient.

Psychodynamic perspective

This perspective can help to treat certain behaviours by delving into the unconscious mind of the client. The assumption here is that behaviours are caused by aspects of the self (wishes, feelings, memories) that are denied consciously, but remain in the unconscious mind and create a variety of symptoms. The following represent methods of treating these symptoms.

■ Psychoanalysis

This is a form of treatment used within the psychodynamic perspective. It usually involves four to five treatment sessions a week, each lasting 50 minutes and can last for as long as five years. The aim of the treatment is to bring the contents of the unconscious into consciousness so the patient is aware of internal conflicts and repressed wishes. In this way, symptoms disappear. The therapy of psychoanalysis includes:

- the interpretation of dreams
- an exploration of factors that influence behaviour.

■ Interpretation of dreams

Sigmund Freud believed dreams to be the 'royal road to the unconscious', i.e. during sleep the unconscious can express itself more freely than during waking. However, in order not to create too much anxiety, the unconscious uses symbolism in dreams. This imagery prevents disturbing and repressed material from entering the conscious mind and thus has the function of 'protecting sleep'. Much repressed material was believed to be connected to sexuality.

A major function of dreams, according to Freud, is **wish fulfilment**. Desires which are unacceptable to the conscious mind cannot be fully repressed and thus are expressed in dreams. However, they are disguised and are shown as **manifest content** (i.e. the actual story of the dream). To understand the real meaning of the dream, an interpretation must be made to find the **latent** (or underlying) **content**. This involves **dream analysis** whereby the analyst and the patient are both involved in working out the meaning of various symbols. When the symbolism of the dreams has been interpreted, its true meaning becomes clear and the patient is able to deal with issues that have been repressed.

Key terms

Wish fulfilment The idea that dreams express unconsciously the things we most desire.

Manifest content The actual narrative (or story) of a dream.

Latent content The underlying meaning (usually symbolic) of a dream. This needs to be interpreted in order to understand its meaning.

Dream analysis A method of looking at dreams in order to understand the contents of the unconscious mind.

■ Exploration of factors influencing behaviour

The primary goal of psychoanalysis is to explore reasons for behaviour. The goal of this treatment is to find ways of reaching the unconscious mind in order to discover what is troubling the patient. Freud believed that memories, events or feelings that will cause us anxiety if we are truly aware of them are pushed into the unconscious. However, they do not just stay there, but emerge as symptoms.

One method used during psychoanalysis is dream analysis, discussed above.

Another way of reaching the unconscious is through **free association**. The idea behind this technique is that, if you say the first thing that comes into your head upon hearing a word, issues in the unconscious will emerge. An example from one of Freud's patients was when he said the word 'shroud' in response to the word 'white'. When explored further it turned out that a close friend of the patient's had died of a heart attack at the same age as the patient was now. His own fear of dying had been repressed but emerged via the response to 'white' of the word 'shroud'. Once this fear had been made available to his conscious mind, he was able to move on with his life.

Key terms

Free association A method used during the process of psychoanalysis to gain access to the unconscious. The patient is encouraged to say the first thing that comes into his or her mind, the assumption being that this reflects unconscious as opposed to conscious feelings, wishes and desires.

Psychoanalysis also examines issues from childhood which may have made such an impact on the individual that, although they are unaware of them, they are still being influenced by them. Once the source of a particular symptom or source of emotional unhappiness has been revealed, this often frees the patient from further symptoms of this type.

Humanistic perspective

The goal of this is to help the individual develop an awareness of barriers to personal growth and self-actualisation

■ Person-centred counselling

This type of counselling was pioneered by Carl Rogers. Rogers believed that the success of any type of therapy depended not so much on the psychological orientation of the therapist (for example, the theoretical perspective or approach they favoured) as the way they behaved towards the patient. Fundamental principles of person-centred counselling include the following.

- **Unconditional positive regard**
  This means that the therapist must show an acceptance of all that the patient thinks, feels, has done, wants, etc. without making judgements. This is the 'unconditional' part. The therapist must also show a totally positive attitude towards, and respect for, the client. 'Unconditional positive regard' thus implies an absence of judgements about the rights or wrongs of the client and a genuine belief that they are a worthwhile person capable of making positive choices and taking positive actions. By viewing the client in this non-judgemental way, the therapist frees the individual to express themselves. The therapist doesn't give advice or make judgments. Instead they hold to a belief that the client, in the right climate, is able to reach an understanding of their situation, and an appropriate decision to choices that confront them, on their own. The task of the therapist is merely to check understanding of the client's problems and help them think through solutions without suggesting a course of action.

- **Self-awareness**
  The crucial aspect of this type of counselling is that the therapist is totally aware of their own feelings and beliefs, is not afraid to acknowledge these, and has no real desire to guide the client towards a specific outcome.

- **Respect for the drive towards healing**
  A final aspect of this therapy is that, regardless of what perspective they have been trained in (for example, psychoanalytic psychotherapy, behavioural therapy, cognitive behavioural therapy, etc.) the therapist holds a firm belief in the capacity of each individual to heal themselves, given the appropriate support.

Reflect

Do you ever feel irritable and jumpy if you have drunk too much coffee? When you feel stressed or overworked or anxious, does your heart race? Do you sometimes have difficulty getting off to sleep if you are worried or angry or anxious? These physiological symptoms demonstrate how closely our behaviours and emotions are linked with our bodily responses.

As mentioned earlier, this perspective assumes that all behaviour is caused by the brain and nervous system. One major treatment involves drug therapy.

■ The use of drugs

Drugs are prescribed for a range of symptoms. For anxiety and stress, anti-anxiety drugs such as the bendodiazepines Valium and Librium may be used. These help to induce a state of increased relaxation which allows people to carry on with their everyday life. Such medication is not recommended for long periods of use as it can lead to tolerance (and so it becomes less effective) or addiction. It is, however, very helpful when used in conjunction with a therapy that helps the individual to find coping mechanisms. Depression can be treated very effectively by a range of drugs, the most frequently prescribed being those that increase levels of the neurotransmitter serotonin (a brain chemical). Prozac is an example of one of these drugs, although there are others. For the condition known as ADHD, an amphetamine-like substance is often used, an example of which is Ritalin. The above are all examples of prescription drugs. Non-prescription drugs which have an influence on our mood and behaviour include alcohol, which initially encourages us to feel disinhibited and carefree but ultimately acts as a depressive, and illegal drugs such as heroin and cocaine, which induce a feeling of euphoria but are highly addictive.

■ Biofeedback

This is mainly used to treat stress-related disorders and illnesses associated with excessive activity within the brain (for example, epilepsy and ADHD). This technique works on changing the way aspects of our body work. It is thus a biological technique.

Biofeedback involves receiving feedback about physiological aspects of the person's state, such as heart rate, blood pressure and temperature, which manifest as visual or auditory signals on a monitor. Adrenaline produced by the body causes sweating, which can be measured by placing electrodes on the skin. This shows changes in skin resistance (known as the galvanic skin response) which then register as a visual signal or tone. If the signal or tone is high, the level of arousal is similarly high. Initially, by a process of trial and error, the individual attempts various relaxation techniques (deep breathing, visualisation, etc.) to reduce the level of signal or tone. As relaxation deepens, blood pressure and heart rate slow down and this is shown (the feedback part of the process) by a lowering of the signal or tone on the monitor. Over time, the individual learns to recognise signs of tension and finds it easier to control physiological functions. This ability to recognise signs of stress (quickened heart rate, etc.) gives the user a greater sense of control over their difficulties as they can quickly work to induce relaxation and remove stress symptoms.

Interventions

This refers to help offered by outside agencies such as GPs, social workers, health visitors, family therapists, psychologists, counsellors and psychotherapists. A whole host of voluntary organisations is also available to offer help to individuals. The purpose of such interventions is to help an individual or group of individuals who are suffering a life crisis or simply feeling uncertain of their future path in life. By intervening at a time of difficulty or crisis, it is hoped to help the individual(s) resolve conflicts that are threatening their ability to cope with life, or that are preventing them from living a satisfying life. These interventions are informed by the theories and treatments of different psychological perspectives.

Use of perspectives to inform development of therapeutic practices

Each psychological perspective has a different way of understanding emotional distress and behaviours that interfere with satisfactory living. For example, the psychoanalytic approach views disorders as arising from unresolved childhood experiences, ego defences and the effect of material trapped in the unconscious mind. By contrast, the cognitive perspective does not concern itself with past experience or unconscious motivations. It focuses on the here and now, seeking to understand emotional distress by tracing it back to thoughts, feelings and behaviour.

Therapeutic practices

A number of therapeutic practices are based on principles of psychology. They tend not to be based on just one perspective, but to use aspects taken from one or more approach. The practice of CBT, for example, began as just a cognitive treatment but, over time, incorporated aspects of behaviourism in its treatment. The goal of all the types of therapy described below is to help individuals identify emotions, beliefs and patterns of behaviour which are causing them distress in life. Sometimes these have originated in childhood – in other situations they may arise from current life events such as bereavement, redundancy or difficulties dealing with changes within the family.

■ How the therapies work

A range of different therapies are covered below, with an explanation of how they work. One common feature is that there must be trust in the therapist or counsellor and confidentiality must be observed at all times. Therapy is not about giving advice or telling people what to do, nor is it about making judgements. Rather it is a process which enables individuals to reflect upon reasons for distress or difficulties in life and to find ways to make changes so that these barriers to living are removed or weakened.

■ Reasons for attending therapy sessions

Although there are sometimes court judgments which require individuals to attend, for example, parenting classes, the basis of successful therapy has to be a desire on the part of the individual to seek help. Many of life's stresses and strains can be dealt with using the support of family and friends but if the source of conflict comes from the family, then professional help may be needed. Individuals with poor social support networks also benefit from therapeutic intervention as the burdens of life's difficulties, when unsupported, can become overwhelming. People also enter therapy when they have a crisis in life, such as an episode of depression, a bereavement or other loss, or when they are concerned that some aspect of their behaviour might be out of control (for example, an inability to control anger).

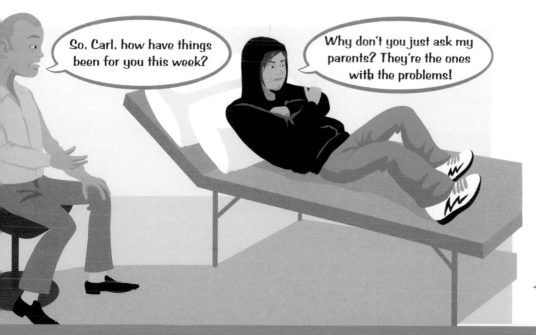

Figure 29.9 A reluctant client cannot benefit from therapy.

Remember!

For an individual to gain benefit from therapy, they must want to attend. The relationship between a therapist and client is an important part of the process and this will not be a happy relationship if the client does not want to attend!

Counselling

Counselling is perhaps the most well known form of therapy. It involves one-to-one conversations with a trained counsellor. Different trainings mean that counsellors may place different emphasis on the way they work but all counselling is aimed to help individuals with emotional difficulties, from depression and anxiety to social phobias or extreme shyness. Issues are explored in a caring and sensitive environment with the counsellor listening carefully. The client is then helped to see things from a different perspective and to consider choices they could make to improve their lives.

Group therapy

This type of therapy is usually entered into by individuals who have difficulties with social or relationship interactions. A therapist, or pair of therapists, works regularly with a group over a period of time. The group will be closed, i.e. it will be the same members every session. Group therapy can trigger very powerful emotions which may well be out of all proportion to the situation in the here and now but which has significant meaning to the individuals. For example, someone who always felt left out within their family or other relationships may suddenly experience tremendous anger if a group member seems to be getting more than their fair share of attention and support. This anger may never have been shown before – it may have been repressed by the individual. Once identified, though, it is then possible to explore the pain of feeling unwanted, not valued or rejected by one's family and also to recognise other situations or patterns of behaviour where they have unconsciously chosen people who will similarly ignore them. At this point, it is possible to make changes.

Family therapy

This type of therapy works by focusing on the way members of a family interact. The aim is to identify dysfunctional interactions and help members of the family to recognise these and change them. It is not uncommon for a family to attend this type of therapy because the behaviour of one family member is causing distress. For example, a teenage daughter may be turning family life upside down by being rebellious, breaking rules, being rude or aggressive towards siblings, etc. The assumption of family therapy is that this behaviour does not just originate in the child but is a result of family dynamics. It may be, for example, that parents have demands and expectations that are unrealistic for an adolescent who is seeking to find their own way in life and develop a new identity. By recognising patterns of behaviour and expectations from all family members that may be contributing to the situation, it is possible to re-negotiate relationships so they become more positive.

Bereavement therapy

Also known as grief counselling, this type of therapy is used to help people overcome the process of mourning a loss. In 1972 Dr Murray Parkes (cited in Kennedy, 1997) sees grief progressing in four stages.

- Numbness – this is in the early stage of grief where we simply cannot bear to recognise the reality of loss. The bereaved person may seem to be coping very well, doing normal everyday things and even comforting other people. This phase will last until the person is able to confront the truth that they really have lost their loved one. The next stage is:
- Pining – this is expressed by deep, grief-filled emotions of longing for the lost person. We may find ourselves searching in crowds or even apparently seeing them, only to find that it is a stranger who resembled our loved one in some way. There is a terrible yearning involved for the person we have lost and a longing to have them back again. The next stage, which does not occur for everyone is that of:
- Depression – the symptoms of depression are very similar to the feelings and behavioural changes associated with grief. For some people, however, this depression is more than part of the normal grief process and professional help may be needed.

- Recovery – this final stage is associated with finding ways to keep the loved person with us in some way – for example, spiritually. During this phase the individual pieces their life back together again and develops a new identity (for example, as a widow).

The key to successful bereavement therapy is to help the bereaved person through their loss, letting them talk about all their feelings – including anger – without making judgements. This is not a time for advice, although practical support and guidance may be offered. Acknowledging that grief is painful but also recognising the strengths the bereaved person has, and helping them to work out what to do in the future, is a vital part of this treatment.

■ Addiction therapy

Because there are so many types of addictions and because people with addiction problems may also have underlying mental health problems, this type of therapy often involves many agencies and a variety of treatments in addition to therapy. Long-term usage of substances causes the brain to change its functioning so there is a very real physical dependence on substances, from nicotine to cocaine. Medication can be offered to individuals with disorders such as depression, anxiety disorder, manic depression or other psychotic disorders. Using these treatments when indicated increases the success of such therapies.

The principles of operant and classical conditioning have also been used effectively in the treatment of addictions. Many cues such as environmental settings (pubs, places associated with taking drugs) trigger cravings because there is such a strong association formed over time that the biological urges are activated. Principles such as systematic desensitization can help people with addiction problems to 'unlearn' this automatic response to such cues. Via operant conditioning, the individual can set up a new repertoire of behaviours that are not associated with satisfying an addiction and this provides an alternative lifestyle which is associated with being and staying healthy. Treatment is long-term and can involve regular sessions following a particular programme. However, residential treatment is often necessary. In either case, treatment for up to a year is often needed for successful rehabilitation.

■ Behaviour modification programmes

Behaviour modification is based on the principles of operant conditioning. Behaviour that we want to see more of is reinforced, whereas behaviour that we want to see less of is **extinguished** (to make it stop happening). Suppose a child screams loudly whenever they don't get their her way. This would be identified as the behaviour to be extinguished. The behaviour we would want to see more of is acceptance that we can't get our own way all the time. To extinguish behaviour, we need to stop reinforcing it with attention – responding in an annoyed or angry manner is often perceived by the child as reinforcement, so this must be stopped. The usual method of doing this is to ignore the child. Reinforcement for the behaviour we want to see more of is, however, both powerful and essential in behaviour modification. In this case, the minute the child stops screaming they need to be reinforced. Over time, the length of screaming episodes will reduce and will eventually be replaced by more acceptable behaviour.

Key terms

Extinguish To cause a reduction in behaviour by no longer providing reinforcement.

■ Ethical issues

Anyone working in a professional or voluntary capacity with individuals must conform to a set of ethical guidelines. These are set out in the British Association of Counselling and Psychotherapy guidelines. These state that:

The fundamental values of counselling and psychotherapy include a commitment to:

- *Respecting human rights and dignity*
- *Ensuring the integrity of practitioner–client relationships*
- *Enhancing the quality of professional knowledge and its application*
- *Alleviating personal distress and suffering*
- *Fostering a sense of self that is meaningful to the person(s) concerned*

- *Increasing personal effectiveness*
- *Enhancing the quality of relationships between people*
- *Appreciating the variety of human experience and culture*
- *Striving for the fair and adequate provision of counselling and psychotherapy services.*

Take it further

Use the following websites to investigate in more detail cognitive behavioural therapy and behaviour modification programmes.

www.rcpsych.ac.uk/mentalhealthinformation/
therapies/cognitivebehaviouraltherapy.aspx

http://add.about.com/cs/discipline/a/behavior.htm

Assessment activity 29.5

P5 Use examples to explain the contribution of psychological perspectives to the management and treatment of two specific behaviours.

1 Explain how cognitive behavioural therapy can be used to treat the frustration and anger associated with many learning difficulties. Explain how operant conditioning can be used to treat and manage the behavioural symptoms of ADHD. **P5**

Grading tip for P5

To achieve P5 you need to re-read the sections on two behaviours (frustration, anger and attention seeking behaviour, and ADHD) and the sections on cognitive behavioural therapy and operant conditioning. Think carefully about the target behaviours you want to reduce or change (for example, flying into a rage, being attention seeking and disruptive) and then use the principles of these two methods to treat and manage these two behaviours.

29.4 The contribution of psychological perspectives to residential care provision

Behaviour of individuals in residential care settings

Concept of role

Roles, sometimes called social roles, are expectations and norms associated with a particular social situation, occupation or role in life. We all have a different number of roles and these vary according to what we are doing at the time. As a student, you will take the role of student. As a son or daughter, you will take the role of child in contrast to the role of parent played by your parents or guardians. You may also be a sister, brother, aunt, uncle, niece, nephew, grandchild, etc. If you have a part-time job you will be an employee and have to adapt to the expectations of the role according to your employment (waitress, cashier, shop assistant, car mechanic, etc.). As a friend you might find that you have the role of 'the one we can always depend on' or 'the lively party-goer'.

We seem to absorb the rules, norms and expectations of behaviour that accompany these various roles without any conscious learning. They are important, however, in guiding behaviour. Someone who is a successful businessman with a wife and children living in an affluent part of the country and carrying an important status in the community will have a large part of their self-concept defined by aspects of the role they take. Loss of role can lead to loss of identity, stress and a sense of helplessness and hopelessness.

Conformity to social roles

Reflect

You take on many different roles within your life, for example, as a student, friend, son, daughter or sibling. When you enter a job situation or go on work experience, what aspects of that role do you take on? How do you know how to behave in order to fit that role?

We all have a very strong awareness of the sorts of behaviour, attitudes and emotions that are expected of different roles. For example, an individual may be very strict in the classroom and insist on high standards of behaviour but then behave quite differently when out with friends.

Philip Zimbardo (1973) conducted a study to examine how much roles influence behaviour within prisons (cited in Cardwell, Clark & Meldrum, 2003). He interviewed a group of young male students and chose those of good psychological and physical health to take part in the study. A basement in the University of Stanford (where he worked) was converted into a mock prison and the students were randomly allocated to take on the role of either prisoner or guard. To encourage identification with roles the guards were given uniforms

and dark sunglasses, while the prisoners were given identical 'convict' clothes and only ever addressed by a number. In a very short period of time the guards became quite brutal in their treatment of the prisoners including humiliating them as a punishment for not obeying orders. The prisoners' response to this treatment was very dramatic. A number became very distressed and passive as a response to this aggression and the study had to be stopped within three days because the prisoners were clearly suffering psychological harm. This study powerfully showed the influence social roles can have on how we behave.

Furthermore, shared beliefs about the attitudes, values and behaviour that accompany particular roles play a very powerful part in influencing us to adapt to the roles we play.

The way in which our attitudes, behaviour and beliefs change when we are in contact with others is called 'social influence' and it has a very powerful impact upon behaviour, as is shown in the following sections which discuss attitude change and behaviour change due to different types of social influence.

Conformity to minority influence

We are all influenced by others all the time. People put forward views we may not have heard, or may disagree with. They behave in ways we may be influenced by or react against. When we conform to minority influence, it is because we believe a minority group to have superior information or knowledge than we do. In a residential care setting it may be custom and practice to impose a fairly rigid set of rules on how a unit is run, in the interests of providing an atmosphere of security and stability. Suppose that two care workers go on a training course where they are shown evidence that convinces them that such rigid rules may actually increase insecurity and lead to people feeling helpless and lacking control. They may argue at a staff meeting in favour of adapting the rules and routines to include more freedom in specific areas. If the arguments they put forward are well thought out, consistent and reasonable, they may well sway the minds of the majority who become converted to this new way of doing things. This is called minority influence.

An important experiment was carried out in 1969 by a French psychologist, Serge Moscovici (cited in Cardwell, Clark & Meldrum, 2003). He arranged for groups of six people to view a series of 36 slides, all coloured blue, but with tints that made the colour vary slightly. In both groups there were two confederates (people working for the experimenter who had been given instructions beforehand on what to say) although the other participants were not aware of this. Each participant stated out loud what colour they judged the slide to be. In one group, the two confederates judged all 36 slides as green (the consistent group). In a second group, the two confederates judged 24 to be green and 12 to be blue (the inconsistent group). It was found that in the consistent group, 8.42 per cent of answers from the real participants were green, while in the inconsistent group only 1.25 per cent said green.

This shows that a judgement or view being consistently expressed by a minority can sway the opinion of some of the majority.

Reflect

Have you ever been in a situation where most of the people you are with hold one view but you don't agree? You may well have found yourself joining in and assuming their views when in fact they are not your own. This is a form of conformity and is a very common feature of social life.

Conformity (majority influence) involves an individual temporarily changing their behaviour or stated views in order to be in line with other group members. Unlike the example given above of minority influence, where people genuinely changed their view because they were convinced that the two confederates were right in judging the slides as green, in majority influence it is much more likely that an individual changes their behaviour or views only temporarily. They are motivated by staying in line with the group, not rocking the boat

and not seeming foolish by disagreeing with others. Privately, however, their views and beliefs do not change.

Psychologist Solomon Asch conducted an experiment to investigate majority influence. Like Moscovici, he used confederates but this time there was only one genuine participant (who thought the others were genuine participants like him). All were seated in a room where they could clearly see a vertical line known as a standard line (see Figure 29.10). They were then shown three comparison lines and asked to judge out loud which of the three lines was the same length as the comparison line.

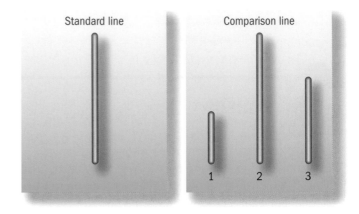

▲ Figure 29.10 Lines used in Asch's task on judging the length of lines compared with a target line.

Altogether, these two cards were shown eighteen times and Asch asked the confederates to give the wrong answer twelve times. He found that the genuine participants gave the *same* wrong answer as the confederates 37 per cent of the time. When they were interviewed afterwards, many of the participants were clear that they thought the others were wrong and trusted their own judgement, but they did not feel comfortable about speaking out and 'rocking the boat'.

This is really quite a surprising finding as the people taking part didn't know one another and there would be no negative consequences if they had simply stated what they believed to be true. It does, however, show how groups have enormous power to shape and change our behaviour.

Obedience

Reflect

How often have you been in a situation where you see a police officer and this prompts you to assess whether you are behaving in a 'respectable' way and not doing anything illegal? If you are learning to drive, you may be very conscious of the presence of a police car in your rear view mirror. This may trigger a set of questions such as, 'Did I indicate? Was I speeding? Was I in the correct lane for that roundabout?', etc. We are so strongly socialised to obey that the mere presence of an authority figure encourages us to check that our behaviour is correct because we do not want to be reprimanded or punished for lack of obedience!

In social psychological terms, obedience refers to a situation where an individual follows orders (sometimes against their morals or better judgement) simply because the order is given by someone of higher authority than themselves. We are socialised from an early age to obey others and this becomes more or less an automatic response.

A very famous experiment in social psychology was undertaken by Stanley Milgram in 1963. Milgram was unhappy with the explanations of the Holocaust currently circulating in society. These focused on an abnormality in the personalities of a whole generation of German society and explained the cruelties of the Holocaust as only being possible in this particular time of history and among this particular group of people. Milgram believed, instead, that there are certain aspects of a situation that can induce any one of us to obey unjust authority and act against our moral code.

To investigate this, he carried out a series of experiments designed to identify the features of a situation that will create obedience and compare them with features that reduce obedience. We shall focus on his first experiment, conducted when he was working at Harvard University in 1963.

This first study involved 40 male volunteers from a variety of occupations who answered an advertisement to take part in an experiment, supposedly designed to test the effects of punishment on learning and memory. The participants were aged between 20 and 50 and were paid $4.50 for taking part.

Upon arrival, each participant was told there were two people involved; a teacher and a learner. The allocation to roles was rigged so the naïve participant was always in the role of 'teacher', while the 'learner' was a confederate of the experimenter.

The stated objective of the task was to learn word-pairs. The learner was to be 'punished' if he gave an incorrect answer by being given an electric shock (although in fact the shocks were fake – the learner didn't receive any). The teacher was administered a 15 volt shock prior to start of the experiment to show him what the 'learner' would experience if he got an answer wrong.

The learner was then strapped to a machine which (supposedly) gave similar electric shocks and the teacher witnessed this. The teacher (the real participant) was then placed in a separate room so he could not see the learner. The teacher read out a list of word pairs (for example, blue–girl and fat–neck). This was followed by a number of other words, one of which was the second member of the original pair. The learner had to choose the correct word by pressing one of four switches which turned on a light on a panel in the teacher's room. Each time the learner made a mistake, the teacher had to deliver a shock. With each successive mistake a further shock was delivered, 15 volts higher than the previous one. The shock generator had a series of switches which increased in 15 volt increments – from 15 volts to 450 volts (potentially fatal).

If the 'teacher' expressed disquiet and wanted to stop, the experimenter was instructed to administer a number of prompts.

'Please continue' (or 'please go on');

'The experiment requires that you continue';

'It is absolutely essential that you continue';

'You have no other choice; you must go on'.

At 180 volts, the 'teacher' hears the 'learner' yell 'I can't stand the pain!' At 315 volts the learner screams loudly and shouts that he won't answer any more. All is silence after this.

To the surprise of everyone involved (including Milgram!) every single one of the participants (those taking the role of 'teacher') gave shocks up to 300 volts. If these were genuine, there was the potential to kill the 'learner'. Furthermore, 68 per cent of the participants gave shocks right up to the maximum of 450 volts!

You will no doubt be relieved to hear that following the experiment, a full debriefing was held where the 'teacher' met the 'learner' and learnt for the first time that no shocks had actually been administered. He was reassured that he had caused no harm to anyone and told that he had taken part in an important experiment that could shed light on aspects of human behaviour that were essential to know about.

The whole set-up of Milgram's experiment was very artificial and unlike normal, everyday settings, so it could be argued that his findings about obedience should not be taken too seriously. However, another experiment was carried out by Charles K. Hofling and his colleagues in 1966 in a hospital setting with very similar findings. Hofling's set up was that nurses were telephoned by an unknown doctor and asked to administer an unfamiliar drug to a patient. The dosage of the drug, Astroten, ordered by the doctor was twice the safe dosage and nurses would be acting against hospital regulations by administering a drug not recognised on the ward list. It was also against hospital policy to administer a drug without signed authorisation from a doctor and to take orders over the telephone. To the surprise of the researchers, 21 out of the 22 nurses who were given this order were on the verge of administering the drug when they were stopped and the purpose of the order explained to them (cited in Cardwell, Clark & Meldrum, 2003). These findings suggest that Milgram's original experiment had tapped something very real about human behaviour. When we are ordered to do something by someone in a position of responsibility, we are likely to do it, even if it means breaking rules or acting against our better judgement!

Attitude change

We have seen in the section on minority influence above that we may change our attitudes if we are exposed to different opinions put forward by people we are convinced by. In Moscovici's experiment, the consistency of the judgements made that the slides were green not blue was influential in changing the judgements of other members of the group.

A psychologist called Leon Festinger developed a theory of attitude change called 'cognitive dissonance'. This basically means that, when there is a vast difference between our beliefs and thoughts, attitudes or behaviour, we feel uncomfortable. We experience dissonance (a state of extreme discomfort when we become aware that we hold contradictory ideas). If, for example, I see myself as a kind and tolerant person but snap at a colleague or friend in an intolerant and unkind way, I will experience dissonance. The way to free myself from this uncomfortable experience is to change one of my thoughts (cognitions). I can either revise my view

---

Public Announcement

WE WILL PAY YOU $4.00 FOR ONE HOUR OF YOUR TIME

Persons Needed for a Study of Memory

"We will pay five hundred New Haven men to help us complete a scientific study of memory and learning. The study is being done at Yale University.

*Each person who participates will be paid $4.00 (plus 50c carfare) for approximately 1 hour's time. We need you for only one hour: there are no further obligations. You may choose the time you would like to come (evenings, weekdays, or weekends).

*No special training, education, or experience is needed. We want:

Factory workers	Businessmen	Construction workers
City employees	Clerks	Salespeople
Laborers	Professional people	White-collar workers
Barbers	Telephone workers	others

All persons must be between the ages of 20 and 50. High school and college students cannot be used.

*If you meet these qualifications, fill out the coupon below and mail it now to Professor Stanley Milgram, Department of Psychology, Yale University, New Haven. You will be notified later of the specific time and place of the study. We reserve the right to decline any application.

*You will be paid $4.00 (plus 50c carfare) as soon as you arrive at the laboratory.

- -

TO:

PROF. STANLEY MILGRAM, DEPARTMENT OF PSYCHOLOGY, YALE UNIVERSITY, NEW HAVEN, CONN. I want to take part in this study of memory and learning. I am between the ages of 20 and 50. I will be paid $4.00 (plus 50c carfare) if I participate.

NAME (Please Print) ....

ADDRESS ....

TELEPHONE NO. .... Best time to call you ....

AGE .... OCCUPATION .... SEX ....

CAN YOU COME:
WEEKDAYS .... EVENINGS .... WEEKENDS ....

 Figure 29.11 The advertisement placed by Milgram to request volunteers for his experiment into obedience.

of myself as mostly kind and tolerant, or justify my behaviour as being in the best interests of my colleague. Either way, this involves attitude change.

Other research by social psychologists has found that there are certain aspects of a message that can persuade us to change our attitudes. We are more likely to be persuaded by an individual whom we perceive as trustworthy, knowledgeable and, interestingly enough, attractive! It seems that these are characteristics that make it less easy to dismiss a message and increase the attention we pay. Sadly, one of the best examples of such persuasiveness on a very large scale is the figure of Adolph Hitler who achieved massive support among the people of Germany. Clearly, persuading people to change their attitudes is not always beneficial.

Factors influencing hostility and aggression

We have seen earlier (on pages 341–42) that prejudice can be explained in a number of ways, including the authoritarian personality, and we have looked at explanations of aggression and violence. Hostility towards others can also be explained using the authoritarian personality explanation. Other factors that influence hostility can be explained from the psychodynamic perspective. Freud would argue that when we refuse to acknowledge (deny) aspects of ourselves that, for whatever reason, we find unacceptable, we often project these onto others. So an individual who is feeling angry and aggressive and spiteful might not acknowledge these feelings, but instead project them onto someone else and believe that others are behaving in an angry, aggressive and spiteful way towards them. Other factors that increase aggression include what are known as environmental stressors. Factors such as heat, unpleasant noise levels and crowding can induce feelings of frustration and aggression in many of us. You may have found yourself walking along a crowded shopping street feeling annoyed with the people who are getting in your way. It is also less easy to hold onto your temper if you are in a hot, crowded underground train.

Effects of residential care on individuals

Effects of institutionalisation

■ Loss of identity

Although we all vary, many of us see our job, status, financial position, appearance, etc. as crucial aspects of our identity. We take pride in being able to earn a living, be a successful worker, a good housewife, an attractive woman. When we enter an institution, many of these personal aspects of ourselves no longer count. Things that once set us apart in the outside world may no longer be seen as important. With this loss of status and difference can come a sense that our identity is slipping away. We are now just a patient or a resident. We saw this happening in Philip Zimbardo's prison study (see page 355) and it can happen in long-term residential care when we take on the category of 'patient' or 'client' rather than Sally Brown, wife of the local GP and ex-primary school teacher. Such a loss can be experienced as deeply distressing and people may lapse into depression and helplessness.

■ Learned helplessness

Reflect

Have you ever experienced a situation where you are waiting for a train in order to get somewhere important? If the train is late, you probably experience increasing anxiety and frustration. Suppose you also don't have your mobile phone on you so you can't ring to explain your lateness. There is literally nothing you can do to make the train arrive! If you were taking a bus a short distance you could at least walk to your appointment but in this situation you have no control: you are helpless.

Learned helplessness is a term used to describe a state of mind where someone has, over a period of time, learnt that nothing they do, no matter how hard they try, can change events. Once they have developed learned helplessness, they will simply stop trying to change things. They may lapse into apathy and not take advantage of opportunities where they might be able to control events. This state of learned helplessness is thought to be a possible contributing cause of depression.

■ Stress

Many people find the experience of institutionalisation extremely frustrating. Often it is hard to find privacy and peace and quiet, or to create a sense of one's own space. We may have to follow routines that don't suit us, to live with people we would not normally choose to spend time with, to eat food we may not have chosen. All these frustrations can lead to feelings of intense stress.

Practices in residential care settings

Policies, procedures and behaviour of staff in residential care settings can have beneficial or damaging effects on residents. If the set-up is such that the main goal is to keep order and avoid disruption, this may result in residents feeling disempowered (having power taken away from them) which has a negative effect on health and well-being. Policies and procedures which promote independence can, on the other hand, protect residents against some of these potentially negative effects.

Promoting independence and empowerment

■ Respecting individual rights

When you are working in a busy institution it may become too easy to forget that the people you are working with are individuals with their own needs and desires. Some people can be difficult and challenging; others might be quiet, not standing up for themselves when it might benefit them to do so. It is important to remember that we all have certain very basic but crucial rights. We all have the right to:

- protection
- dignity
- self-determination (where possible)
- independence
- emotional well-being

- intellectual stimulation
- respect for culture, race, religion.

Giving people choices over simple things such as what they watch on television, choice of meals, what activities they join in, etc. helps them to maintain a sense of dignity and independence. Similarly, showing expectations that someone will succeed, rather than automatically jumping in to help or do something for them, helps to promote a sense of independence and to maintain self-esteem.

It is important that people are treated as individuals, not just one of many people to be cared for. This can help to prevent lapses into learned helplessness, or loss of identify or stress. Care workers work within a framework of values known as the value base of care.

■ Care Value Base

This consists of a set of guidelines and values to help care workers foster the equality, diversity and rights of clients. It also ensures that the human needs of their clients are met. Care workers must do more than just look after the physical needs of their clients: they need also to consider their social, emotional, spiritual and psychological needs. A set of principles has been drawn up, known as the Care Value Base, which must underpin everything that is done in health and social care. The core values are:

- promote anti-discrimination
- promote effective communication
- preserve confidentiality
- promote the rights and responsibilities of all
- promote and preserve equality and diversity.

Theory into practice

Use the Internet or other sources to investigate how one institution puts the Care Value Base into practice. Ask for a copy of their code of practice or policies designed to promote independence. Compare this with your work placements. Are they broadly similar or does one appear to do a better job of this than another?

Assessment activity 29.6

P6 Describe the contribution of psychological perspectives to the promotion of good practice in residential care services.

1 When a group of people live in close proximity, it is inevitable that tempers will flare from time to time as different personalities clash and people become annoyed by situations or events in their day. Explain how the principles of cognitive behavioural therapy and the idea of unconditional positive regard from the humanistic approach can be used effectively to improve harmony in a residential care setting.

Grading tip for P6

Cognitive behavioural therapy is very useful in helping us identify and recognise negative thoughts. If the person using this also adopts the principle of unconditional positive regard (i.e. makes no judgement about hostile or critical attitudes being expressed) it is possible for individuals to learn to be more tolerant. You need to describe how this can take place. Refer to the Care Value Base.

D2 Evaluate the contribution of psychological perspectives in terms of informing and influencing the health and social care sectors.

2 Within the health and social care sectors, behaviour change is often an important priority. For example, encouraging people to eat more healthily and to take up exercise, or helping individuals develop independence and high self-esteem so they are better able to look after themselves and live life independently. Create a detailed information leaflet explaining how staff can use techniques from psychological perspectives (for example, CBT and/ or social learning theory principles) to encourage behaviour change. Compare at least one of these perspectives to the more familiar technique of giving information and advice and explain why this is a useful perspective to use.

Grading tip for D2

To achieve D2 you need to be sure you evaluate. You could do this by creating 'How will this help?' and 'But what's the down side?' questions that might be asked by someone who is unsure about using these new methods.

Knowledge check

1 Who developed the theory of observational learning?

2 How many developmental stages does Piaget suggest there are?

3 Name two psychologists associated with the humanistic school of psychology.

4 Who believed that self-efficacy was an important component of one's sense of self?

5 Who coined the term the 'looking-glass self'?

6 Which psychologist is associated with operant conditioning?

7 What psychological perspective sees development as progressing through a series of psychosexual stages?

8 Which two psychologists carried out an observational study into how infants form attachments?

9 Who developed the maternal deprivation hypothesis?

10 Whose psychological theory of prejudice suggests that this is to do with the authoritarian personality type?

11 What psychological perspective involves the interpretation of dreams as part of its treatment (the psychoanalytic perspective)?

12 Which psychologist is associated with the treatment known as person-centred counselling?

13 Which psychologist investigated obedience in a hospital setting?

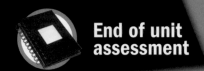
Preparation for assessment

When examining the development of individuals over time, Freud maintains that a child goes through two stages of psychosexual development between birth and the age of about 3. Bowlby, on the other hand, explains development through these life stages as being continuous.

1   Summarise the views of Bowlby on continuity and Freud on discontinuity in relation to the continuity v discontinuity debate in psychology. **P1**

2   Describe key features of the nature v nurture development as it relates to the temperament v maternal sensitivity hypothesis explanations of individual differences in attachment. **P1**

3   Describe one nomothetic approach and one idiographic approach to studying child development within psychology. **P1**

   You should note that, to achieve P1, you need to give a detailed and accurate description of these three debates.

4   Describe key features of the temperament hypothesis and the maternal sensitivity hypothesis as they relate to explanations of individual differences in attachments. Analyse these two approaches from the perspective of nature and nurture. **M1**

   In order to achieve M1 you need to state the strengths and weaknesses of each explanation for individual differences in attachment.

   Prepare for your assessment of P2 by considering the following scenario and the question that follows.

   In the early years of his life John was a quiet, shy child. When he began nursery at the age of two, he found it difficult to adapt and would cry a lot when his mother left. He seldom played with the toys or joined in with the activities at the nursery and never played with the other children.

   He was very clingy when he returned from nursery at the end of the day. Now, at the age of eight, John

has changed and is very boisterous and aggressive. His mother describes him as 'a handful' and explains that she is afraid to leave him alone with his younger sister Sinead (aged three) because he is so aggressive towards her. John is beginning to refuse to go to school and is very rebellious about following the rules of the house.

5   Choose three of the principle psychological perspectives to explain John's behaviour when he was two and now when he is eight years old. Include social learning theory, psychodynamic theory and attachment theory in your answers. **P2**

   To achieve P2 you need to review the three psychological perspectives suggested and apply theories of development to explain John's development.

   Prepare for your assessment of P3, M2 and D1 by considering the following text and the questions that follow.

   John Bowlby, the founder of attachment theory, has stated that, 'what is believed to be essential for mental health is that an infant and young child should experience a warm, intimate and continuous relationship with his mother (or permanent mother-substitute – one person who steadily 'mothers' him) in which both find satisfaction and enjoyment.'

6   Select research into individual differences in attachment to explain how behavioural differences can be seen in children who had different experiences in early life. You may want to look at research into individual differences in attachment, types of romantic attachment relationships with partners in adult life, children with experience of early deprivation and children who spent part of their early lives in orphanages. **P3**

7   It has often been found that people who are securely attached in infancy go on to be more popular, sociable and self-assured and to form more stable adult relationships than those who have been deprived or suffered privation (being unable to form a bond). Use information from your research findings to explain how secure or insecure attachment can explain why some people are more likely to become depressed or delinquent than others. Make a judgement about how well each piece of research explains such behaviours. **M2**

8   Explain how well the four pieces of research account for the development of behaviour and make clear and specific references to aspects of behaviour that may be caused by other factors (for example, environment). Weigh up the strengths and weaknesses of each piece of research and draw a conclusion about which two are the most useful to explain how attachment influences development. **D1**

In order to achieve P3, M2 and D1, you may find it helpful to draw up a table with each piece of research on one row and two columns to the right. Fill in one column with positive contributions made by each piece of research and the second column with any shortcomings you have identified. This could form the basis of an essay and will enable you to justify your points.

Prepare for your assessment of P4 and M3 by considering the following scenarios and the questions that follow.

Sonja is 15 years old and her form tutor is worried that she seems to be becoming seriously withdrawn and socially isolated. She seldom spends time with her friends outside lessons and is often seen just sitting gazing into space. Whereas she used to be quite motivated to do well in lessons, now she often does not work. When asked why she just says, 'What's the point! I won't be able to do it anyway!' Sonja's teacher has spoken to her mother about her concerns and they are both worried that Sonja is showing signs of depression

Alice has a phobia of water. Her mother always says this began when Alice was little and standing on a cliff top looking at the sea. As Alice ran towards the edge to get a clearer view, she tripped and nearly fell. She was saved by her father grabbing her dress and dragging her backwards.

9   Explain Sonja's behaviour using the cognitive approach. **P4**

10 Use the principles of classical conditioning to explain Alice's phobia. **P4**

11 Analyse the role of the behavioural perspective in understanding Alice's phobia and the cognitive perspective in understanding Sonja's depression. **M3**

To achieve M3 you could consider how well each perspective describes phobias and depression. If you feel there are aspects the perspective is unable to explain, you could suggest an alternative.

Prepare for your assessment of P5, P6 and D2 by considering the following scenarios and the questions that follow.

Josie is 45 years old and a partner in a small practice of solicitors. She divorced 18 months ago and is finding it increasingly difficult to manage both her workload and looking after her two children, aged six and three. Her ex-husband frequently telephones her at night and is verbally abusive towards her. Increasingly, Josie feels stressed and is beginning to find it hard to sleep. Her GP is worried that her blood pressure might be getting too high.

Daisy is seven years old and has recently entered a local authority residential home for children after her mother died early of motor neurone disease. Apart from an aunt who lives in Australia, Daisy has no other living relatives. She has never known her father.

Daisy is prone to fierce temper tantrums. If she doesn't get her way all the time she screams and smashes furniture and other objects. She is very jealous of any attention paid to the other children and has been observed hitting them and taking away their possessions when she thinks no one is looking.

12 Biofeedback emerged from the biological perspective. It works on changing the way the body works. Explain how biofeedback might benefit Josie in managing her levels of stress. **P5**

13 Explain how the principles of learning theory (operant conditioning and observational learning) could be used to help reduce Daisy's negative behaviour and replace it with more positive behaviour. **P5**

   To achieve P5 you need to use examples from the case studies to illustrate your answer. If you also know about examples from elsewhere, you may include these as long as you show clearly how the perspectives can be used to manage and treat them.

14 Social learning theory draws attention to the importance of modelling in learning new behaviour, while operant conditioning offers a way to change and manage behaviour. Describe how these two approaches can be used to create a set of rules, and guidance to staff, on how to minimise conflict and disharmony and enhance respect and choice for individuals in residential care. **P6**

15 Psychological perspectives give us a range of 'tools' to understand the behaviour of individuals and groups of individuals. For example, the biological approach explains how people behave when they are under stress while the humanistic perspective gives insight into why people may develop low

self-esteem. Use these two perspectives to describe how individuals working within the health and social care sectors can become more effective in understanding and working with clients and patients if they are given training in these approaches. Use specific examples to illustrate your answer. Explore the strengths and weaknesses of each perspective you discuss and suggest which you think is the most effective overall. **D2**

You may want to consider how behaviours of individuals under stress can make life difficult for members of staff in a hospital and the extent to which people with low self-esteem can become aggressive as a result of their negative feelings. This will help you to consider improvements to the situation if staff receive appropriate training in the use of psychological perspectives.

Resources and further reading

American Psychiatric Association, *Diagnostic and Statistical Manual of Mental Disorders (DSM-IV-TR)*, fourth ed. Virginia: USA

Belsky, J., Fearon, R.M. (2002) 'Early attachment security, subsequent maternal sensitivity, and later child development: Does continuity in development depend upon continuity of care giving? *Journal of Attachment & Human Development* vol 4 no 3, 361–87

Birch, A., Malim, T. (1988) *Developmental Psychology: from infancy to adulthood*. Bristol: Intertext

Bowlby, J. (1988) *A Secure Base: Clinical Applications of Attachment Theory* Bristol: JW Arrowsmith

Bowlby, J. (1965) *Child Care and the Growth of Love* London: Penguin Books

Bowlby, J. (1979) *The Making and Breaking of Affectional Bonds* London: Tavistock Publications

Cardwell, M., Clark, L., Meldrum, C. (2003) *Psychology for AS Level,* third edn. Hammersmith: Collins

Cardwell, M., Flanagan, C. (2003) *Psychology AS: The Complete Companion* Cheltenham: Nelson Thornes

Donaldson, M. (1978) *Children's Minds* London: Flamingo

Ewen, R.B. (1993) *An Introduction to Theories of Personality*, fourth edn. Hove: Lawrence Erlbaum Associates

Eysenck, M. W., Flanagan, C. (2001) *Psychology for A2 Level* Hove: Psychology Press

Gross, R. (2001) *Psychology: The Science of Mind and Behaviour,* fourth edn. London: Hodder & Stoughton Educational

Haralambos, M. et al (2000) *Psychology in Focus for AS Level* Ormskirk: Causeway Press

Haralambos, M., Rice, D. (2002) *Psychology in Focus A2 Level* Ormskirk: Causeway Press

Holmes, J. (1993) *John Bowlby and Attachment Theory* London: Routledge

Kennedy, E. (1997) *On Becoming a Counsellor: A Basic Guide for Non-professional Counsellors* New York: Seabury Press Inc.

Moxon., D., Brewer, K. & Emmerson, P. (2003) *Psychology AS for AQA A* Oxford: Heinemann

Sarafino, E.P. (1998) *Health Psychology:Biopsychosocial Interactions*, third edn. New York: John Wiley & Sons

Shaffer, D. R. (2002) *Developmental Psychology, Childhood and Adolescence,* sixth edn. Belmont, Ca: Wadsworth

Useful websites

British Association for Counselling and Psychotherapy
www.bacp.co.uk

National Institute of Child Health and Development (NICDH)
www.nichd.nih.gov

Websites related to self-harming
www.selfharm.net
www.wellcome.ac.uk

GRADING CRITERIA

To achieve a pass grade the evidence must show that the learner is able to:	To achieve a merit grade the evidence must show that, in addition to the pass criteria, the learner is able to:	To achieve a distinction grade the evidence must show that, in addition to the pass and merit criteria, the learner is able to:
P1 describe three debates in developmental psychology **Assessment activity 29.1 page 313**	**M1** analyse one debate in developmental psychology **Assessment activity 29.1 page 314**	
P2 explain the principal psychological perspectives as applied to the understanding of the development of individuals **Assessment activity 29.2 page 316**		
P3 describe four key pieces of research into the role of attachment in behaviour acquisition **Assessment activity 29.3 page 339**	**M2** analyse the contribution made by the four pieces of research to the understanding of the role of attachment in behaviour acquisition **Assessment activity 29.3 page 339**	**D1** evaluate the contribution made by the four pieces of research to the understanding of the role of attachment in behaviour acquisition **Assessment activity 29.3 page 339**
P4 explain two specific behaviours using psychological perspectives **Assessment activity 29.4 page 343**	**M3** analyse the role of psychological perspectives in understanding the two specific behaviours. **Assessment activity 29.4 page 343**	
P5 use examples to explain the contribution of psychological perspectives to the management and treatment of two specific behaviours **Assessment activity 29.5 page 354**		

GRADING CRITERIA (*Cont.*)

To achieve a pass grade the evidence must show that the learner is able to:	To achieve a merit grade the evidence must show that, in addition to the pass criteria, the learner is able to:	To achieve a distinction grade the evidence must show that, in addition to the pass and merit criteria, the learner is able to:
P6 describe the contribution of psychological perspectives to the promotion of good practice in residential care services. **Assessment activity 29.6 page 361**		**D2** evaluate the contribution of psychological perspectives in terms of informing and influencing the health and social care sectors. **Assessment activity 29.6 page 361**

Glossary

A&E This is a shortened term which refers to the accident and emergency department of a hospital. Patients are admitted here by ambulance, via their GPs or can walk in by themselves for treatment.

Absolute poverty A term introduced by Seebohm Rowntree, referring to people on a level of income below that which will maintain 'physical efficiency'.

Accommodation A process that goes alongside assimilation and allows an individual to modify their understanding of concepts in order to create a new type of understanding.

Accountability Being responsible and required to account for your own conduct.

Acid A substance giving rise to hydrogen ions in solution.

Active transport The movement of materials against a concentration gradient using energy from ATP.

Actualising tendency An innate (inborn) tendency to become all that we can be; to use all skills and qualities, both psychological and physical, to the full.

Advocate An independent representative who can speak or act on a service user's behalf, ensuring that their wishes and feelings are promoted.

Affectionless psychopathy A serious psychological condition where the individual shows no conscience and is unable to form intimate relationships with others.

Afferent arteriole The arteriole preceding the glomerulus.

Amino acids The nitrogenous end products of protein digestion normally used to build up new structural and physiological body proteins such as enzymes and hormones.

Anions Negatively charged ions like chloride and hydroxyl.

Anal expulsive A personality type originating in the anal stage when the infant rebelliously expels their faeces anywhere. Adults fixated at this stage tend to be messy and creative.

Anal retentive A child in the anal stage who feels pressured by their parents into being potty trained may rebel by 'refusing to go'. This is associated with later personality traits such as obstinacy and miserliness.

Antidiuretic hormone (ADH) A pituitary hormone causing tubular cells to become more permeable to water.

Assimilation The process of adapting to new situations and problems by using existing schemata to make sense of incoming knowledge.

ATP Aderosine triphosphate; a chemical whose role in the cell is to store energy and release it for use when necessary.

Autolysis Self-destruction of the cell by lysosomes.

Axons These are processes leading nerve impulses away from the cell body.

Base Chemically a purine or pyrimidine structure such as adenine, guanine, thymine, cytosine and uracil.

Birth rate The number of live births per thousand of the population over a given period, normally a year.

British Medical Association (BMA) This is the professional body for the medical profession. It represents their interests at a national level, for example in negotiations with the government over changes in management of the profession.

Bowman's capsule The cup-shaped beginning of a nephron in the kidney.

CAPD (Continuous ambulatory peritoneal dialysis) A form of dialysis carried out by running dialysing fluid into the peritoneal cavity of the abdomen for several hours and then running the fluid to waste and replacing with 'clean' dialysate.

Care planning The joint planning of an individual's treatment and/or care that involves all concerned.

Carrier molecules Molecules that bind to others facilitating their transport.

Cations Positively charged ions like sodium and hydrogen.

Census A compulsory and detailed count of the population in the UK held every 10 years.

Centration A tendency to focus only on certain key elements of an object without seeing its other properties (for example, using height to judge volume).

Cholesterol A type of fatty steroid present in cells.

Chromatin A complex of DNA and protein that forms chromosomes during cell division.

Chromosomes Thread-like structures seen during cell division composed of DNA and proteins.

Clinical diagnosis A diagnosis made on the basis of signs and symptoms.

Codon A sequence of bases on mRNA which correspond to a particular amino acid.

Colostomy This is the same as an ileostomy except that the artificial opening is from the colon. The artificial opening is known as a stoma and faeces are evacuated into a bag attached to a belt or by adhesive.

Concentration gradient The difference between opposing concentrations.

Consequence Something that happens as a result of your behaviour.

Conservation Technical term for an ability to recognise that objects do not change when they are moved into different positions or their shape is changed.

Continuity A view of development which sees growth and development occurring slowly and continuously, for example, height.

Core conditions These are the essential ingredients/requirements for a person-centred approach.

Countercurrent mechanism A process involving active transport of sodium ions from the descending limb of the loop of Henlé of a nephron to the ascending limb.

Cristae Internal folds or shelves of mitochondria holding an orderly arrangement of enzymes for ATP production.

Cyanosis Bluish colour of the skin and mucous membranes indicating poor oxygenation of blood.

Cytology The study of cell structure.

Cytoplasm (cytosol) Material found between the cell membrane and the nucleus.

Death rate The number of deaths per thousand of the population over a given period, normally a year.

De-centration The ability to move away from one classification system to another. An object is no longer judged by its external properties, such as height.

Dehydration This is the loss of fluid or water from the body. It can have serious consequences and can occur for many reasons including severe infection which causes sweating and vomiting or spending long periods of time in hot conditions without drinking.

Dendrons These are processes taking impulses towards the cell body.

Depression Extreme sadness or melancholy. Reactive depression occurs as a result of illness. Some types of depression have no known cause.

Diagnosis The process by which the nature of the disease or disorder is determined or made known.

Differential diagnosis The recognition of one disease from a number presenting similar signs and symptoms.

Diffusion The movement of molecules from a region of high concentration to a region of low concentration.

Disclosure Revealing information that is held about a person.

Discontinuity A view of development which involves stages. Each stage is qualitatively different from the preceding and the next stage.

Discrimination Treating a person differently (usually less favourably) because of particular personal characteristics, for example, their age, race, colour or gender.

Dissociate To split into ions.

DNA Short for deoxyribose nucleic acid responsible for transmitting inherited characteristics.

Dream analysis A method of looking at dreams in order to understand the contents of the unconscious mind.

Echoic A sound made in imitation of a sound that has been heard (a bit like an echo).

EEG or electroencephalogram This is a tracing of the electrical activity of the brain. An abnormal rhythm may be found in epilepsy, dementia (Parkinson's disease) and brain tumours.

Efferent arteriole The arteriole leaving the glomerulus.

Ego The part of the psyche that attempts to mediate between the demands of the id for instant gratification and the superego for restraint. The ego operates on the reality principle and tries to steer a course that will keep the person on an even keel.

Egocentrism An inability to see things from the perspective of others.

Emigration The movement of people from their home country to make a permanent residence in a different country.

Empowerment When an individual is encouraged to make decisions and to take control of their own lives.

Endocytosis Transport of materials from the outside of a cell to the inside.

Endoscopy This is a clinical investigation to make a direct observation of a hollow organ or tube. The endoscope is a flexible or rigid tube fitted with light-transmitting fibres. It can incorporate a camera, scissors and biopsy forceps.

Epidemiology The study of diseases in human populations.

Equality of opportunity A situation where everybody has the same chance of achieving and acquiring the way of life valued in a society

Equilibrium The state of having no net movement of molecules because the concentrations have evened up.

Erythropoietin A hormone produced by the kidneys which stimulates the production of red blood cells.

Ethics The moral principles which guide a person's behaviour.

Euphoria An inflated sense of well-being when circumstances do not warrant it.

Evaluation A judgement of the worth of something.

Exocytosis The reverse of endocytosis, i.e. transporting materials from inside the cell to the outside.

Expectations These are things that we would hope, expect or like to receive. We are not necessarily entitled to them though, and have no right to demand them.

Extinguish To cause a reduction in behaviour by no longer providing reinforcement.

Facilitated diffusion Diffusion down a concentration gradient that is dependent on energy-using carrier molecules or channel membranes.

Filaments Protein filaments of two types, actin and myosin, are contained in a myofibril. Contraction is achieved when these slide between each other.

Fistula An artificial connection made between an artery and a vein for attachment to a kidney machine.

Formative evaluation This evaluates a project as it progresses.

Free association A method used during the process of psychoanalysis to gain access to the unconscious. The patient is encouraged to say the first thing that comes into his or her mind, the assumption being that this reflects unconscious as opposed to conscious feelings, wishes and desires.

Glomerulus The tuft of capillaries located within the Bowman's capsule of a kidney nephron.

Glycerol A sugary alcohol.

Glycolipid Phospholipid with a sugar chain attached.

Glycoprotein Cell protein with a sugar chain attached.

Golgi body A series or pile of flattened membranes which lie close to the cell nucleus.

Haemodialysis The removal of metabolic waste products from the blood via a kidney machine because the kidneys are seriously damaged.

Health Development Agency (HDA) A national health agency set up in 2000 to provide information about what works in terms of health promotion activity. This in turn enables evidence-based practice in health promotion. Its role has subsequently been taken up by NICE.

Health education An aspect of health promotion which largely relates to educating people about good health and how to develop and support it.

Health protection The measures taken to safeguard a population's health, for example, through legislation, financial or social means. This might include legislation to govern health and safety at work, or food hygiene, and using taxation policy to reduce smoking levels or car use by raising the price of cigarettes or petrol.

Health Protection Agency (HPA) An independent organisation dedicated to protecting people's health in the UK.

Homeostasis Maintaining a constant internal environment around cells.

Humanistic approach This focuses on treating people with dignity, respect and as unique individuals with individual needs.

Hydrophilic Having an affinity for water.

Hydrophobic Lacking an affinity for water.

Hypothalamus Part of the brain involved in water balance.

Id The part of the psyche that is determined to get its own way. It contains all the drives without knowing any bounds – aggression, sexuality, happiness. It operates on the pleasure principle.

Ideal self An internal view of ourselves as we would like to be. This provides a standard against which we can judge ourselves.

Idiographic This approach to development involves the study of all the unique characteristics of one particular individual.

Ileostomy An artificial opening from the ileum to the abdominal wall to evacuate faeces and bypass the large intestine.

Immigration The arrival in a country of people who have left their home country and who wish to make the new country their permanent place of residence.

Immuno-suppressant Specific types of medication to suppress or reduce the immune response. Given to prevent rejection.

Incidence The rate of a disease at a given point in time.

Inclusive technology A range of technological communication aids primarily for individuals with learning difficulties and/or disabilities.

Infant mortality rate The number of deaths of babies under the age of one year, per thousand live births over a given period, normally a year.

Internal environment This is the physical and chemical composition of blood and tissue fluid which surrounds body cells.

Ionisation The process of forming ions.

Irrational thoughts Thoughts which have no real basis in fact or which do not accurately reflect reality.

Kinetic energy The energy of motion.

Labelling A term closely linked with stereotyping where the stereotypical characteristics are applied to a person and their individuality is ignored.

Language acquisition device A device believed by Chomsky to be an innate, pre-programmed system that prepares us to develop language. The device is thought to be located somewhere within the brain.

Latent content The underlying meaning (usually symbolic) of a dream. This needs to be interpreted in order to understand its meaning.

Latent learning This refers to the situation where a new behaviour has been learnt by being observed, but is not necessarily performed.

Life chances The opportunity to achieve and acquire the way of life and the possessions that are highly valued in a society.

Life expectancy A statistical calculation which predicts the average number of years a person is likely to live. This is usually based on the year of birth but can be calculated from any age.

Lumpectomy An operation to remove a suspect lump which is then sent for microscopic examination.

Lysosomes Membranous vesicles filled with digestive enzymes.

Macroscopic Concerning changes that can be seen without the aid of a microscope.

Mand A verbal or non-verbal request or command that is regularly reinforced with a predictable consequence. For example, when a child gestures to a parent with their arms open, it is reinforced by the parent picking the child up.

Manifest content The actual narrative (or story) of a dream.

Marginalisation Individuals or groups of people who feel on the edge of a society and excluded from the way of life and the status enjoyed by others.

Maternal deprivation hypothesis A belief that deprivation results from long periods of separation, or many short periods of separation from the mother, particularly in the early years of life. Bowlby believed this would inevitably lead to damage to later personality.

Maturation The biological changes that take place as the child develops. Intellectual growth and change cannot take place until this maturational process reaches a stage where the child is ready to move on.

Membrane potential The potential difference across a cell membrane caused by different ions.

Meritocracy A society where social position is achieved by ability, skill and effort rather than ascribed at birth. High achievements are open to all.

Microscopic Concerning changes that cannot be seen without using a microscope.

MMR vaccine A vaccination against measles, mumps and rubella.

Morals The rules created by the society we live in, that decide what is right and wrong, good or bad. Issues such as sexual behaviour, criminality and honesty are linked to moral values.

Morbidity This refers to the number of people who have a particular illness during a given period, normally a year.

Mortality Deaths due to a particular condition.

Motivation This is the key factor that determines whether someone will put what they have learnt into practice. Motivation is mostly governed by the individual's own emotions, thought processes, wishes etc.

mRNA Messenger RNA that carries the code for the synthesis of a protein and acts as a template for its formation.

Mucopolysaccharide A molecule made from protein and long sugar chains; it is one of the most important biological molecules.

Multi-disciplinary team A team of people drawn from a range of disciplines or services, for example, health care, education and social service professionals all working together towards a common goal.

Multiple deprivation A situation where many factors linked with poverty and deprivation come together, for example, long-term unemployment, poor housing, pollution, low incomes and poor health.

Muscle wasting Observable diminishing muscle mass.

Myofibrils Bundles of parallel myofibrils are contained in a muscle fibre.

National Institute of Health and Clinical Excellence (NICE) The independent organisation responsible for providing national guidance on the promotion of good health and the prevention and treatment of ill health.

National Statistics Office (NSO) The national body which compiles information on the UK population and which is responsible for carrying out the census every 10 years.

Nature All aspects of a person that are inherited or coded for in the genes.

Needle biopsy This is when a fine needle is inserted into a lump or organ to remove material for microscopic examination. Needles may have cutting tips to remove small sections of tissue or have a hollow needle for removing fluid (containing cells). The material is prepared for microscopic examination. The search is for abnormal cells which might be enlarged, peculiarly shaped or have actively dividing nuclei.

Negative thoughts Thoughts which are self-critical.

Net migration The difference between the number of immigrants and the number of emigrants in a country over a given period, normally a year.

Neurotransmitter A chemical which is released into the minute gap between the next neurone or muscle cell which allows onward progress of the impulse.

Nissl granules Characteristic dark granules found in the cytoplasm of neurones.

Nomothetic This approach is concerned with investigating a group of individuals to see what traits and behaviours they have in common.

Nuclear pore Gap in the nuclear membrane of a cell.

Nucleoli Dark spots inside the nucleus of a cell, probably the site of ribosome synthesis.

Nucleoplasm Soft featureless material contained in the nucleus.

Nucleotide Structural units of DNA and RNA consisting of a base, sugar and phosphate grouping.

Nucleus Membrane-surrounded organelle in a cell, containing genetic material.

Nurture Influences from the environment which shape development and behaviour.

Obesity A Body Mass Index in excess of 30.

Observational learning A type of learning where we do not experience a consequence directly but learn from watching others.

Oedema The accumulation of tissue fluid around the body cells.

Operation The process of working things out. In the early stages of life this is by touching objects or using fingers to count. In later stages it is being able to do this in your head.

Osmoreceptors Modified neurones sensitive to the osmotic pressure of blood.

Osmosis The movement of water molecules from a region of high concentration to a region of low concentration (of water molecules) through a selectively permeable membrane.

Osmotic potential The power of a solution to gain or lose water molecules through a membrane.

Osmotic pressure The pressure exerted by large molecules to draw water to them. Plasma proteins in blood plasma have an osmotic pressure necessary to return tissue fluid.

Outcome evaluation This seeks to establish the worth of work when it is finished.

Outcome measure An indicator of success for a health promotion activity.

Pain threshold The level at which the agony becomes unbearable. Individuals have different pain thresholds and the levels can be affected by past experiences of pain.

Peptide bond This is a chemical bond formed between the amine and carboxyl groups of two amino acids by the removal of the component of water.

Perinatal mortality rate The number of deaths of babies who die during their first week of life per thousand live births over a given period, normally a year.

Phagocytosis The engulfing and destruction of cell debris and foreign bodies by mobile cells which produce arm-like extensions to surround the material.

Phonemes Units of sound used within a language.

Phospholipid A molecule consisting of glycerol, phosphate and lipid chains.

Picture chart scale This is very useful when there is a language barrier. For example, a patient with limited use of English can look at a row of faces from very smiley to very sad and point to the one that shows how they are feeling.

Pinocytosis A process similar to phagocytosis but involving pinching off a vesicle filled with tissue fluid to take into the cell.

Pituitary gland An endocrine gland chiefly controlled by the hypothalamus in the brain.

Pleasure principle A drive towards self-gratification. It has to be kept in check by the ego and superego.

Pneumoconiosis Industrial disease caused by inhaling dust particles over a period of time.

Polar Carrying an electric charge, positive or negative.

Poverty line A term introduced by Seebohm Rowntree and still used by policy makers to refer to the level of income necessary to keep people out of poverty.

Prejudice A fixed set of attitudes or beliefs about particular groups in society which people are normally unwilling, unable and often uninterested in changing.

Prelinguistic Literally meaning 'before language', this refers to all types of communication used before language takes over. It includes things like pointing and turn-taking.

Primary research This is information collected by you during the course of your investigation. It might consist of observations or interviews.

Privation This occurs when a child forms no bond at all with a care giver. Children in orphanages where there is a very low staff-to-child ratio have been found to suffer from privation because they have no interaction with others.

Proximity A state of being close. In terms of attachment, proximity is very important to give the infant a sense of security. When proximity is broken, and the infant is farther away from their care giver than they are able to bear, they will show signs of distress.

Punishment An undesired consequence of behaviour.

Racism Discrimination against a person on the basis of their race background, usually based on the belief that some races are inherently superior to others.

Reality principle An awareness of what is socially acceptable and necessary for the individual to negotiate safely through life. This is the prime function of the ego.

Reconstituted family This is usually two adults living together, one or both with children of their own from another relationship, living together as one family.

Referral This means handing over to another professional (usually a specialist) or type of service such as physiotherapy.

Reflexes These are automatic responses to stimuli. The patellar or knee-jerk reflex is a common reflex that doctors use as a test. It reveals damage to the nervous pathway and also whether the speed of nervous impulses is increased or decreased.

Reinforcement When a consequence is experienced as desirable or pleasurable.

Reinforcer Something that acts to reinforce behaviour. This could be a treat, praise or thanks or a simple smile.

Relative poverty A level of income that deprives a person of the standard of living or way of life considered normal in a particular society.

Remanded To be kept separate from society for a period of time, usually in a prison or young offender's institution.

Renin An enzyme released from the kidneys when blood pressure is low. It causes blood pressure to rise.

Resolution. The capability of making individual parts or closely adjacent images distinguishable (in the absence of good resolution, stronger lenses make images blurred).

Resources These are things that are needed to enable the services to run, for example, money, staff, time, skills, accommodation and equipment.

Respite A break or a time of relief from the demands of care.

Reversibility An ability to reverse, in one's mind, something that has just happened. For example, knowing that if water is poured into a new beaker it can be poured back and stay the same.

Ribosome A tiny cell organelle responsible for protein synthesis.

Rights These are things that everyone is entitled to receive without question.

RNA Ribose nucleic acid, associated with controlling the chemical activities within the cell.

rRNA Ribosomal RNA, the type of RNA found in the ribosomes.

Rough ER Endoplasmic reticulum studded with ribosomes.

Salt A substance produced by the action of an acid and a base.

Sarcolemma The special name given to the cell membrane of a muscle fibre.

Sarcoplasm The name given to the cytoplasm of a muscle fibre.

Schema A type of mental shortcut to understanding physical and mental objects, thoughts, situations and events in the world. It is built up from previous experience. For example, an interview schema contains information about what to wear and how to behave at an interview Plural: *schemas, schemata*.

Screening The identification of unrecognised disease or defect by the application of tests, examinations and other procedures which can be applied rapidly. Screening tests sort out apparently well people who may have a disease from those who do not.

Secondary poverty A term used by Seebohm Rowntree, referring to a situation where people had sufficient money but were in poverty because they spent it on non-essentials.

Secondary research This is information collected by other people and used by you in your investigation. It might include published data and statistics, information about the same or related topics or different case studies. Secondary data should always be referenced and acknowledged.

Selective reabsorption The process whereby some materials are reabsorbed back into the capillary network but not others.

Selectively permeable membrane A membrane such as the phospholipid bilayer which allows some molecules to pass through by osmosis but not others.

Self-actualisation The achievement of the actualizing tendency. People who have achieved self-actualisation include Albert Einstein.

Self-assigned class The social class to which people think they belong or with which they identify.

Sign An objective indication of a disorder noticed by a doctor (or nurse) (*see* **Symptom**)

Single assessment The assessment of an individual's needs is carried out by one professional/co-ordinator on behalf of a multi-disciplinary/agency team.

Smooth ER Endoplasmic reticulum without ribosomes.

Social class The form of stratification that describes the social hierarchies in most modern industrialised societies.

Social exclusion The situation for people who suffer from a combination of linked problems such as unemployment, poor housing, high crime rates and poor health.

Social mobility The process of moving from one social stratum to another. Social mobility can be upward or downward.

Social releasers These are things an infant does that cause others to respond instinctively with care-giving behaviour.

Social stratification A term borrowed from geology (i.e. the earth's strata) which describes the hierarchies in society and how some groups have more status and prestige than other groups.

Stereotyping Defining a group of people (for example, women) as if they all share the same characteristics and ignoring their individual differences.

Strategy A long-term plan, a way of working.

Stroke A cerebral vascular accident (CVA) is commonly referred to as a stroke. It is a bleed that happens in the brain which affects people differently depending on the severity of the bleed.

Strong acid An acid which greatly dissociates.

Superego The part of the psyche that develops last (about 3-5 years of age). It is composed of all the morals and requirements of socialisation. Resembling a conscience, the superego is the part of the psyche that governs reason and restraint.

Symptom This is a sign noticed by the patient.

Synaptic knob The swollen end of the axon which terminates close to other neurones or muscle cells.

Tact response Reinforcement of a child when it recognises that a word (the tact) is being used to name a given object.

Tissue-typing Identifying the protein markers on cell membranes to determine compatibility for transplantation.

Transcription The process of forming mRNA from a template of DNA.

Translation The process of forming a protein molecule at ribosomes from an mRNA template.

tRNA A small molecule of RNA which transfer amino acids to the ribosome to be made into protein.

Ultrafiltration The process driving a protein-free filtrate from plasma from the glomerulus.

Urea A nitrogenous substance resulting from the liver breaking down excess amino acids from the digestion of proteins. Nitrogenous material not required for metabolism cannot be stored in the body. If allowed to accumulate, urea is toxic to body tissues and can result in death.

Vesicles These can also be called cysts, vacuoles etc. and usually mean fluid-filled sacs or pouches.

Victim blaming People frequently simplify health choices by blaming the person who chooses to adopt an unhealthy behaviour for making that choice. In reality things are rarely that simple. For example, people cite lack of time due to work pressures as the major reason why they don't take enough exercise.

Voluntary sector Agencies which obtain their funding from charitable giving, specific funding from public sector organisations such as PCTs or through the National Lottery.

Weak acid An acid which does not dissociate very much.

Wish fulfilment The idea that dreams express unconsciously the things we most desire.

Working document This is an ongoing piece of work that people add things to as circumstances change.

World Health Organisation (WHO) Established on 7 April 1948, it was a response to an international desire for a world free from disease, and since then 7 April has been celebrated each year as World Health Day.

Index

Key words have **bold** page numbers. Tables and illustrations have *italic* page numbers.

A

absolute poverty **259**

abuse (children)
  alleviating the effects of 73–4
  behaviour as a result of 63
  in care setting 55
  and childhood disability 59
  consequences of 64, *64*
  disclosure 70–3
  indicators of 61–3, *62, 63*
  injuries *54*
  models of *64*
  observation of children 70
  in and outside the family 54–5, 57
  potential locations 54–5
  pre-disposing factors of abuser 57–8
  and pre-maturity of children 59, *59*
  predisposing factors related to children 59–61
  procedures when discovered 68–71
  psychological perspectives on 342
  recognition of 65, 70
  strategies to minimise 66–8
  types of *59, 60*, 60–1, *61*

abuse (vulnerable adults)
  Care Homes Regulation (2001) 100
  decision-making processes and forums 101–2
  domestic violence 94–5
  historical view of 90–1
  indicators of *95*, 95–6
  legislation to prevent 105–7
  multi-agency working 101–2
  National Service Framework 100
  by other service users 92
  policies and procedures for protection from 103–4
  potential for in different contexts 97–8
  predisposing factors for 98–9
  Protection of Vulnerable Adults Scheme (POVA) 100
  self-harm as a result 94
  and standards of care 106
  strategies to minimise 100–4
  types of 91–5
  working practices to minimise *103*

access to leisure and recreational facilities 137–8

access to services
  effect on life chances 268
  as influence on health 134–5, 267

accommodation **317**

accountability **25**

Acheson report into health inequalities 119–20, 128, 268

acid-base balance 182–3

acids **180–1**

active transport **173**

actualising tendency **325**

acupuncture 229

addiction 342, 347–8, 353

adenosine triphosphate **164**

ADHD. *see* attention deficit hyperactivity disorder

adoption *46*

adult services users, professional relationships with *84*

advice from professionals 228

advocates **5,** 7–8, 104

A&E **6**

affectionless psychopathy **334**

afferent arteriole **187**

ageing population, implications of 253–4, *254*

aggression 343, 359

aids 226

aims of a health education activity 298

Ainsworth, Mary 337–8

amino acids **215**

anal expulsive **330**

anal retentive **330**

anions *180,* **180**

antidiuretic hormone (ADH) **193**

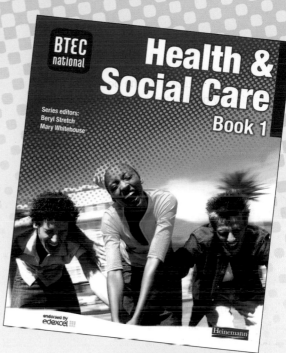
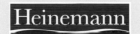

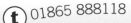 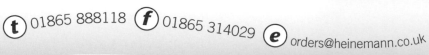 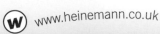
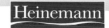